THRIVING IN A TOXIC WORLD

TOOLS FOR FLOURISHING IN THE 21ST CENTURY

William Randall Kellas, Ph.D.
and
Andrea Sharon Dworkin, N.D.

Professional Preference
Olivenhain, CA

This book is not intended to replace the advice of your own doctor or to diagnose or prescribe, but rather to impart knowledge and understanding so you can make decisions that are right for you. You are ultimately responsible for your decisions and your own well-being. It is strongly suggested that you seek the advice of a practitioner or clinic that is in accord with these ideas.

Publisher's Cataloging in Publication
(Prepared by Quality Books Inc.)

Kellas, William Randall
    Thriving in a toxic world: tools for flourishing in the 21st
century / William Randall Kellas and Andrea Sharon Dworkin.
    p. cm.
    Includes bibliographical references and index.
    ISBN 0-9636491-1-6

    1. Health. 2. Nutrition. 3. Emotions--Health Aspects. I.
Dworkin, Andrea Sharon. II. Title

RA776.K45 1996   610
                        QB196-40536

Acknowledgments

This book and its companion volume *Surviving The Toxic Crisis* are a compilation of the knowledge, skills, clinical experience, and personal experience of the two authors. However, these books would not exist if it were not for the direct and indirect contributions of many others.

The chapters in both of these books cite about 1200 references. Each of these references is a book or article which itself is the product of the training and experience of one or more authors, and of the many reference sources they themselves used.

We would like to thank the doctors, dentists, and other practitioners at Comprehensive Health Centers for their input.

The artwork in this book is from several sources:

- Ed Silas Smith, who did many of the drawings.
- Nancy Henderson, who did many of the drawings in this book, especially in the Introduction chapter.
- The clipart files of CorelDraw 5, copyright Corel Corporation, 1994.
- Andrea S. Dworkin has done the design, book layout and computer graphics.

We are grateful to Oralee Archer, Ann Buller, and William Watt Lawrence, MS, for their editing and proofreading.

> We can see so far because we stand on the shoulders of giants.

The pioneering work of many people has helped to make our work, and these books, what they are:

- Stephen Lawrence, DDS, who reviewed the Mercury and Nickel chapters.
- John Yiamouyiannis, PhD, who reviewed the Fluoride and AIDS chapters.
- Sherman Brees, MFC, who reviewed the Emotions Plus chapter.

Dan Gole, DDS	Devi Nambudripad, LAc
Dave Kennedy, DDS	John Davis, inventor
David Olinger, DC	Carl Mayer, PhD, JD
Suzanne Fuselier, DC	Hal Huggins, DDS
Lowell Ward, DC	Jim Kennedy, DDS
Joe Smith, DDS	Carol LaBate, DDS
Joseph Lytle, DDS	John Rothschild, DDS
Jim Dobson, PhD	Tim LeHay, PhD
Alvin Dettloff, DC	Jeffrey Bland, PhD
Bill Timmins, ND	Chris Katke, Metagenics
Elias Illyia PhD	Rick Myatt, pastor
Susan Carlson	Terry Lemerond, Enzymatic Therapy

Last of all, we are grateful to those patients at Comprehensive Health Centers and elsewhere who have so much to teach those who will listen.

About the Authors

This book, several years in the making, is the melding of the skills, knowledge, and dedication of two gifted people. They both have scientific backgrounds consisting of five college degrees between them and considerable practical experience. This book and its companion volume *Surviving The Toxic Crisis* are their first books written together.

Both authors have personally triumphed over chronic illness using principles and methods described in these books.

William R. Kellas (Bill) has a Bachelor's degree in Business/Physics with a Premed minor and a Ph.D. in Nutritional Biochemistry. Over a decade ago he worked for IBM and became enormously successful in his field by looking for and working with the root causes of business problems as he now seeks out root causes of illness. However, his health was rapidly deteriorating. In the late 1970s he was diagnosed as having ankylosing spondylitis, a crippling autoimmune disease; his body was almost literally disintegrating. Although he appeared to be on a fast track to a wheelchair, he refused to accept the no-hope verdict offered by the medical establishment. He researched and tried progressive treatments, developed a deep understanding of how the body works, and over time has regained his health.

Bill's desire to use his knowledge to help others and his belief "To whom much is given, much is expected" led to his forming Comprehensive Health Center (CHC) in Encinitas, California. This clinic, which started in 1984 with two people, has grown to the point where it now employs about thirty people, including MDs, chiropractors, nutritionists, immunologists, naturopaths, and other progressive practitioners, and support staff. CHC also has proximity to a progressive dental center.

In addition to helping patients for the past ten years, he has written the *Toxic Immune Syndrome Cookbook*, has worked on this book and its companion volume for several years, hosts the syndicated radio program called *Health Talk: A Second Opinion* which originates in Southern California and is simulcast across the country, lectures throughout the country to both medical/dental and lay audiences, and is planning to coauthor other books on progressive health care with Andrea.

He lives in Olivenhain, California with his wife and three children.

Andrea Sharon Dworkin has a Doctorate in Naturopathic Medicine (N.D.). She also has Bachelor's and Master's degrees in Chemistry, which gives her a strong background in Toxicology and an understanding of how chemical toxins and nutrients affect the body. She is currently working on her Ph.D. in Nutrition, which she should complete in 1997.

Like Bill Kellas, Andrea has overcome personal health challenges. Years of working in chemistry laboratories in both school and work environments took their toll. The combination of chemical exposure and demanding schedule left her with debilitating chronic fatigue and life-threatening multiple chemical sensitivities. After about 18 months of treatment and healing with Dr. Bill Kellas and the CHC team, Andrea regained her health. She is strongly motivated to use her skills and knowledge to help others as she has been helped. She currently works as a practitioner and writer at Comprehensive Health Center.

This book and its companion volume are her first books. Other books in the progressive health care field and other fields are in the planning stages.

Andrea lives in Oceanside, California. In addition to consulting with patients, writing books, and studying nutrition and natural healing methods, she is an artist in various media.

Preface

Do they say you're not sick but you know you're not well?

Do you want to maintain your health to the greatest extent possible? The key is your body's environment.

Two controllable things must be considered in recovering and maintaining one's health:

- **Suppressors** - Those things that can interfere with health, such as toxins and structural misalignments, must be identified and removed from the environment and the body. These include the primary toxic suppressors such as chemicals and the secondary suppressors such as microorganisms which move in when the body is weakened by the primary suppressors.

- **Supporters** - Those things such as nutrients and necessities like air, water and sleep which support the body must be provided.

Surviving The Toxic Crisis focuses on the suppressors: how they can be identified, avoided, and removed from the body as the first necessary step to attaining or maintaining health.

Thriving In A Toxic World focuses on the supporters. The book also discusses how the body works, the mental/emotional/spiritual connection, and specific topics such as cancer, evaluating the validity of a scientific study, and complications from medical treatment.

The books *Surviving The Toxic Crisis* and *Thriving In A Toxic World* were originally written as one book, but the sheer volume of information necessitated the splitting into two books. These two books can each stand alone but work best together to provide the full picture. They are a compilation of what has proven successful in preventing and treating chronic illness and supporting the body's optimal function in a clinic that integrates medical, dental, chiropractic, nutrients, herbs, and other modalities.

These are possibly the only two books you'll need to survive the 21st century.

THRIVING IN A TOXIC WORLD
Table of Contents

Introduction
and
Overview

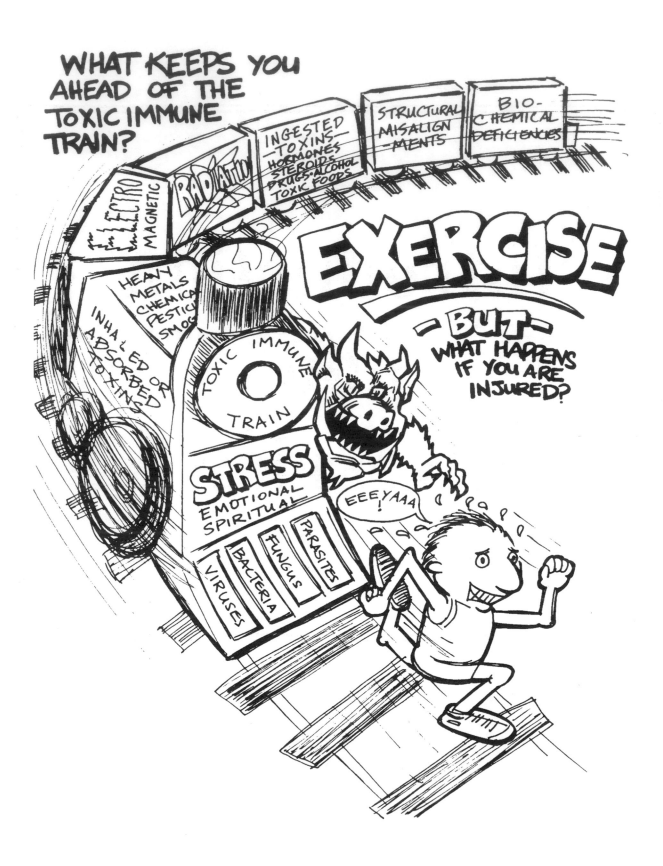

INTRODUCTION AND OVERVIEW

Getting the Train Back On Track

Topics of interest in this chapter:

- *There are root causes for your symptoms, and these root causes and their treatments are the focus of this book.*
- *The body's systems are interconnected, and one problem can affect all parts of the body.*
- *Why looking at the total person is the only way to achieve true healing.*
- *Why books on single problems or solutions are usually not adequate.*
- *What is comprehensive integrated health care, in contrast with today's system of specialization.*
- *How you got to your present state of ill health, and what can be done about it.*
- *How this book is set up.*

Do they say you're not sick but you know you're not well?
You don't feel quite right even though you have been told that all your medical tests are normal. You may have many of the symptoms shown in this graphic.

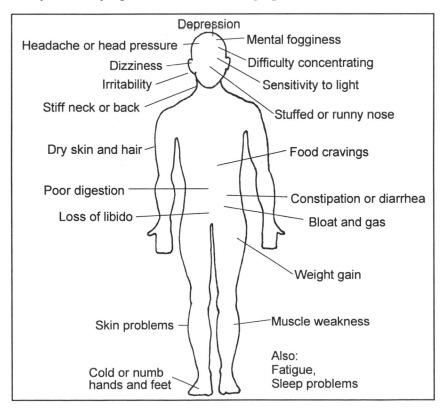

Depression
Headache or head pressure
Mental fogginess
Dizziness
Difficulty concentrating
Irritability
Sensitivity to light
Stiff neck or back
Stuffed or runny nose
Dry skin and hair
Food cravings
Poor digestion
Constipation or diarrhea
Loss of libido
Bloat and gas
Weight gain
Skin problems
Muscle weakness
Cold or numb hands and feet
Also:
Fatigue,
Sleep problems

> **You don't have to be tired, stiff, or forgetful as you grow older!**

You may have felt this way for a long time. Do you want to find out why? Do you feel that your stiffness, fatigue, forgetfulness and grey hair are an inevitable part of aging? Not so. This book will give you insight into the causes of your symptoms and the treatment of those causes.

Have you already been to a doctor, or to many doctors?

Maybe you have gone to a doctor, only to be told:

- "The tests don't show anything."

- "It might be" - fill in the blank - "and here's a prescription for it just in case it is." *Antibiotics are routinely prescribed this way.*

- "It's idiopathic." *This is a term meaning "of unknown cause". The only difference between "It's idiopathic" and "We haven't got a clue" is about fifty dollars, the cost of the office visit. Unknown cause usually means unknown cure.*

- "It's all in your head."

- "It's genetic."

- "Nothing can be done so you'll have to learn to live with it." *They may be so sure that there is no treatment that they advise you not to seek alternative treatment elsewhere.*

- "You have..." list of symptoms you came in with in the first place. *They restate the obvious, in Latin or Greek:*
  high blood pressure = hypertension
  high cholesterol = hypercholesterolemia
  tiredness = chronic fatigue
  This is not a diagnosis, it's an expensive word.

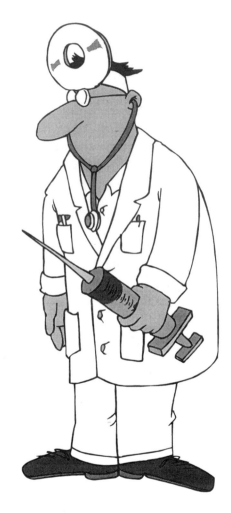

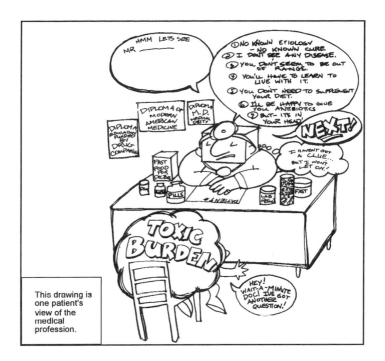

This drawing is one patient's view of the medical profession.

Did any of these help you?

In all fairness, many doctors may be able to help you feel better using symptom-suppressing methods. Other doctors are root cause oriented and may use many of the methods in this book.

Most chronic patients have gone to about ten doctors and/or other practitioners and have not received the degree of help they are looking for. Isn't it time you got some help?

It has been said that the definition of insanity is doing the same thing over and over and expecting different results. It's time to try a different approach.

Why has this book been written in this form?

After all, there are numerous books that address many of the issues that are touched on here. There are:

- *Books about yeast*
- *Books about mercury fillings*
- *Books about food additives*
- *Books about Chronic Fatigue Syndrome*
- *Books about body structure and Chiropractic*
- *Books about allergies*
- *Books about microorganisms*
- *Books about many single subjects*

And many of these books contain excellent information. However, the body's systems and these topics are complex and interrelated. This means that it is unlikely that a book about a single problem, no matter how well written and lengthy the book may be, will cover everything that is wrong with *your* body. Not only can several problems exist at once, but since all of the body's systems are interlinked, one problem may be making another worse and vice-versa.

For example:

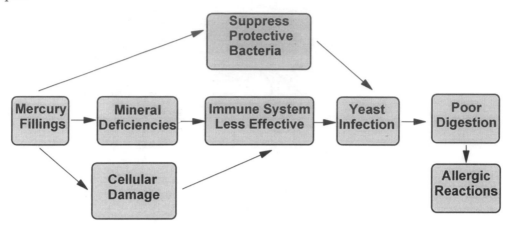

This book provides an overview of the body's systems and the various problems that can cause symptoms, and how these are all interrelated.

How is your body like a clogged pipe?

Picture an old rusty plumbing pipe which is so clogged that water no longer runs through it. There may be rust, hair, grease, and limestone and calcium deposits contributing to the problem of blockage that is keeping the water from running, just as you may have several problems contributing to your symptoms.

Suppose you wanted to make water flow through the pipe again. You put in something to dissolve limestone and calcium deposits, and yet the water does not flow. You eliminate the rust and clear out the grease, and still the water doesn't flow. Last of all you remove the hair ball and now your pipe is clear. Finally, the water flows freely. It looks like the first three treatments did nothing and the last one was the one that worked, but in actuality all four treatments played an equal part in restoring the pipe's functioning. It was purely chance which one was the last one and got the credit.

Similarly, if you have multiple problems causing your symptoms, it is important to treat all or most of them to get relief. The problems should be treated in a logical order based on importance. This book discusses the many problems and treatments in totality, not in isolation.

What are symptoms?

Symptoms are early warning signs of the body systems affected. Symptoms are things you can see (rashes) or feel (headache), and include the items on the list on the first page of this chapter.

Problems are the causes of symptoms. For example, a poorly functioning gallbladder is a problem that can cause the symptoms of nausea when eating fatty food, hormone imbalance, or chemical sensitivity. Explanations of the links between problems and their attendant symptoms are provided throughout this book.

This book may even make you aware of symptoms that you didn't realize you had.

Why would it be to your advantage to worry about things that never bothered you before?
When these symptoms can point the way to finding out what is really wrong and where you may be heading if you do nothing, eliminating this root cause can clear up symptoms that *do* bother you. For example:

- White spots beneath the nails and loss of taste and smell can be early warning signs of zinc deficiency, which can in turn be caused by mercury in tooth fillings or cadmium in cigarettes. These toxic metals fight with beneficial zinc for bio-chemical binding sites in the body like players in a game of musical chairs fight for chairs.

- If cologne smells like bug spray, this can be a sign of deficiency of healthy oil which leads to the absorption of chemicals through the skin and resultant chemical sensitivity.

> **Does your cologne smell like bug spray? It's not your imagination!**

* * * * * * * *

This book, in conjunction with ***Surviving The Toxic Crisis***, is intended to be an overview of the concepts behind the many toxic burdens that might be the root cause of your particular collection of symptoms. Nutrient deficiencies may be contributing to your problems as well, and these are discussed in the section on Supporters. After reading these books, you will most likely have a much clearer idea of what may be ailing you, or ways to avoid being made ill. You can then choose to visit a doctor or clinic that is oriented towards comprehensive integrated medicine which looks at the total person.

This is recommended, as no book, including this one, can diagnose your symptoms sight unseen. The book ends with a list of references for each chapter, including books which cover the subject in greater depth, so you can read more about what you are now fairly sure is one of your problems. In addition, recommended books, groups, and other sources are listed in the back of each chapter where relevant.

You can follow the treatment suggestions outlined in these chapters if your doctor agrees and it is something you can do fairly easily and without risk, such as dietary changes, low-dosage vitamin supplements, or exercise.

How is this book set up?
The purpose of this book is to aid in understanding how your body works and how it can be affected by the toxic suppressors around you, as well as the way nutrients support your body's functions and how the healing protocols work to get you well.

For example, if you are simply told that a certain poison affects the kidneys, you will not be receiving any useful information if you don't know what the kidneys do or why they are important to your total health. For example, the toxic metal mercury, found in metal tooth fillings, interferes with your kidneys' balancing of certain vital minerals in the body. A knowledge of basic body systems and chemistry allows you to understand why so, you can make an informed choice about replacing your mercury fillings.

You then become an active partner in your own preventive and healing health care rather than a passive recipient of instructions. You can in many cases figure out what to do based on genuine understanding of your total health picture, and have more insight into your unique health needs.

Section One: How It All Works

To this end, the first section of the book is **How It All Works**. This section provides background information which leads to an understanding of the concepts discussed throughout this book and explains topics such as:.

- *What is a cell?*
- *The parts of the body, its junctions and how they work together.*
- *The immune system and why it is key to your health.*
- *How testing and studies are really done and why they are often biased.*
- *What exactly is cancer anyway, can we avoid it, and are doctors treating it the right way.*

Sections Two: Supporters

This section deals with ways to support your body and immune system nutritionally and biochemically.

Section Three: Emotions Plus. Your Life View - Toxic or Terrific

This section takes a look at how the mind and emotions along with spiritual aspects of our lives can have an affect on the physical and can be a key to physical healing. The cumulative effect of stressors, both physical and emotional, contribute of the state of total physical and emotional overload. This chapter shows you how to recognize unhealthy patterns and replace them with healthy ones.

Section Four: Pulling It All Together

This section explores some general testing techniques such as blood tests and allergy tests, and discusses what happens at a typical doctor's visit and how you can best help your practitioner. In addition, this section discusses maladies whose incidence seems to be growing and for which the medical establishment has few answers - chronic fatigue, fibromyalgia (all-over pain), environmental illness (EI), brain fog and others. The book is summarized and an existing clinic which provides answers is discussed.

There are References and Resources listed at the end of most chapters for further information on the subject of the chapter (Numbered references within the chapter are found at the end of the book). A glossary, a list of abbreviations used in the book, and a list of sources for many of the supportive products named are also provided.

This book is not intended to replace the advice of your own doctor or to diagnose or prescribe, but rather to impart knowledge and understanding so you can make decisions that are right for you. You are ultimately responsible for your decisions and your own well-being.

COMPREHENSIVE INTEGRATED HEALTH CARE
AN EXPLANATION OF THE CONCEPT

What is comprehensive integrated health care?

The focus of this book is on a comprehensive integrated approach to health care, which has as a basic philosophy getting to the root cause in fostering healing, rather than prescribing symptom-suppressing medicine. It gives you the best of both worlds -- excellent medical care with a natural approach that boosts the immune system and supports the body's own healing mechanisms. This type of comprehensive health care has sometimes been called alternative, complementary, or progressive medicine.

Comprehensive integrated health care goes one step further, as stated, combining natural, supportive health care undergirded with solid medical knowledge that is more preventive in nature, but also seeks to turn chronic health problems around before they reach acute proportions that require heroic medical intervention. It can best be understood by contrasting it with the type of medicine most of us are more familiar with.

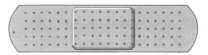 The Segregationists: Symptom-suppressing medicine, sometimes called allopathic or drug-oriented medicine, is the focus of mainstream medical care. Allopathic medicine is characterized by:

- Looking at the individual organ or system where the problem appears to be. 73% of allopathic physicians are specialists. The way some allopathic doctors treat parts of the body is like an architect designing each building component separately.

- Running tests to verify the disease or syndrome (collection of symptoms) for insurance purposes or to protect against malpractice suits, then prescribing a drug.

- Separating the mind from the body, considering only one of them significant, and treating either one or the other.

- Using drugs, surgery, or radiation to attack disease, even though some of these methods weaken an already suppressed immune system.

- Aiming for relief of symptoms if the disease is not readily apparent or easily treatable.

- Removing the symptom so the body doesn't know it's out of alignment, thereby allowing the underlying problem to get worse. This is like disconnecting the "idiot light" on your car's dashboard.

The integrationists: In contrast, comprehensive integrated health care is characterized by:

- Getting to the root cause of symptoms rather than just aiming for relief.

- Looking at the total person and his or her patterns rather than just separate organs, parts, or symptoms, as these are all interrelated. For instance, a small gland in your neck (the thyroid), microorganisms in your digestive tract, misalignment of the vertebrae of your spine, or allergies can be causing your weight gain, versus being told your weight problem is caused by overeating. A blood clot in the brain or low sodium or potassium levels can cause weakness in your leg.

- Looking at the body and mind as being interconnected, rather than separate.

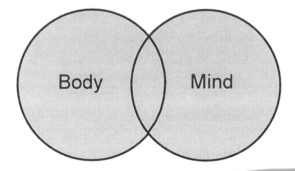

- Physical problems such as toxic waste build-up, meningeal contraction, hormonal imbalance or allergies can cause mental symptoms such as depression, fatigue, and irritability. Emotional problems such as job stress can increase the body's need for nutrients such as vitamin A and the B vitamins, and this vitamin deficiency can, in turn, adversely affect every organ in the body.

- Focusing on the total person rather than on the disease or condition.

- Simply put, working with the body by increasing that which is beneficial and decreasing that which is not. However, this is not always easy.

- Often including the person's spiritual beliefs and general outlook on life to see the total picture.

- Seeing the body as being synergistic. In synergism, the whole is greater than the sum of its parts.

- Assuming the body was designed correctly, and studying how to keep it that way rather than how to change or override it.

Comprehensive and allopathic (drug, or symptom-suppressing) methods are not necessarily in opposition. For some people, the best course of treatment lies in choosing the best combination of remedies from both types of medicine. For example, a cancer patient may benefit from surgery or drug chemotherapy (allopathic) to kill the cancer cells quickly, combined with nutritional supplements such as antioxidants, adaptogens like ginseng which increase cellular capabilities, superfoods such as Life Solubles rice protein and bran and Chlorella, thymus glandular extract to restabilize immune function, and biofeedback (comprehensive) to support the patient's immune system and minimize side effects.

How do allopathic and comprehensive integrated medicine define health?

Allopathic medicine tends to look at health as being the absence of specific named disease, while comprehensive integrated health care goes beyond this point to where the person feels as well as is optimally possible. A person who feels generally tired and rundown but has no clearly defined disease that can be named (cancer, arthritis, etc.) is considered to be well only in the allopathic (treatment) model. The comprehensive integrated (self-responsibility) model goes much farther, as shown in this graphic:

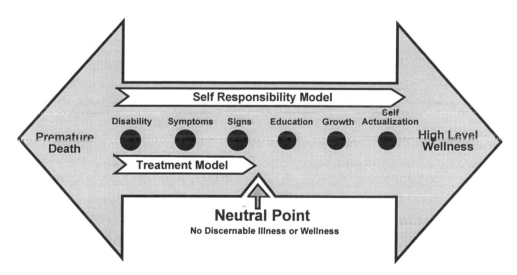

We aren't saying that you shouldn't take a prescription drug or ever have surgery. However, it is generally best to start with the least harmful therapies first, then move to the more drastic ones if needed.

Is comprehensive integrated health care always better than allopathic medicine?

Western (allopathic) medicine is among the best in the world for acute and trauma care, such as heart attacks, critical injuries, and some severe infections. However, it has a very poor track record in dealing with chronic and degenerative diseases such as immune system malfunctions (allergy, autoimmune disease, AIDS), diabetes, obesity, and chronic fatigue.

Comprehensive integrated health care has better solutions for these problems, through dealing with root causes and prevention, versus heroic measures necessary when the system goes awry and the problem now has become life threatening. Indeed, an ounce of prevention is better than a pound of cure, especially when the pound of cure may carry with it side effects that require many more pounds of cure!

It is estimated that 54% of heart disease, 37% of cancer, 50% of cerebrovascular disease such as stroke, and 49% of atherosclerosis (hardening of the arteries) is preventable through lifestyle modification [1,2].

Acute infectious illness, such as diphtheria, whooping cough, polio, and smallpox, has almost become a thing of the past due to improved sanitation and allopathic medicine. However, chronic degenerative diseases have been steadily increasing in the last hundred years or so. These include cancer, heart disease, and diabetes. Treatment of chronic disease accounts for 85% of our health care expenses [3].

For example, degenerative diseases are now our first, second, third, and fourth leading causes of death. Coronary heart disease and Alzheimer's disease, both major problems today, were virtually unknown in 1900 [4]. Statistics reveal that 2700 Americans are killed by heart disease each day, or two per minute, and 1000 are permanently disabled each day by heart disease [5].

In 1900, cancer killed one person in thirty; today it kills one in five. One out of three people will get cancer sometime in their life, and 80% will die of it. Cardiovascular disease caused one death in seven in 1900, versus one death in two today. The five most prevalent diseases today are all degenerative: heart disease, cancer, diabetes, obesity, and osteoporosis [6]. About 15% of the world's population have osteoarthritis [7], and 70 million Americans have arthritis.

American men are ranked 8th healthiest among industrialized nations, but American women only rank 15th. We don't need to change how we finance health care, but rather how we approach preventive and chronic treatment. We have destroyed our heritage of basic health care - the remedies your grandmother swore by - to the point that it is theoretically illegal to claim that chicken soup helps to cure a cold!

Chronic degenerative disease, which takes years to develop and to show its effects, is best prevented and treated by comprehensive integrated health care which combines the best of both disciplines to the benefit of the patient.

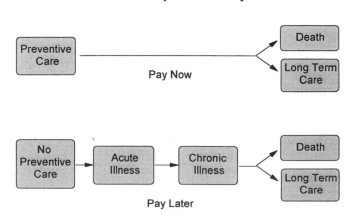

Your Choice - Pay Now or Pay Later

Is the concept of comprehensive integrated health care becoming more prevalent?
Yes, and it's quickly gaining ground! Harvard Medical School, known for its conservative allopathic approach to treatment, held a 3-day symposium called "Alternative Medicine: Implications for Clinical Practice" in March 1995. The course director, David Eisenberg states, "We need to apply to alternative medicine the same rigorous criteria and open-minded skepticism that characterize our research of more mainstream medicine." [8,9]

A study in the *New England Journal of Medicine*, which is a major allopathic medicine journal, showed 1/3 of those surveyed chose complementary medicine over conventional / allopathic medicine [10].

Do you remember the childhood poem about the blind men and the elephant? One blind man felt the ears and thought the elephant was a fan. The one who felt the tail thought the elephant was like a rope. And the one who felt a leg was convinced the elephant was like a tree. Since each of them focused on only one part of the elephant without realizing that it was part of a whole, they were very much mistaken in their evaluation of what an elephant actually is.

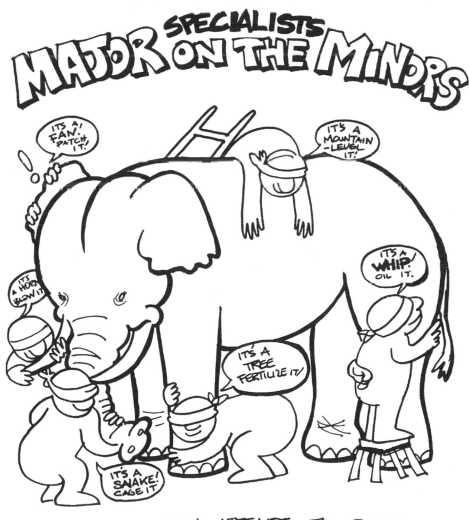

THE BLIND MEN ATTEMPT TO IDENTIFY THE WHOLE OF THE ELEPHANT BY LOOKING AT ONE PART.

How does this relate to our discussion? Since allopathic (drug) doctors are often specialists (73% of the total are specialists), they may focus on only one organ or system, even though the presenting problem affects not only the entire body but the mind as well. Such doctors may come up with a diagnosis that, like the description of an elephant given by any one of the blind men, is a bit shortsighted because they are seeing only one aspect of an integrated whole.

What kinds of doctors are there?
There are basically two types of doctors:

- *Those who believe that drug companies know what is wrong with you, or...*

- *Those who believe that **you** know what is wrong with you, once you tune in to what your body is really saying.*

Is medicine an absolute concept?
Different cultures, even when they are as similar as American and European, have vastly different outlooks on medicine and on what is emphasized. For example, the French are healthier overall, they focus on the health of the liver more, and they have a more casual attitude about dirt and germs as compared with their American counterparts. In Britain, physicians receive the same salary regardless of how much or how little treatment is given, with less treatment given in most cases than by American doctors, who are generally paid by the treatment. The British focus more on quality of life and less on simple longevity as compared with Americans. In Germany new drugs must only be shown to be harmless, not necessarily effective, to be approved [11].

The differences between the American outlook and that of Eastern or less technologically oriented societies would likely be even greater than the differences between America and Europe, or between different European countries. A cross-cultural perspective says that medicine is not always a constant or absolute.

The comprehensive integrated approach is not just replacing drugs with herbs, but rather a rethinking of the entire process and integrating the best of both as well as other therapies in a cohesive plan based on setting priorities and beginning with the root cause.

Today the horizons are widening on a more integrated approach to the medical care and resolution of a whole new set of health problems unique to our contemporary society which require a unique and contemporary solution. Comprehensive, integrated health care provides the vehicle that will take us there.

All Aboard!

Prepare to journey through the maze of the disease of the 21st century -- Toxic Immune Syndrome -- and learn some survival techniques that will equip you to thrive in a toxic world.

References and Resources

- The Burton Goldberg Group, *Alternative Medicine: The Definitive Guide*, Future Medicine Publishing Inc., Puyallup WA, 1994.

  *This excellent guide to alternative / progressive medicine is highly recommended for further understanding of the issues in this book. In addition, books, journals, and organizations pertinent to each chapter are found at the end of each chapter. Specific sections of **Alternative Medicine** will be referenced where applicable at the end of chapters in this book.*

- *Townsend Letter for Doctors is a monthly journal with many articles pertaining to issues raised in this book. Although the journal is geared towards progressive doctors and practitioners, much of the information would be understandable to the layperson.*

- Airola, Paavo, *How To Get Well*, Health Plus Publishers, Phoenix AZ, 1974.

- **American College of Advancement in Medicine**, P.O. Box 3427, Laguna Hills CA 92654. Phone 714-583-7666. *Provides worldwide listing of practitioners trained in nutritional and preventive medicine.*

- Austin, P., *Natural Remedies: A Manual*, Yuchi Pines Institute, Seale AL, 1983.

- Beasley, Joseph, *The Betrayal of Health*, Times Books, NY, 1991. *The effect of lifestyle and nutrition choices on health.*

- *Better Health Through Natural Healing: How To Get Well Without Drugs or Surgery*, McGraw-Hill, NY, 1985.

- Chopra, Deepak, *Quantum Healing: Exploring the Frontiers of Mind/Body Medicine*, Bantam Books, NY, 1989.

- Dirchfeld, Friedhelm and Wade Boyle, *Nature Doctors: Pioneers in Naturopathic Medicine*, Medicina Biologica, Portland OR, 1994.

- Goodheart, RS and MD Shils, *Health and Disease*, Lea and Febinger, Philadelphia PA, 1980.

- Heimlich, J., *What Your Doctors Won't Tell You*, Harper Perennial, NY, 1990.

- Hirschberg, Caryle and Marc Ian Barasch, *Remarkable Recovery*, G.P. Putman's Sons, NY, 1995. *Looks at survivors of cancer and other illnesses who were given a death sentence by their doctors. Discusses the many types of treatment, primarily "alternative", that the survivors credited with their recovery.*

- Moyers, Bill, *Healing and the Mind*, Doubleday, NY, 1993.

- Page, Melvin, *Degeneration and Regeneration*, St. Petersburg Beach, FL, 1949.

- Payer, Lynn, *Medicine and Culture: Varieties of Treatments in the United States, England, West Germany and France*, Henry Holt and Co., NY, 1988.

- Pizzorno, Joseph E. and Michael T. Murray, *A Textbook of Natural Medicine*, John Bastyr College Publications, Seattle WA, 1989.

- Pizzorno, Joseph E. and Michael T. Murray, *Encyclopedia of Natural Medicine*, Prima Publishing, Rocklin CA, 1991.

- Shannon, Sara, *Good Health In A Toxic World: The Complete Guide to Fighting Free Radicals*, Warner Books Inc., NY, 1994. *Fighting free radical damage. Has over 150 pages of resources and references.*

- Shreeve, Caroline M., *The Alternative Dictionary of Symptoms and Cures*, Century Hutchinson Publishing, London England, 1986.

- Simonton, O. Carl and S. Matthews, *Getting Well Again*, Jeremy P. Tarcher, Los Angeles CA, 1978.

- Sinclair, Brett Jason, *Alternative Health Care Resources*, Parker Publishing Co., West Nyack NY, 1992. *A directory of self-help groups, professional care providers, scientific journals, lay magazines and newsletters, and institutes / foundations. These are listed by subject heading.*

- Thomas, John, *Young Again!*, Plexus Press, Kelso WA, 1995. *Techniques and information to maintain youthfulness, including detoxification procedures, colon cleansing and nutrition.*

- Weil, Andrew, *Natural Health, Natural Medicine: A Comprehensive Manual for Wellness and Self-Care*, Houghton Mifflin, Boston MA, 1990.

- Wigmore, Ann, *Be Your Own Doctor: A Positive Guide to Natural Living*, Avery Publishing Co., Garden City Park NY, 1983.

CHART OF TOXICITIES AND DEFICIENCIES

A Good Place To Start

What is the purpose of this chart?
This chart lists symptoms and the various toxicities and deficiencies that can cause those symptoms. If you have a particular symptom or problem, you can look it up and find a listing of those things (toxic excess or deficiency) that may be responsible.

How is this chart used?
The symptoms are grouped into categories based on the body system affected. For convenience, the symptoms are in alphabetical order within their category. The symptom is in the center; toxins which can cause the symptom are listed in the left-hand column, and nutrient deficiencies associated with the symptom are on the right.

Look up the problem that is of concern, note the possible causes, and then you can read about these causes in greater detail in the appropriate book chapters. The Tables of Contents and Indexes for both books will aid in locating the information.

In general, deficiencies are covered in *Thriving In A Toxic World*, while toxicities are covered in *Surviving The Toxic Crisis*.

What do the abbreviations on the chart mean?
The abbreviations and their meanings are listed below by category.

Minerals and metals are listed here together, as some of them can function as a necessary mineral whos deficiency can cause symptoms as well as a metal which is toxic in excess. The abbreviations are taken from the Periodic Table of the Elements. Minerals are discussed in *Thriving In A Toxic World*, while metals are covered in *Surviving The Toxic Crisis*.

The elements listed are:

Ag	Silver	Al	Aluminum	As	Arsenic
B	Boron	Ba	Barium	Be	Beryllium
Bi	Bismuth	Ca	Calcium	Cd	Cadmium
Cl	Chlorine	Cr	Chromium	Cu	Copper
F	Fluorine, Fluoride	Fe	Iron	Hg	Mercury
I	Iodine	In	Indium	K	Potassium
Li	Lithium	Mg	Magnesium	Mn	Manganese
Mo	Molybdenum	N	Nitrogen	Na	Sodium
Ni	Nickel	P	Phosphorus	Pb	Lead

S	Sulfur	Sb	Antimony	Se	Selenium
Si	Silicon	Sn	Tin	Sr	Strontium
Tl	Thallium	V	Vanadium	Zn	Zinc

Vitamins are discussed in *Thriving In A Toxic World* and include: A, B1, B2, B3 (niacin), B5, B6, B12, B15 (pangamic acid), PABA, inositol, choline, biotin, folic acid, B vits. (B vitamin complex), C, bioflavonoids, D, E, vit. K.

Amino Acids are discussed in *Thriving In A Toxic World*. The ones in the chart are:

Arg	Arginine	Cys	Cysteine	GABA	
Glu	Glutamine	His	Histidine	Iso	Isoleucine
Lys	Lysine	Met	Methionine	Phe	Phenylalanine
Tau	Taurine	Try	Tryptophan	Tyr	Tyrosine
Val	Valine				

Sulfur aminos are the sulfur-based amino acids which are particularly important in detoxification.

Toxins, discussed in *Surviving The Toxic Crisis*, include the following as abbreviations:

BHT	Butylated hydroxytoluene, a food preservative
CMV	Cytomegalovirus
CO	Carbon monoxide, a deadly gas
EBV	Epstein-Barr virus
EMR	Electromagnetic radiation
NSAIDs	Non steroidal anti-inflammatory drugs
PCBs	Polychlorinated biphenyls, a type of plastic
TCE	Trichloroethylene, a solvent
TMJ / TMD	Temporomandibular joint dysfunction

The most likely causes for any one symptom are in **bold** print.

A suggestion for using this chart: As you go through these charts, write down the causes of all your symptoms on a separate sheet of paper. If certain causes (mercury toxicity, for example) are listed more than a few times, this is an indication that a major area needs to be dealt with.

It is possible for a nutrient to be both a toxicity and a deficiency. For example, either a deficiency or an excess of iodine (I) can cause symptoms of low thyroid function.

References are found in the relevant chapters in both books.

Mouth and Teeth

Toxic Excess	Symptom	Deficiency
Se, Hg, mouth infection	Bad breath, garlic breath odor	Vit. B3, P
As, Hepatitis B	Bitter taste	
Hg	Bleeding gums	**Vit. C**
Mo, Ni, tobacco	Cancer of the esophagus, oral cancer	Cu, Fe
Mg, Mo, Se, sugar	Dental cavities	Ca, Cu, Fe, Na, P, Vit. C, fiber
Pb, **Hg**	Discoloration of gum margins	Fe
I	Greasy taste	
Ni, Cu, **battery effect (voltage)**	Grinding of teeth	Cu, K
Fe	Inflamed tongue	
As, Hg, Ni	Inflammation of mouth (stomatitis)	Vit. C, bioflavonoids
TMJ/TMD, whiplash, teeth grinding	Jaw pain or popping	
Hg	Leukoplakia (white patches in mouth)	
F, Hg	Loose, brittle teeth	Ca, Mg
Hg, Cd, Cu, Fe, tobacco	Loss of taste	**Zn**
Hg, Pb, Se	Metallic taste	Fe
F, Ni	Mottling of teeth	Ca, Mg
F, Herpes, Hg, Ni	Mouth sores and cracks	Vits. B2, B6
Ag, Hg, Ni, Be, Cu, Sn, allergy	Periodontal disease, gingivitis	Mg, P, vits. E, B3, C
Battery effect, pesticides, F, Hg	Salivation, excessive	
Se	Throat pain	
TMJ	Tooth pain	Ca, B, Mg, vit. C, omega 3 oils

Gastrointestinal

Toxic Excess	Symptom	Deficiency
As, Ba, Ca, Cd, F, K, Li, Hg, Ni, Pb, Zn, pesticides, microorganisms, caffeine, structural	Abdominal pain, rigidity, cramps	Ca, Cu, Fe, I, K, Mg, Mn, Na, Zn
Mg	Abrasive stool	Ca, Na, P
Fe	Achlorhydria (insufficient HCl)	Cl, Cu, HCl, vit. B3
Hg, parasites	Alternating constipation and diarrhea	Cu, Zn, Fe
Cu	Anal cramps	P, Zn, cys, met, glutathione
As, Ca, Cd, Cl, F, Fe, Hg, Mg, Mn, Na, Ni, P, Pb, Zn, giardia, round-worm, fungus, h.pylori, pesticides	Anorexia (appetite loss)	Ca, Cu, Co, Fe, I, K, Mg, Mn, Na, P, **Zn**, vits. A, B1, C, biotin, protein
Roundworm, bacteria, fungus	Appendicitis	Cu, fiber
Ni, aspirin, h.pylori	Bleeding in GI tract	
Hg, alcohol, microorganisms, al-lergy	Bloating, bulging abdomen	Cu, Fe, Zn, glu, glutathione, metallothionein
Ni	Cancer of intestine	S, glutathione, metallothionein
Al, Hg, Ni, structural	Colitis	K, Se, fiber
Al, As, Ca, Cd, Cu, Fe, Hg, I, K, Mg, Na, Pb, F, microorganisms	Constipation	Ca, Cu, Fe, I, K, **Mg**, Mn, Na, P, Zn, B vitamins, tau, choline, fiber
Ni, Se	Degenerative GI conditions	S, Se
As, Ba, Cd, Cl, Cr, Cu, F, Fe, Hg, K, Li, **Mg**, Ni, Pb, S, Si, Zn, caf-feine, aspartame, microorganisms	Diarrhea	Ca, Cu, Fe, I, K, Mg, Mn, Mo, Na, P, Se, Zn, vits. K, B3, pro-tein, oils
Cl, F, I, Hg, Ni	Disruption of intestinal and colon flora	Cu, biotin, folic acid
Al, Cu, Mg, Na, Ni, allergy, micro-organisms, excess protein / carbo-hydrates	Flatulence (gas)	Ca, K, Na, P
Alcohol, microorganisms, aspirin	Gastritis (stomach inflammation)	Sulfur aminos, glutathione
AS, B, F, Hg, Ni, Pb, Se, Zn	Gastroenteritis	Sulfur aminos, glutathione
Ag, Cu, Cr, Ni	GI tract damage and irritation	Ca, Fe
Al, Cl, Fe, fungus	Heartburn, hyperacidity	Cl, Cu, B3, HCl
Hg, Ni, chemicals	Hemorrhoids	Fiber, vits. A, C, E, bioflavonoids
Cl, Hg, Ni	Impaired digestion	Cl, Cu, HCl, vitamins C, B3, B5
Mn, Na	Impaired protein digestion	Ca, **Cl**, Cu, Fe, I, K, B3, HCl
Cu, Fe, Mg, Mn, Ni, allergy, micro-organisms	Indigestion, dyspepsia, painful digestion	Ca, Fe, I
Ni, microorganisms, klebsiella, al-lergy, chemicals	Irritable bowel	Cu, Se, fiber
Ni, microorganisms, pinworms, allergy, chemicals	Itchy anus	
Cu, Hg, F, Ni, Pb, microorganisms, air pollution, TCE, caffeine, aspar-tame, gallbladder problems	Nausea	Cu, Na, B3
Hg	Nutritional disturbances	any
Be, Cu, Ni, Sn	Pain in GI tract	Cl, B vits., vit. C
Al, Cr, Fe, Hg, Ni, NSAIDs, micro-organisms, **h.pylori**, giardia, roundworm, fungus	Ulcers, hiatal hernia	Ca, Fe

Mental and Behavioral

Toxic Excess	Symptom	Deficiency
Al, Hg, Ag, Al, Bi, Hg, organics, alcohol, concussion, whiplash	Amnesia, memory loss	Mg, vit. B1, folic acid, choline
Ag, Ba, Hg, Mn, Mo, Pb, alcohol, toluene	Anxiety	Ca, Cu, Fe, I, K, Mg, Mo
As, Cd, Hg, In, Na, Sb, Se, Sn	Apathy, lethargy	Cl, Cu, Fe, I, K, Mn, Na, Zn, B6, glu, tyr
Hg	Behavioral changes	Oils, GABA, glu, tau, try
Ag, Al, As, Ca, Cl, F, Hg, K, Mn, Na, Pb, Tl, giardia, toluene, organics, aspartame, toxoplasmosis, TMJ, EMR	Brain fog, confusion, disorientation, impaired concentration, indecisiveness	Ca, Cu, Fe, I, K, Mg, Mn, Na, vitamins B5, B6, glu
Hg	Compulsions	
Methylene chloride	Delusions and hallucinations	
Ca, Fe, Hg, Li, Mg, Mn, Ni, Pb, Se, Zn, alcohol, EMR, aspartame	Depression	Ca, Cu, Fe, I, K, Li, Mg, Na, P, vit. A, PABA, vits. B5, B6, biotin, phe, try, tyr, GABA
Hg	Discouragement	
Alcohol, formaldehyde	DTs	Vits. B1, B6, fatty acids, choline
P, Pb, Zn, alcohol	Emotional instability, excitable	Ca, Cu, Fe, K, Mg, glu, try, GABA
Ag, Hg, methyl chloride, EMR, aspartame, Lyme disease	Forgetfulness	Ca, Fe, I, P, Mg, Mn
Cu, Hg, Mg, Pb, sugar, pesticides	Hyperactivity, hyperkinesis	Ca, Fe, K, Na, P, oils (GLA), glu, try, GABA
Ca, Cd, Cl, Hg, I, Mg, Mn, Ni, Pb, Sb, Se, toluene, EMR, pesticides	Irritable, moody	Ca, Cu, Fe, I, K, Mg, Mn, Na, Zn, PABA, glu, try, GABA
Hg	Lack of self-confidence	
I, Hg, Pb	Loss of alertness, slow mental reaction	
Hg, giardia, marijuana	Loss of motivation	B vits, B5, B6, B12, FA, tyr
Hg, Ni	Manic-depressive illness	Li, Na
Ag, Fe	Mental instability	Ca, K, Mg, GABA, glu, phe, try
Hg, P, Pb, Se	Nervousness	Ca, Fe, Mg, vits. B3, B6, B12, PABA
Hg, chemicals, fluorescent lights	Panic attacks, agoraphobia, phobias	Ca, K, Mg, sulfur aminos, oils
Mg, organics	Personality change	Ca, Na, P
Bi, Hg, Mn, Ni, Zn	Psychosis, psychiatric disorders	Ca, Cu, Fe, I, try, tyr, GABA
Hg	Rage	Ca, Cu, K, glu, try, GABA
Cr, Cu, Fe, Hg, Mn	Schizophrenia	Ca, Fe, I, Zn
Hg	Shyness, timidity	
Cu	Sociopathic behabior	
As, Ca, Pb, Sb, CO	Stupor, giddiness	Fe, I, oxygen, glu, tyr
Ag	Thought processes blocked	Glutamine

Brain and CNS

Toxic Excess	Symptom	Deficiency
Hg, Al, solvents, rear molar voltage	Alzheimers disease, senile dementia	Mn, choline
Hg, EMR, chemicals	Amyotrophic lateral sclerosis (ALS)	Vit. B6
Cu, Pb	Autism	Mg, choline
Hg	Black and white dreams	Ca, Mg
Pb	Brain capillary permeability impaired	Fe
Hg	Brain damage	Vit. B12
Pb, alcohol	Cellular degeneration and brain cell death	Fe, vit. B6
Cd, Ni	Cerebral hemorrhage	Cu, Fe, Mn, Zn
Cr, K, Mn, Zn, TCE, pesticides	CNS depression and disturbance	Ca, Cu, Fe, I, Na, vit. B6
Ni, atropine, strychnine, caffeine, amphetamine, cocaine	CNS stimulation	K, GABA
Alcohols, glycols	CNS stimulation, then depression	Vit. B6
Ca, F, Hg, Li, Mg, Na, Ni, Pb, toluene, fluorescent lights, inhaled chemicals, microorganisms	Convulsions, seizures	Ca, Fe, K, Mg, Mn, Na, P, oils, GABA
Hg, Pb, solvents, detergents, aspartame	Demyelination of nerves, multiple sclerosis	Fe, vit. B6, oils
	Difficulty remembering dreams	Vit. B6
Ag, As, Fe, K, Hg, Mn, Na, Ni, Pb, Sb, Se, acetone, pesticides, aspartame, inhaled chemicals, h.pylori, giardia	Dizziness, vertigo	Ca, Cu, Fe, I, K, Mn, Na, vits. B2, B5, B6, PABA, oils
Hg, I, Pb, pesticides, EMR	Down syndrome, retardation, learning disabilities	Ca, Fe, Mg, vit. B6, oils
S, Tl, carbon dioxide, CO, giardia, fungus, allergy, sugar	Drowsiness	Ca, Cu, Mo, Se, oxygen
B	Edema (swelling) of brain	
Ag, Pb	Encephalomalacia (brain softening)	Fe
Ni, meningeal contraction from toxins, chemicals, allergy, microorganisms	Head pressure	K
Ag, Al, As, Ca, Cd, Fe, F, Hg, I, K, Mo, Mn, Na, Ni, Pb, S, Sb, Sn, CO, Vit. A, toluene, pesticides, alcohol, caffeine, aspartame, EMR, structural, TMJ, microorganisms, allergy, nasal/meningeal, chemicals	Headaches	Ca, Cu, Fe, I, K, Se, Zn, oxygen, PABA, vit. B3
Hg, Mn, Pb, Tl, organics, pesticides	Incoordination, motor difficulty, ataxia	Ca, Cu, Fe, I, Mn, vit. B6, choline, inositol, oils
Ca, Cu, Hg, K, Mn, Ni, Pb, pesticides, caffeine, aspartame, EMR, B6	Insomnia, sleeping trouble	Ca, Cu, Fe, I, **K**, Mg, Mn, Na, Pb, Zn, B vits., vit. A, tyr, try, oils
Ni, EMR, structural, TMJ/TMD, giardia, microorganisms, allergy	Neckaches	Ca, I, K, Vit. C, bioflavonoids
As, Cl, Hg, Mg, Pb, Sb, Sn, organics, pesticides, allergy, microorganisms	Nerve inflammation and irritation	Ca, Fe, I, Na, P, vits. B6, B12, choline

Mn, Na	Neurological excitability	Ca, Fe, I, K, vit. B6, choline
Hg, K, MMn, Ni, P, Se, Sn, Zn, pesticides	Paralysis	Ca, Cu, Fe, I, Mg, Na
Mn, Hg, EMR, voltage from metals in mouth	Parkinsons disease	Ca, Fe, I, vit. B6, choline
Al, Hg	Sclerosing (hardening) of brain tissue	Se, vits. A, C, E, biotin, choline, oils
I, Pb, pesticides, allergy, microorganisms, structural	Slow mental reaction	Mg, Mn, B vitamins, PABA, FA, glu
Ca, F, P, Ni	Tetany	Ca, Fe, Mg
Hg, Ni, Pb, alcohol, TCE, pesticide, allergy	Tremors, shaking, muscle twitches	Ca, Cu, Fe, Na, Mg, P
As, Ag, Ba, Cd, Cu, F, Fe, Hg, Mn, N, Na, Ni, P, Pb, Sn, allergy, microorganisms, pesticide	Weakness	Ca, Cu, Fe, I, K, Mg, Mn, Na, Se, Zn, B vitamins, vits. A, C, E, bioflavonoids, sunlight

Bones and Joints

Toxic Excess	Symptom	Deficiency
Ca, Cu, F, Fe, Hg, Mn, Ni, Pb, S, Se, giardia, Lyme disease	Arthritis	Ca, Cu, Fe, I, Mg, Mo, P, Se, oils (GLA), cys, his
Cd, F, Hg, aspartame, Lyme disease	Bone and joint aching and pain	Vit. C
Ca	Bone spurs	
F, P, Pb, Sr	Brittle bones	B, Ca, Fe, Mg, Mn, Mo, V
Ca	Bursitis	
Ca, F, Mg	Calcification of bones and joints	Ca, Mg, Na, P
F	Collagen problems	Lysine
F	Exostosis (bony growth)	Ca, Mg
Fe	Hyperplastic bone marrow (excess cells)	
Al, Mn, Pb, Se, F	Impaired bone formation	B, Ca, Fe, I, Mn, Mo, V, vit. D
F	Increased skeletal density	Ca, Mg
Cd	Long bone pain, leg pain	**Ca**
Pb	Opaque lines on bones in x-ray	
Al, Ca	Osteomalacia (bone softening)	Ca, vit. D
Al, Ca, F, Hg, steroids	Osteoporosis, bone loss	B, Ca, Cu, Mg, lysine
F	Osteosclerosis (bone hardening)	Ca, Mg
Ag, Hg	Rheumatism	Cu, K
Ca	Rickets (bone deformity)	**Vit. D**
	Stiffness of back, neck, and joints	Ca, K, Mg, Mn
I	Tenderness of lower ribs	
Ag, Hg	Vertebral pain	K

Muscles

Toxic Excess	Symptom	Deficiency
F	Decreased oxygen consumption in muscle	Ca, Mg
	Fat deposits in muscles	Vit. E
Hg, EMR, e. histolytica	Fibromyalgia	
Mn	Hyporeflexia (diminished reflexes)	Ca, Fe, I
Ca	Increased lactic acid in muscles	
Mn	Motor difficulty	Ca, Fe, I
Ag, Al, Ba, Cd, Mn, Ni, Pb, S, Sn, microorganisms	Muscle and joint pain and stiffness	Ca, Cu, Fe, I, K, Mg, Mn, Mo, Se, Zn, biotin
Al, As, Ca, Cd, Cu, F, I, Hg, K, Mg, Mn, Na, Ni, P, Pb	Muscle spasms, cramps	Ca, Cu, Fe, I, K, Mg, Mn, Na, P, Zn, vit. E
Ag, Al, As, Ca, Hg, K, Mn, Ni, P, Pb, cologne, pesticides, EMR, microwaves	Muscle weakness	Ca, Cl, Fe, I, K, Mg, Na
F	Muscular hyperirritability	Ca, Mg
Fe, Mn	Myasthenia gravis (muscle weakness)	Ca, Fe, I
F, Hg, I	Numbness and tingling in hands	Cu, Na, oils
Al	Paralytic muscle conditions	Mn
	Restless legs	K, Vit. E
Se	Stiffness	
Ba, Bi, Cu, F, Hg, I, Mg, Pb, Zn, alcohol	Tremors	Ca, Cu, Fe, Mg, Na, P

Liver and Gallbladder

Toxic Excess	Symptom	Deficiency
Fe, Ni, Pb, Zn, **alcohol**	Cirrhosis	Cu, Fe, vits. E, A, oils
Se	Degenerative liver	Mo, vits. C, E, A, oils, tau, glutathione
Fe, microorganisms	Deposits in liver and spleen	Vits. C, E, A, tau, glutathione
Ag, B, alcohol, pesticides, methotrexate (cancer drug), tetracycline	Fatty liver	Oils (omega 6), choline, olive oil, tau
Hg, Ni, microorganisms	Gallbladder problems	Vit. B6, tau, choline
Ca, Cl, F, Hg, Vit. C	Gallstones, kidney stones, sludge	Ca, Mg, fiber
As, Ba, Cu, Fe, Pb, Sn, alcohol, solvents, virus, microorganisms	Hepatitis	Cu, Zn, vits. E, A, C, oils, lys, bioflavonoids
Cu	Hepatosis (noninflammatory liver disease)	Zn, vit. C, lys
Be, acetaminophen (Tylenol), aflatoxin, pesticides	Liver cell necrosis	Vits. A, E, oils, glutathione
As, Cd, Cl, Cu, Fe, Mo, Se, Si, chloroform, e. histolytica, flukes, h.pylori, fungus, virus, microorganisms	Misc. liver damage	Cu, Fe, I, Mn, Zn, leu, iso, val, vitamins A, D
Ca, Cd, Cu, F, Fe, Hg, K, Mg, Na, Ni, Pb, Se, Zn	Nausea related to liver/gallbladder	Ca, Cu, Fe, K, Mg, Mn, Na, P, Zn, vit. B6, choline, tau
Ba, Ca, Cd, Cr, Cu, F, Hg, Ni, Pb, Zn	Vomiting related to liver/gallbladder	Ca, Cu, Fe, Mg, Mn, vits. B5, B6, choline, lecithin, tau, sulfur aminos

Blood Disorders

Toxic Excess	Symptom	Deficiency
Cl, Hg, I	Acidity of blood (acidosis)	Ca, S
Al, Cd, Cu, Fe, F, Hg, I, Mo, Mn, Na, P, Pb, V, Zn, microorganisms, allergy	Anemia	Ca, Co, Cu, Fe, I, K, Mg, Mn, Zn, vitamin B6, folic acid
Ba, Cd, Cr, Hg, Mg, Ni, Zn, root canals, microorganisms	Arteriosclerosis, atherosclerosis	Mg, vits. A, E, C, bioflavonoids, choline
Ca, Hg, Na, Ni	Blood vessel deposits	K
Chemicals, metals, allergy, micro-organisms	Bruising	Vit. C, bioflavonoids
F, aspirin, om.3 oils	Coagulation problems	Ca, Mg, vit. K
Hg, Mn, Ni, Zn	Decreased hemoglobin	Ca, Cu, Fe, I, vit. C
Cr, Hg	Elevated blood cholesterol	Ca, Fe, Zn, B vits., inositol, choline
Cu, Ni	Hemolysis (red blood cell rupture)	Vit. E, bioflavonoids
Ca, Cl, Ni, NSAIDs, aspirin, allergy, microorganisms	Hemorrhages	Vit. K
Ba, Cd, Fe, Hg, Mn, Na, Ni, Zn, diet drugs, alcohol, caffeine, allergy	High blood pressure	Ca, Cu, Fe, I, K, Mn, Na, Zn, fiber, try, tau, GABA, choline
Ca, Vit. D, allergy, toxicity, inflammation, structure, whiplash, bite	Hypercalcemia (excess blood calcium)	Mg, P
Alcohol, sugar, carbos, sat'd fat	Hyperlipidemia (fat in blood)	Cr, V
Cd, Li, Na, Ni, sugar, carbos, sat'd fat, allergy	Hypernatremia (excess blood sodium)	Cu, Fe, K, Mn, Zn
F, P, Pb, Mg	Hypocalcemia (low blood calcium)	Ca, Mg, HCl, oils, albumin
Hg, K, Mn, alcohol, sugar, yeast	Hypoglycemia (low blood sugar)	Ca, Fe, I, Na, glu, protein
K, Li, sweating, vomiting, gallbladder toxicity	Hyponatremia (low blood sodium)	Na
As, F, Pb, microorganisms, pesticides	Jaundice	Ca, Fe, I, Mg
Hg, Pb, Zn, EMR, EBV, fiberglass, ethylene oxide, benzene, pesticides, microorganisms	Leukemia	Cu
Zn	Leukocytosis	Cu
Hg	Leukopenia (white cell disease)	Cu, Zn, vits. A, C
Fe	Low antibody production	Cu, Zn, vits. A, C
Co, F, Fe, Hg, K, Mg, Ni, Sn	Low blood pressure	Ca, Cu, K, Mg, Na, P
Hg, Pb	Lowered ability to carry oxygen	Fe, vits. B12, B15, FA
Hg, gallbladder microorganisms	Pernicious anemia	Co, vit. B12, FA
Ag, Cd, Hg, Ni, chemicals	Slow healing	Zn, vits. A, C, oils

Cardiovascular (Circulatory) System

Toxic Excess	Symptom	Deficiency
Ni, allergy, microorganisms, chemicals	Arterial inflammation, capillary damage	S, Se, glutathione, vits A,C,E, bioflavonoids
F	Cardiovascular collapse	Ca, K, Mg, P
Cd, Cl, Ni, allergy, microorganisms	Enlarged heart	Cu, Fe, K, Mg, Mn, Zn
F, K	Impaired circulation	Ca, Mg, Na
As, EMR	Irregular heartbeat	I, **Mg**
Vit. K	Phlebitis	Omega 3 oils
Ca, metals in mouth, allergy, structural, whiplash, bite	Plaque on blood vessel walls	Cr, V
Si	Poor development and maintenance of aorta	Se, vits. A, E,C, bioflavonoids, oils, lys, pro
I	Rapid pulse	**K**
Cd, Hg, Ni, tobacco, alcohol	Stroke	Ca, omega 3 oils, lys, pro
Cd, tobacco	Thrombosis	Cu, Fe, Mg, K, Mn, Zn
Ni, metals, chemicals, allergy	Varicose veins	Se, vits. A, E, C, bioflavonoids, fiber, tau
Ag, vit. B3	Vasodilation	I, his, sulfur aminos
Cd	Vascular disease	Cu, Fe, Mn, Zn
Ba, Ca, Cd, Cr, Cu, Fe, Hg, K, Mg, Pb, Se, Ni, diet drugs, amphetamines, cocaine, nicotine, caffeine, metals in mouth, Lyme disease, EMR, CO, hydrogen sulfide	Miscellaneous heart problems	Ca, Cr, Cu, Fe, K, Mg, Na, P, fiber, oils, vitamins B1, B12

Eyes, Ears, Face, Nose, Throat and Speech Problems

Toxic Excess	Symptom	Deficiency
As, Cd, Hg	Anosmia (loss of smell)	Cu, Fe, I, Mn, **Zn**, Vit. A
Pb	Ashen face	Fe
Se, CMV	Blindness	Vit. A
Hg, I, voltage, whiplash, chemicals	Bulging eyes	Cu, I, Zn
Ca, Pb, ammonia	Cataracts	Fe, antioxidants, vit. C, bioflavonoids
Ni, allergy, structural (cranial), whiplash	Clogged sinuses	Ca, Fe
Chemicals, microorganisms, h.pylori, Hg in gallbladder	Cologne smells like bug spray	Oils
Worms, **milk allergy**	Ear infections	Cu, Zn, oils, vit. A
TMJ, whiplash, milk allergy	Earaches	Oils
Si	Eye problems, general	Vit. A, B2
Hg, CO, vit. B3 (niacin), allergy	Flushing of face	Glutathione, sulfur aminos, his, vit. C
Hg, Sn, allergy, voltage, microorganisms	Hoarseness	Ca, I, Zn, vit. A
Microorganisms, allergy, chemicals	Inflamed eyelids	Vit. A
Se, TCE, formaldehyde, air pollution	Irritation and burning of eyes	
Microorganisms	Itchy ears	Cu, lys, vit. C
Cr	Laryngitis	Ca, Fe, I, zn, vit. A
Hg, Ni, microorganisms, TMJ/TMD, CNS chemicals	Light sensitivity, sunlight sensitivity	Vits B1, B6, choline
Whiplash, bite, CNS chemicals, TCE	Loss of facial sensation	
Bi, Co, Cu, Hg, Mn, Na, Pb, TCE, CNS chemicals, pesticides, whiplash, bite	Misc. hearing and vision impairment	Ca, Fe, I, K, Mn, oils, vit. A, B2
As, Cr, Ni, Se, microorganisms, allergy	Nasal irritation	Sulfur aminos
Ni, microorganisms, allergy	Nasal polyps	Sulfur aminos
Ni, voltage	Nasal septum necrosis	Sulfur aminos
	Night blindness	Vit. A
Microorganisms, allergy	Nose picking	
Chemicals, allergy, microorganisms, aspirin	Nosebleeds	Vit. C, bioflavonoids, Vit. K, electrolytes
F, Pb, Se, aspartame, vit. A, ozone, microorganisms	Reduction or dimness of vision	Fe, oils (omega 3), vit. A
Hg, CNS chemicals, allergy, microorganisms	Sensitive eyes	Zn, sulfur aminos, vit. C, antioxidants
Hg, CNS chemicals, allergy, microorganisms	Sensitivity to noise	Zn, sulfur aminos, vit. C, antioxidants
Vit. D, formaldehyde, ozone, allergies	Sore eyes	Zn, sulfur aminos, vit. C, antioxidants

As, formaldehyde, allergy, microorganisms	Sore throat	Ca, I, Zn, vit. A
Hg, Ni, chemicals, microorganisms, whiplash, bite	Speech impairment	Ca, Fe, I
Herpes	Throat infections	Ca, Cu, I, Zn, vit. A, lys
Aspirin, caffeine, TMJ, whiplash	Tinnitus (ringing in ears)	Mn, K
Milk allergy	Tonsillitis	
Hg, Ni, voltage, portable phone	Tumors on face and head	Zn, sulfur aminos, vit. C, antioxidants

Pulmonary (Lung)

Toxic Excess	Symptom	Deficiency
Ba, Co, Cr, Cu, Fe, Hg, Mn, Ni, P, toluene, air pollution, fungi, giardia, **roundworm**, pollen, whiplash	Asthma	Ca, Co, Cu, Fe, I, K, Mg, Zn, vits. B2 and B6, oils, sulfur aminos
Air pollution	Bronchitis	Ca, Co, Cu, Fe, I, K, Mg, Zn, vits. B2 and B6, oils, sulfur aminos
Hg, pesticides, microorganisms, allergy, whiplash	Chest tightness	K, Mg
As, Cd, F, Sn, Zn, pesticides	Cough	Ca, Cu, Fe, I, Mg, Mn, Zn
Cd, Ni, **tobacco**	Emphysema	Cu, Fe, Mn, Zn, sulfur aminos
Co, Fe, Se, Si	Fibrosis of the lung	Sulfur aminos, oils
Roundworm, whiplash	Impaired breathing	Ca, Cu, K, Mg
Cd, Co, Se, e.histolytica	Lung damage	Cu, Fe, Mn, Zn
Be, Cd, sulfur dioxide, microorganisms	Pneumonitis (lung inflammation)	Cu, Fe, Mn, Zn
Si, whiplash	Poor development, maintenance of trachea	Ca, Mn, Zn, vit. C, antioxidants
Cl, Cr, F, Se, pesticides	Pulmonary edema	Ca, Fe, Mg
Ba, F, Fe, K, Se, Si, whiplash	Respiratory failure	Ca, Mg, Na
Pesticides	Shortness of breath, irregular breathing	Cu, K, Mg, P
Asbestos	Silicosis, pneumoconiosis, mesothelioma	Sulfur aminos, oils
Cu, Si	Tuberculosis, susceptibility to	
Pesticides	Wheezing	

Skin, Hair, Nails and Mucous Membranes

Toxic Excess	Symptoms	Deficiency
Cd, Hg, microorgaanisms, sugar, allergy	Acne	Cu, Fe, Mn, Zn, vit. A, B vits., sulfur aminos
Ag, Hg	Blackening of mucous membranes	Sulfur aminos
	Brittle nails	Ca, Vit. A, oils
Ca, Hg, microorganisms, chemicals, allergy	Bruising	Vit. C, bioflavonoids, Vit. E
Lyme disease	Bull's-eye rash	
Cr	Burrows deep in hands, knuckles, nail base	Ca, Fe
F, Ni, microorganisms, allergy	Collagen problems	**Vitamin C, bioflavonoids**
Hg, microorganisms	Cutaneous (skin) eruptions	Sulfur aminos
Cl, F, CO, nitrites	Cyanosis (bluish discoloration of skin)	Ca, Mg, sulfur aminos
Microorganisms, allergy	Dandruff	S, Se, oils (omega 3), B6, B12
Allergy, microorganisms	Dark circles under eyes	
CO	Deeply flushed skin	
As, Co, Cr, Ni, S, Se, Vit. A, formaldehyde	Dermatitis	Ca, Cu, I, Mo, Se, vits. A, B2, B3, B6, fiber
Al, Cl, I, N, S, Se, chemicals	Dry and irritated mucous membranes, skin	Ca, Cu, Mo, I, Na, Se
Cr, Hg, Ni, S	Eczema	Ca, Cu, Fe, I, Mo, Se, vit. A, B vits., inositol, oils (omega 6)
Fe, I, S, Se, Zn	Fingernails misshapen	Ca, Cu, Fe, Mo, Se
Hg, Vit. B3, caffeine, allergy, microorganisms	Flushing	Sulfur aminos, his, vit.C
Fungus, acrylic nails	Fungus infection of nails	Biotin
Cd, Hg, Pb	Grey hair	B vits., PABA, Zn
Microorganisms	Greyish skin color	Biotin, oils, bifidus bacteria
Microorganisms, chemicals, allergy	Hair dry and dull	I, oils, vit. A, B vits., PABA
As, Hg, I, S, Pb, Vit. A, EMR, cancer drugs, microorganisms, allergy	Hair loss (alopecia)	Ca, Cl, Cu, I, Mo, Se, B vits., Vit. C, oils (omega 6), arg, cys
As	Herpes	Cu, I, Zn, vit. A, **lys**, gamma globulin
As, Ni, chemicals, allergy, microorganisms, whiplash, bite	Inflammation of nasal mucous membranes	Ca, I, Zn, vits. A and C, sulfur aminos
Vit. D, B3, chemicals, allergy, microorganisms, whiplash, bite	Itching skin	Sulfur aminos, his
As	Keratosis on palms and soles	I
F	Loss of skin elasticity	Cu, Na, water, oil
Ni, giardia, allergy, microorganisms, chemicals	Mucus in the throat	Sulfur aminos, his, vit. C
Microorganisms	Nailbiting	
Cr	Nasal inflammation and ulceration	Ca, Fe
As, Fe, I, Se	Pallor	Fe, I
S	Poor complexion	Ca, Cu, Se, Mo, oils
S, Zn, chemicals, microorganisms, allergy	Psoriasis	Ca, Cu, Mo, Se, oils
F, Hg, S, Vit. A, cologne, aspartame	Rash	Ca, Cu, Mo, Se

Cr	Rhinitis	Ca, Fe
Cr	Sinusitis	Ca, Fe
Se	Skin eruptions	
	Skin depigmentation	Cu, Zn, biotin
As, S	Skin pigmentation, darkening	Ca, Cu, I, Mo, Se
Cologne, some drugs, chemicals	Sunlight sensitivity on skin	Oils
Cr, Se, chemicals	Ulceration of skin	Ca, Fe
Cd, Hg	White spots on nails	**Zn**, Vit. B with Vit. C
F	Wrinkling	Oils
Se, Vit. A	Yellow skin color	Sulfur aminos, vit. C

Reproductive Disorders

Toxic Excess	Symptoms	Deficiency
Fe, Hg, Ni, Pb, organics, alcohol, tobacco, EMR, Lyme disease	Birth defects, premature birth	Cu, Zn, GLA oils
Hg, I, Ni, whiplash, voltage	Cretinism (diminished thyroid hormone)	Cu, I, Zn
Ni, chemicals	Cystic breast disease	Vit. E
Cd	Decreased androgen activity	Cu, Fe, Mn, Zn
Cd, Hg, Pb, Ritalin (drug)	Delayed sexual maturity	Zn
Cu, fungus	Elevated estrogen	Protective bacteria
Ni, chemicals, microorganisms, allergy, whiplash	Endometriosis	Oils
Cu, Zn, GLA oils, cholesterol	Excessive reproductive hormones	
Microorganisms, allergy, chemicals, whiplash	Hot flashes	Se, vit. E
F, structural (lower back), circulation	Impotence	Mo, Zn, vit. E
Cd, Hg, EMR, Lyme disease, chlamydia, mycoplasma	Infertility, difficulty getting pregnant	Cu, Fe, I, Mn, Zn, oils (omega 6, GLA)
Hg, pesticides, yeast	Inhibited sexual desire, low libido	Zn, GLA oils
Pesticides	Low sperm count	Zn, GLA oils
Hg, pesticides	Low testosterone or progesterone	Zn, oils (omega 6)
Ca, Hg, estrogen birth control pills	Menstrual cramps	**Mg**, K, Na, P, vit. B6
Fe	Menstrual irregularity	Mg, K, Na, P, Zn, vit. B6
	Menstrual problems	Vits. B6, B12, folic acid
Hg, EMR, Lyme disease, chlamydia	Miscarriages, difficulty getting pregnant	Zn, vit. B6, GLA oils
F, I, , Mn, P, Zn	Miscellaneous reproductive problems	Ca, Cu, Fe, I, Mg, Zn, vit. B6
Cu	Postpartum psychosis	Vit. B6, DHEA, try, tyr
Hg, mycoplasma	Premature birth	Zn, vit. B6, GLA oils
Ca, Cd, Hg	Premenstrual syndrome (PMS)	Mg, Zn, vit. B6, Vit. E, GLA oils
Zn, vasectomy	Prostate problems	Cu, **Zn**, gly, vit. B6
Cu	Toxemia of pregnancy	
Trichomonas, yeast, chlamydia	Vaginal discharge	Cu, Zn, protective bacteria
Yeast, vaginal deodorants	Vaginal itching	Vit. B2, biotin
Fungus, trichomonas	Vaginal odor	Cu, Zn, protective bacteria

Kidneys and Urinary System

Toxic Excess	Symptom	Deficiency
Cl, Hg, Ni, protein, chemicals, **metals**	Acid urine (in morning)	Cu, HCl, vit. B3
Hg, pesticides	Albuminuria	Vits. B2, B6
Cl, Hg, **fermentation**, **fungus**, h.pylori, microorganisms	Alkaline urine (in morning)	Cu, HCl, vit. B3
Worms, parasite allergy, melatonin	Bedwetting	Cu, V, Zn, vits. B2, B5, B6, tyr
Ni, mycoplasmas, allergy, microorganisms	Bladder infections	Cu, Zn, vit. A, lys, sulfur aminos
Ag, B, Se	Degenerative kidney changes	K, vit.. B2, oils (omega 6)
Cr, Fe, Hg, K, Mn, Se, Zn	Diabetes (sugar in urine)	Ca, Cu, Cr, Fe, I, Mn, Na, V, Zn, fiber
Ag, Cl, Cr, F	Diminished urine (oliguria, anuria)	Ca, Fe, Mg
Hg, caffeine	Frequent urination	
As, Cd, Hg, I, K, N, Na, Ni, Se	Edema, water retention	I, K, Na, P, protein, vits. B2, B6
As, Cd, Hg, Pb, Ni, Sn, giardia, caffeine	Electrolyte and fluid loss, dehydration	Cl, I, Na, P
Hg	Electrolyte imbalance	
Ca, Cl, F, Hg, Vit. C	Kidney stones	Ca, Mg, fiber
Al, As, B, Cd, Cl, Cr, Cu, F, Hg, K, Mn, Ni, Pb, Se, aspirin, mycin antibiotics, pesticides, organics	Misc. kidney damage	Ca, Cu, Fe, I, K, Mg, Mn, Na, Zn
Cd	Protein in urine	Cu, Fe, Mn, Zn
Na, Vit. D	Thirst	K, oils (omega 6)
Cl, microorganisms, whiplash, low back structural	Urinary tract problems	
I, microorganisms	Violet or yellow-green urine	

Cancer

Toxic Excess	Symptoms	Deficiency (see also Cancer in General)
Ni, dyes, plastics, tobacco	Bladder, urinary tract cancer	
Pb, Sr	Bone cancer	
Hg, Ni, Pb, pesticides, formaldehyde, portable phone	Brain cancer	
PCBs, Ni, alcohol, pesticides	Breast cancer	Fiber
As, Cd, Cr, F, Fe, Ge, Hg, Mo, Ni, Pb, Se, organics, coal tar, saccharin, mineral oil, talc, ozone, dyes, BHT, cancer drugs, radiation, pesticides	Cancer in general	Ca, Cu, Fe, Mg, Zn, vits. C, E, antioxidants, beta-carotene, cys, tau, sulfur aminos, oils (GLA)
Hg, Zn, EBV, pesticides	Hodgkins disease, lymphoma	Cu, sulfur aminos
Pb, formaldehyde	Kidney cancer	K, vit. B2, sulfur aminos
Ni, tobacco, alcohol	Laryngeal cancer	sulfur aminos
Hg, Pb, EMR, EBV, fiberglass, pesticides, ethylene oxide, benzene	Leukemia	Cu
As, Ni, solvents, alcohol	Liver cancer	
As, Be, Co, Cd, Cr, Fe, Ni, **tobacco**, solvents, plastics, marijuana, asbestos, soot, fiberglass, pesticides	Lung cancer	
Tobacco (smoking, chewing), alcohol	Mouth and throat cancer	
Hair dye, pesticides	Non-Hodgkins lymphoma	
Ni	Pancreatic cancer	
Cd, Hg, vasectomy	Prostate cancer	Zn
Cr, Ni, Se, Sr, soot	Sinuses, nasal cancer	
As, soot, formaldehyde, sun	Skin cancer	
Ni, ethylene oxide, plastics, alcohol	Stomach and digestive tract cancer	Fiber
Cd, soot	Testicles, scrotum cancer	

Other Symptoms

Toxic Excess	Symptoms	Deficiency
Cu	Abnormal tissue growth	
Hg	Acrodynia ("pink disease")	
F, Zn	Acute poisoning	Ca, Cu, Mg, sulfur aminos
Na	Adrenal stress	Cu, K
	Airsickness, seasickness	Vit. B1
Se	Alkali disease	
Cu, F, Hg, K, Mg, Mn, Na, Ni, Sn	Allergy	Ca, Cu, Co, Fe, I, K, Mg, Na, P, Zn, vits. A, B1, C, protein, biotin, sulfur aminos, oils
F	Anaerobic glycolysis (degradation of glucose)	Ca, Cr, Mg, V
Cd, Hg	Antibody suppression	Cu, Fe, Mn, Zn
Pb	Atrophy of organs or tissue	Fe, sulfur aminos, oils
Al, Hg, Ni	Aversion to meat	
	Beriberi (deficiency disease)	Vit. B1
Se	Blisters	
I, Na, whiplash, giardia, fungus, h.pylori	Bloating	Cl, Cu, K, vit. B3
Se	Body odor	Zn, vit. B12
Hg, caustics, UV light (as from sun)	Burns	Oils
Ni, Se	Cellular degeneration	Sulfur aminos
I, F, Sn, whiplash, fungus, microorganisms	Cold hands and feet, sensitivity to cold	Na
B, Cl	Congestion of all body organs	Sulfur aminos, oils
Cu	Cystic fibrosis	Sulfur aminos, oils
Al	Debility	
Cd, Hg	Decreased body temperature	Cu, I, Zn
F	Decreased phosphatase	Ca, Mg, P
Cu	Decreased retinol (Vit. A)	Vit. A
Ni	Degeneration of protoplasm	Zn, sulfur aminos, oils
Fe	Deposits in the lymph	
Steroids	Depressed adrenal function	Cu, K, Na
Cu	Depressed glutathione reductase	Zn
Cl, Hg	Detox and cleansing problems	Fiber, oils, sulfur aminos
I	Disturbed metabolism	Cl, Cu, I, Zn, vit. B3
Si	Enlarged spleen	Sulfur aminos, oils
Cd, Cu, F, Hg, Pb, Se	Enzyme system inhibition	Ca, Fe, Mg, Zn
Se	Exudative diathesis (fluid accumulation)	
Pb	Ferritin migrates to mitochondria	Fe
As, B, F, Hg, Mn, S, Zn, microorganisms, pesticides	Fever	Ca, Cu, I, Mg, Mo, Se, Zn
Be, Si	Foreign body granulomas in breast and liver	
Al, Cd, Cu, Hg, Pb, parasites, organics	Frequent colds and infections	Cu, Fe, Zn, lysine, vits. A, C, B5, oils (omega 6)

As, S	Garlic smell to body	I, sulfur aminos, oils
Mn, allergy, microorganisms, pesticides, whiplash	Glandular swelling	Ca, Fe, I, sulfur aminos
Cr	Glucose intolerance	Ca, Fe
As, F, I	Goiter, thyroid gland enlargement	Ca, **I**, Mg, sulfur aminos, oils
Pb, meat purines	Gout	Cl, Cu, Fe, folic acid, vit. B3
Cu	Grippe (acute infectious disease)	Zn
Alcohol, fungus, h.pylori	Hangover	Vits. B1, B12
Ca	Hormone imbalance	
Hg	Hyperthyroid	I
F, Cl	Hypothyroid	Cu, I, Mn, Zn
Cd, Ritalin (drug)	Impaired growth	Cu, Fe, Mn, Zn
Ag, Ni, microorganisms, fungus, whiplash	Inability to handle stress	B vits., vits. A and C
Cd	Itai-itai disease in Japan	Cu, Fe, Mn, Zn
Cr	Kwashiorkor	Ca, Fe
Hg, Ni, chemicals, allergy, whiplash	Lupus	B vits, vit. A, antioxidants
Cl, dyes, chemicals	Lymph problems	Oils
Pb, S	Malaise (flu-like feeling)	Ca, Cu, Fe, Mo, Se
Ca, Cl	Mineral deposits	Sulfur aminos, oils
Ca	Night sweats or cramps	
Al, Ca	Numbness	Na
I	Obesity, weight gain	I, fiber
Co, Sn	Pain sensitivity	Phe, try
Alcohol	Pancreatitis	
As, Hg, Sb	Paresthesia (abnormal sense of touch)	I
Fe	Phytates decrease absorption	
I	Polio in summer	
F, Fe, Se, Si	Premature aging	Mo, Se, sulfur aminos, oils, antioxidants
Hg	Prostration, exhaustion	Na
F	Protoplasmic poisoning	Ca, Mg
Ca	Scar formation	
	Scurvy	Vit. C
Cr, F, I, P, Zn	Stunted growth	Ca, Co, Cr, Cu, Fe, Mg, Zn, Vits. B2, B12, folic acid, protein, oils
	Suppressed immune system	Ca, Cu, Zn
Hg, microorganisms	Swollen lymph glands	Sulfur aminos, oils
As, F, Co, Cu, I, Mn, Pb, structural	Thyroid dysfunction	Ca, Cu, Fe, I, Mg
Mn	Transmanganin	Ca, Fe, I
Zn	Vitamin A storage impaired	Cu
Cd, Cl, F, Hg, Pb	Weight loss	Ca, Cu, Fe, Mg, Mn, P, Zn
Cu	Wilson's disease	Sulfur aminos, vit. C, antioxidants

How It All Works

TOXIC IMMUNE SYNDROME

Unscrambling the Disease of the 21st Century

What is Toxic Immune Syndrome?

There are certain conditions, not even clearly recognized as diseases, that have become more prevalent and more widely recognized in the past decade. These include:

- *Chronic Fatigue Syndrome*
- *Multiple Chemical Sensitivity, or Environmental Illness*
- *Allergies and sensitivities*
- *Brain fog*
- *Fibromyalgia*
- *Some degenerative or autoimmune diseases*
- *Conditions caused by blocked filters, such as skin and bowel problems and asthma*

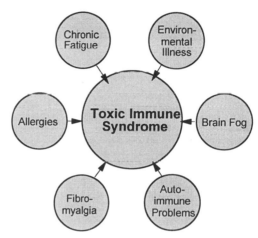

Autoimmune diseases such as arthritis and lupus, and allergies of all types, discussed in the Immune System chapter, are becoming much more prevalent as well.

It is not unusual for more than one of these to be present. In all of them, the cause is often a body that is overwhelmed by any of the toxic suppressors described in this book, alone or in combination. This is called Toxic Immune Syndrome. **While chronic fatigue, chemical sensitivity, or fibromyalgia is a description of the symptoms, Toxic Immune Syndrome describes what is actually going on (the cause).**

The idea of Toxic Immune Syndrome causing a wide variety of ailments, especially CFS and AIDS, is discussed in a two-part article with a total of 106 medical / scientific references. In these articles TIS is referred to as Syndrome of Immune Dysregulation (SID), but the basic premise is the same [1,2].

Chronic Fatigue Syndrome

What is the Chronic Fatigue Syndrome part of Toxic Immune Syndrome?

Chronic fatigue syndrome (CFS) also goes by several other names:

- *Chronic Epstein-Barr virus syndrome (CEBV)*
- *Chronic Fatigue and Immune Dysfunction Syndrome (CFIDS)*
- *The "Yuppie flu"*
- *Myalgic encephalomyelitis, or M.E. This term is more common in Europe.*

> **Chronic fatigue is the way Toxic Immune Syndrome manifests itself in some people.**

CFS is called a syndrome, or collection of recognizable symptoms that usually occur together, rather than a distinct disease. CFS affects about 3 million Americans and about 90 million people worldwide [3]. Although it has been reported in all age groups, chronic fatigue syndrome is most prevalent in the 20-40 age range. Women sufferers outnumber men two to one, and 95% of the victims are Caucasian [3,4].

Doctors may disagree on the definition of Chronic Fatigue Syndrome. Some define it as a clearly delineated set of symptoms, or the presence of a certain number of symptoms from the lists on the next few pages. Others consider any debilitating fatigue lasting at least several months to be CFS regardless of the presence or absence of other symptoms.

What are the symptoms of chronic fatigue syndrome?
There is some dispute as to which patients should be diagnosed as having CFS. The definition can be as simple as a feeling of long-term tiredness and listlessness that is severe enough to have a significant impact on the sufferer's life.

Do you have the following symptoms? You may have the Chronic Fatigue Syndrome part of Toxic Immune Syndrome.

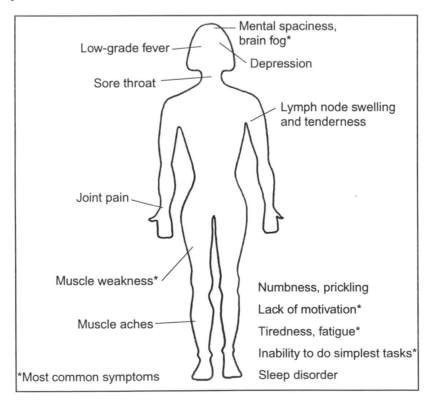

The most common description of symptoms is a feeling of:

- *tiredness*
- *muscle weakness*
- *lack of motivation*
- *dragginess*
- *mental spaciness*
- *inability to do the simplest daily tasks*

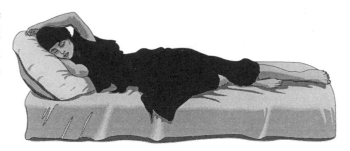

Depression, which may be magnified by the EBV or other virus (CMV, herpes etc.) and may be a side effect of having to put up with the other symptoms, is also common. The severity of symptoms ranges from inconvenient to completely debilitating. The symptoms can last for six months or more and then improve, or may get progressively worse, or may vary in intensity from day to day or month to month. Stress, either emotional or physical, usually worsens the illness. Sufferers often can't work or can work only part-time, causing stress over financial issues, which exacerbates symptoms in a vicious cycle.

One source [4] defines a CFS patient as having at least six of the following symptoms for at least four months:

- *Fatigue*
- *Sore throat*
- *Muscle aches*
- *Low-grade fever*
- *Headache*
- *Sleep disorder*
- *Joint pain*
- *Depression*
- *Lymph node swelling and tenderness, especially side of neck and under arms*
- *Numbness, prickling, or heightened sensitivity*
- *Difficulty in concentrating, remembering, and expressing ideas, sometimes called brain fog*

These symptoms sometimes occur following apparent recovery from an acute viral infection or flu, and especially mononucleosis. Some victims cannot completely overcome the infection; their immune systems can only control it intermittently. The chronic syndrome that develops affects about 5% of those who develop mononucleosis, which is itself caused by the Epstein-Barr Virus (EBV). The symptoms can last for years unless the overwhelmed immune system is assisted by measures discussed throughout this book.

Other symptoms attributed to CFS are:

- *Irritability*
- *Mood swings*
- *Decreased libido*
- *Gastrointestinal symptoms*
- *Heart rhythm disturbances*
- *General muscle weakness*
- *Sensitivity to light and noise*
- *Changes in taste, smell or hearing*
- *Neck and low back pain*
- *Liver and spleen swelling and tenderness*

- *Weight gain*
- *Hot flashes, night sweats*
- *Recent onset of food and environmental sensitivities*
- *Lightheadedness, feeling "spaced out"*

This list of symptoms does not convey what it is really like to have one's life defined by chronic fatigue. CFS has been described as feeling as if one is two months from death with cancer or AIDS, but the feeling continues daily for years. Since there is often no objective evidence of illness (like a rash or fever), and there is no definitive blood test for CFS, the sufferer may find that nobody takes them seriously. Just because they look fine doesn't mean that they are. They may be told to "snap out of it," to get counseling (when they *know* the problem is physical), or to "just learn to live with it". Doctors tell them that nothing is wrong, and their family may accuse them of being lazy. The feeling that there is no support and no help often worsens the disease in a vicious cycle.

The fatigue goes beyond simple tiredness. The person with CFS may be tired but can't rest, and often feels just plain awful, but may have a difficult time pinpointing just what feels so awful. Sometimes something as simple as doing the laundry, making lunch, or climbing the stairs seems insurmountably difficult. Added to this is the nagging uncertainty as to whether life will ever be normal again.

Two indicators of CFS are decreased brain circulation after exercise and decreased cortisol levels in the blood after exercise [5].

How does CFS start?

For some people, CFS seems to begin with mononucleosis or the flu, or may develop after a concussion, whiplash injury or some other stressful event. In these cases the actual onset of CFS is clearly defined and a particular day can even be pinpointed. A person may feel fine in the morning, have typical flu symptoms by afternoon, and five years later the situation is unchanged. They just never got better. For other people, the onset is so gradual that it is difficult to determine what *year* the illness started.

Even if the flu, mononucleosis or EBV infection appeared to precipitate the fatigue and other symptoms, it is likely that the infection is the last straw on an already overloaded toxic scale. The immune system is so overwhelmed that these or other symptoms finally tip the scales, allowing the virus to thrive.

What can contribute to the fatigue?

The list of possible causes can be quite long, and these causes can exist alone or in combination. Nearly any toxicity or deficiency can cause fatigue, and this fatigue can last for years if the underlying cause isn't identified and treated.

Some of the more common contributors to the symptoms are [6]:

- *Primary suppressors*
  Chemicals, chemical sensitivity, drugs

> *Metal toxicity, especially mercury from dental amalgams or nickel from*
>   *stainless steel root canal posts*
> *Electromagnetic radiation*
> *Unresolved emotional and/or spiritual issues*
> *Adrenal insufficiency from stress or stimulants such as caffeine*

- *Nutritional deficiencies*

- *Secondary toxic suppressors - Microorganisms*
    Viruses
    Infection of any type
    Yeast overgrowth

- *Symptoms that make matters worse*
    Allergies
    Anemia
    Depression
    Hypoglycemia
    Hormonal factors - fatigue may be worse premenstrually
    Thyroid problems, especially hypothyroidism

A large percentage of adults with CFS (about 80%) have a history of frequent and recurrent antibiotic treatment in childhood or the teen years [7].

Melatonin, which comes from the stimulation of the pineal gland in the brain by sunlight, is released at night to help regulate sleep cycles. A vicious cycle often develops in CFS patients. They are tired, stay in bed all day with the curtains closed, often wear sunglasses when they do go out because their eyes are sunlight sensitive due to toxins, do not produce enough sunlight-stimulated melatonin, do not sleep well, and are tired the next day. Insomnia and poor quality sleep are common in CFS.

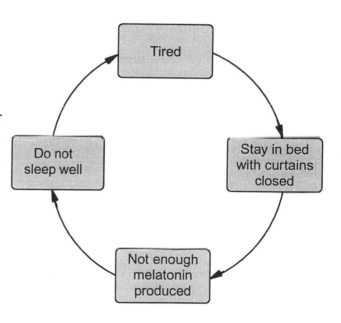

Patients who have come to a comprehensive clinic with CFS, and in many cases in addition to fibromyalgia and brain fog, had a wide range of problems. When their particular major problem was treated, along with other supportive therapies, their health improved considerably. In these as in most cases, however, there is more than one cause, and treatment is like going through several layers of clouds before you break through to blue skies.

- A woman in her late 30s changed the lights in her home and office before getting well. After working through some of her main issues, this was a seemingly insignificant thing that was affecting her health. But it made the difference in finally getting well.

- A man in his early 40s had whiplash, and was helped by getting a structural realignment and then balancing the bite. A bite that was off contributed to an alignment that was off and continually had a negative effect on his health.

- A woman in her 30s had giardia and chemical sensitivity cleared. She had to deal with both of these issues before she got well. She did get well.

- A man around 40 had a concussion and whiplash, and his bite was off. These problems were resolved by dealing with structural problems, then balancing the bite.

- A woman of 50 who had fibromyalgia and allergies got well. By getting to the root causes, and working through the issues pinpointed, the supportive therapies available helped her resolve her health problems and she felt like she got her life back.

- A man around 30 had helicobacter pylori but didn't know this was the root cause of his ulcer-like symptoms and digestive problems. Once this root cause was pinpointed, he got the proper treatment and he got well.

- A woman in her 40s who had a weight problem in addition to CFS due to gluten allergy (celiac disease) got well. Through proper testing, which pinpointed the gluten problem, she was able to go on a program which addressed all the issues and resulted in restoring her to a state of health she had begun to feel could never be hers.

- Two women, one around 30 and the other around 50, had yeast problems and got well by getting the type of therapy that dealt with the root cause rather than just getting a prescription for the most obvious manifesting symptoms. They eradicated the root cause of their problems.

In all these cases, as throughout the book, getting to the root cause rather than giving out a prescription to deal with surface symptoms made a positive impact on the state of their health. It made the difference between taking vigorous actions to deal with the situation once and for all, and letting the situation drag on and perhaps lead to even more debilitating and possibly life threatening health problems down the road.

> **The affluent may be more prone to CFS because they have more access to the causative toxins.**

Why is CFS sometimes called the "Yuppie flu"?
Most people with the syndrome appear to be well educated and affluent, thus the source of the nickname "Yuppie flu". This may be due to the fact that people in this socioeconomic group are most likely to seek medical treatment for a condition whose symptoms are chronic and yet can be vague.

The correlation of CFS with the more affluent may also be due to the fact that such people are most likely to be able to afford toxin-inducing luxuries such as microwave ovens, antibiotics, mercury fillings, root canals and capped teeth, as well as expensive but often ineffective health care. Other immune system suppressors common among the affluent include Cesarean section births, no breastfeeding, recreational drugs, and birth control pills. Since the disease tends to hit hard-driving Type-A "yuppies", burnout where the adrenal glands are overworked due to mental stress is probably also a major player.

How can you tell the difference between CFS and depression?

Since both fatigue and a loss of interest and motivation are major components of both CFS and depression it is often hard to tell them apart; in fact, they may be nearly indistinguishable. The importance of distinguishing between them lies in the focus of treatment - physical causes or counseling. This may in fact be an academic distinction only, since the mind and body are so intrinsically interlinked.

Depression is usually the more accurate diagnosis if there is a clear emotional precipitating event - a death in the family or job loss, for example. Depression is sometimes called frozen anger, and is more likely if the event (death or loss) is accompanied by anger or a feeling of abandonment.

However, most of the time feelings of depression do not have a clear cause. One easy way to distinguish between physical fatigue and emotional depression is to do something that is mildly strenuous but enjoyable, such as a walk in the park or a shopping trip. Such an excursion will often cause emotion-based depression and

> Is it physical illness or depression? Here's one indicator.

fatigue to lift at least temporarily, while fatigue and depression with a primarily physical cause will often worsen.

Is the Epstein-Barr virus (or other virus) involved in CFS?

There is some disagreement among professionals as to the extent to which the Epstein-Barr virus is responsible for the syndrome. Some feel that EBV causes the syndrome. Others feel that since EBV is not present in all chronic fatigue patients, and is also present in those who do not suffer from chronic fatigue syndrome, it is not the causative agent, although it may have a contributory role. The idea that EBV causes CFS is favored by fewer people than in years past as other causes are discovered.

> There is no one cause for Chronic Fatigue Syndrome -CDC-

Even the conservative Centers for Disease Control (CDC) now admits that there is no one cause for CFS, concluding it's the last precipitating thing that pushed your health over the edge.

About 80% of patients have IgE mediated (airborne) allergy. It is possible that this allows the Epstein-Barr virus to gain a foothold. It is also possible that the allergic reactions themselves can cause the symptoms, regardless of the presence of EBV. It is our experience that the many toxic suppressors described in this book accumulate until they finally exceed the health threshold, causing both the chronic fatigue symptoms and the EBV infection through immune suppression.

Does CFS ever get better?

CFS may get better on its own, or may worsen if untreated. In some people, the fatigue may come and go in cycles, with improvement or relapses lasting for months. The outlook for partial or full recovery is optimistic if the sufferer is able to find and be treated by a knowledgeable practitioner (see "The Perfect Clinic" chapter). The likelihood of recovery decreases after the first five years of illness [8]. Don't give up hope, however. No matter how long you have been sick, you can begin to make a come back. You just need the right approach and the direction which a knowledgeable practitioner can provide.

What can be done?

Nearly any toxicity, structural misalignment, nutritional deficiency, microorganism or yeast overgrowth, and/or illness can contribute to fatigue. Treatment thus consists of first finding out the root cause(s) of the fatigue and then treating those causes. Treatments normally prescribed for fatigue and depression are primarily drugs, but such treatments often only serve to cover up or suppress the symptoms and may make the problem worse in the long run. And there may be more than one root cause. These must all be dealt with in the proper order, much like peeling away an onion, layer by layer.

Go through this book and its companion volume *Surviving The Toxic Crisis* chapter by chapter to try to pin down the primary causes of your illness, whether chronic fatigue or otherwise. Do you have most of the symptoms listed at the beginning of any one chapter? Do you have numerous mercury fillings, a history of drug, medication or alcohol use, a heavy exposure to pesticides, or a poor diet? The suggestions in these chapters would be a good place to start. Even better would be to go to a clinic that deals with chronic problems. They would be more experienced at doing the detective work needed to pinpoint the root causes and can usually short-cut the process to getting your health back on track.

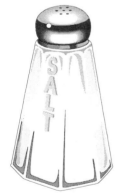

Since yeast overgrowth is a common contributor to fatigue, eliminating sugar and other yeast feeders (see chapter on Yeast Infections in *Surviving The Toxic Crisis*) is a good place to start.

Sodium (salt) deficiency and its accompanying low blood pressure has been shown to be related to CFS [9]. Salt, preferably mineral salt, Real Salt or sea salt, can help alleviate some of the symptoms, although it is not a cure. If salt makes a difference in your energy level, this can be an important clue to an alert health professional.

Chronic fatigue patients in one study were given amino acid supplements for three months. The particular amino acid mixture was individualized according to each patient's fasting blood plasma values. The most commonly deficient amino acids were phenylalanine and tryptophan. Up to 75% of the patients reported a 50-100% improvement in their symptoms, and some experienced a substantial increase in energy within several days to two weeks [10].

Environmental Illness

What is Environmental Illness?

Environmental Illness (EI), also called Multiple Chemical Sensitivity (MCS), is an immune system disorder characterized by heightened reactivity to many different chemicals, usually by inhalation. Such a person has been described as "allergic to the 20th century". A National Academy of Sciences workshop estimated that 15% of the U.S. population are chemically sensitive to some degree [11]. The term Universal Reactor is also used. Many of the chemicals that the person is sensitive to would be toxic to anyone, but someone with EI would have a more immediate and severe reaction and/or would react to a much smaller amount than would affect the average person.

EI can dramatically limit the life of the person who has it. Such a person must weigh the advantages of every shopping trip or social outing against the possibility of becoming ill from diesel fumes on the highway, cologne, formaldehyde, or other chemicals that may be encountered. Some EI sufferers can become apprehensive about leaving their homes, a condition called agoraphobia (literally, "fear of the marketplace"), while others may have to leave their homes to escape the mold and new house chemical toxins within.

What kinds of chemicals can the person be allergic to?

Although nearly everything is, strictly speaking, chemical, the term as used here refers to substances which have been created through modern technology versus those naturally occurring in nature. Thus the term includes but is not limited to:

- *Solvents, paints*
- *Formaldehyde from carpet etc.*
- *Pesticides*
- *Food additives*
- *Gasoline, diesel fumes*
- *Cologne*
- *Air pollution, smog*
- *Drugs, alcohol*
- *Cooking gas*
- *Chlorine in water*
- *Soaps, detergents*
- *Plastics*
- *Cigarette smoke*
- *Pencil lead, ink, newsprint*
- *Laminants, glues from particle board and other sources*
- *Dental metals and materials, including mercury and nickel*

The term chemical as used here excludes natural materials such as foods, mold, pollen, and pet dander, although allergies or sensitivities to these things often exist along with the multiple chemical sensitivities.

What types of symptoms occur with EI?

Symptoms can be roughly broken down into acute or chronic. Acute symptoms are easily recognizable and come on almost immediately after exposure to the chemical. Because of the rapidity and distinctness of the symptoms, it is usually fairly easy to determine the chemical(s) responsible. Symptoms can include [12]:

- *Seizures*
- *Headache*
- *Asthma*
- *Nausea*

- *Abrupt drop in blood pressure, leading to dizziness and a prickling feeling in the face*

- *Hypersensitivity to odors - the person may smell the chemical before anyone else can*

- *Emotional reactions, including sudden tears or anger*

- *Confusion and brain fog, discussed later in this chapter, that comes on suddenly*

- *Panic attacks, agoraphobia*

- *Fear of any new assault or stress - an "I can't handle one more thing" feeling*

With chronic symptoms it is usually more difficult to pin down the cause of the symptoms. Such symptoms are usually more vague, and may not come on immediately after exposure, so the sufferer may not even realize that s/he is chemically sensitive, much less the particular chemical(s) involved.

Chronic symptoms include:

- *Fatigue*
- *Muscle weakness*
- *Fibromyalgia, or overall pain, discussed later in this chapter*
- *Brain fog*
- *Lowered immunity to illness*
- *Emotional reactions including depression, irritability or anxiety*

Acute reactions may become chronic as the body adapts (or more accurately maladapts), or chronic reactions may become acute as the body's tolerance is stressed. As the sensitivity progresses, reactivity may change from hyper (overreactivity) to hypo (underreactivity). For example, the person may go from anxious and manic to depressed and apathetic, or the immune system may go from allergic (overactive) to suppressed (worn out or burned-out).

Neurotransmitters called GABA and NMDA influence the degree to which a person tends toward hyperactive or hypoactive responses. More NMDA shifts the balance towards hyperactivity, while more GABA relative to NMDA does the opposite. Paradoxically, since CFS seems to more closely resemble coma than hyperactivity, more NMDA relative to GABA is associated with CFS, as shown in this chart.

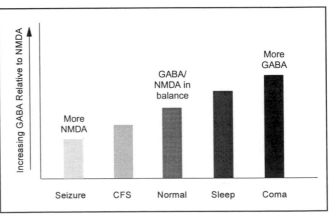

What brings on Multiple Chemical Sensitivity?

MCS/EI usually starts when the body's detoxification pathways are overwhelmed by more chemicals and other burdens (emotional or structural, for example) than it can handle. For some people the precipitating event is a single massive exposure, such as an industrial accident (rare) or having one's house sprayed for termites or other bugs (quite common). With other people, the exposure is so prolonged and so subtle that it is difficult to pinpoint a year of disease onset. Sometimes the sensitivity begins when there is an apparently unrelated trauma, such as a car accident, surgery, childbirth, or emotional trauma. Gallbladder problems brought on by helicobacter, giardia or fungus, which themselves are set up by mercury dental fillings among other causes, can set the stage for intolerance to oil-soluble chemicals by leaving you so oil-deficient that your cells start soaking up oil-based chemicals like a sponge.

What determines who will become chemically sensitive?

Reactivity is dependent on the interaction of these various factors:

- Genetic tolerance - some people can handle more than others. What may appear to be genetic (some babies seem to be born allergic) may be due to the pre-birth toxic load of the mother (mercury, microorganisms, etc.) or to C-section birth or lack of breastfeeding.

- Total body burden, including non-chemical problems such as structural trauma (e.g., whiplash, concussion), emotional problems, and microorganism infestation (e.g., helicobacter, giardia, roundworm, fungus).

- Total toxic or chemical load.

- Competition for removal of chemicals and toxins by the same biochemical pathways.

- How long the chemical stays in the body, doing its damage.

- Synergism (or 1+1=3) - some chemicals worsen the effects of others.

An example of synergism is the taking of the ulcer medication, like Tagamet, which can inactivate the body's detoxifying Cytochrome P-450 system. If the person then is exposed to the pesticide Malathion, which the body usually deals with via the Cytochrome P-450 system, the person can get very sick. Tagamet and Malathion together, therefore, are much more toxic than either one by itself. In another example, yeast puts out the toxic byproduct acetaldehyde (acetyl aldehyde), and a body which is busy coping with acetaldehyde is likely to be much less tolerant of the common and chemically related toxin formaldehyde. The detox pathway for aldehydes is already full.

What changes can be expected with MCS?

Types of symptoms, severity of symptoms, and amount of chemical needed to precipitate a reaction not only varies between individuals, but can vary from day to day in the same person. This is probably due in part to the daily variation in total toxic burden. Different toxins are eliminated by way of different detoxification pathways, and one pathway may be more overloaded than another on any given day, explaining some of the day-to-day variation [13].

Women are often more sensitive during certain parts of their menstrual cycle, especially just before and at the beginning of their periods.

Over time, an untreated chemical sensitivity will often worsen, especially if the triggering chemicals are not identified and avoided. Sensitivity can spread to other chemicals, other reactions, and other organs or systems.

What can be done?
The first step is to identify the chemicals involved. Keep a diary of exposures and reactions. Then reduce or eliminate exposure to the greatest extent possible. Elimination of other toxic suppressors can also help reduce chemical sensitivity by reducing the total body load.

Suggestions for detoxifying chemicals - sauna therapy is especially useful - are outlined in the chapter on Chemical Toxicity in *Surviving The Toxic Crisis*. NAET allergy testing and treatment, developed by Dr. Devi Nambudripad [14,15] can also help to identify and eliminate chemical allergies.

Allergies

What other types of allergy are prevalent?
Chemical sensitivity is not the only type of allergic condition. Allergies in general are on the increase. This includes sensitivities to foods, pollen, pet dander, mold, and others.

Why are allergies on the rise?
One reason for the apparent increase in allergies lies in the fact that we are more and more overloaded with toxins and body stressors, i.e. Toxic Immune Syndrome. As discussed in the Immune System chapter, allergy is essentially an overwhelmed body overreacting to things that are otherwise relatively harmless. The immune system is not in error; it is simply doing the best it can to deal with the combination of self and non-self.

How do we know toxins are involved?
The relationship between toxic overload and allergies has been amply demonstrated by many patients who became less allergic in general after undergoing detoxification through sauna, chelation, diet, or other means.

Allergic or toxic?
Toxins may be involved in another sense. A reaction to a certain substance or food may appear to be an allergy but does not actually involve the immune system. Instead, certain detoxification pathways may be overloaded by toxins, and the slight amount of toxic substances in many foods

may then not be detoxified by the relevant pathways. The result: a toxic reaction from the food that may look like an allergic reaction [16].

A knowledgeable practitioner can look at the types of food that you are reacting to and be able to tell which detox pathways are blocked. From there s/he can infer what types of toxins are causing a problem.

For example, do you react to:

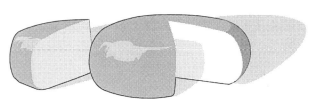

- *Red wine, cheese, bananas or chocolate*
- *MSG, often found in Chinese food*
- *Onions or garlic*
- *Caffeine*
- *Alcohol*
- *Grapefruit or other citrus*
- *Foods with the preservative sodium benzoate*
- *Sulfites in dried fruit, wine, and some salad bars*

If the answer is yes to any of these food groups, or if your urine has an unpleasant odor of sulfur after you eat asparagus, you may have a blockage or overload of the associated detox pathway.

What can be done for allergies?

There are many treatments for specific allergies. One such treatment is Nambudripad's Allergy Elimination Treatment (NAET) developed by Dr. Devi Nambudripad [14,15]. Her treatment is based on the idea that, although some substances are inherently toxic, others are toxic or not depending on how the brain perceives it.

The brain has thus been programmed, for whatever reason, to see something which is normally harmless to most people as being toxic. It follows that the brain can be reprogrammed, and if the brain is reprogrammed, it will no longer see the substance as harmful. The programming is much like the way colostrum from breast milk programs a baby's immune system to recognize self and non-self and to know the dangers in its mother's environment, similar to the way in which a computer needs the appropriate software before it works properly.

The testing part of the treatment involves muscle testing, in which a muscle will test weak if the body/brain is reacting adversely to a substance. The treatment involves unblocking acupressure points corresponding to the various organs while the patient is holding a vial of the substance being treated for. The substance is then avoided for 25 hours, after which the patient is retested. Allergies have been permanently cleared in this manner.

High doses of vitamin C (up to 16 grams daily, or to bowel tolerance) can lead to relief for allergy symptoms [17]. The herbs echinacea, goldenseal root, astragalus root, and Brazilian ginseng help strengthen and normalize immune response and thus offer allergy relief [18].

Fibromyalgia

What is the fibromyalgia part of Toxic Immune Syndrome?

Fibromyalgia, the most recent basket diagnosis, is a condition characterized by pain in the muscles, joints and tissues. The word fibromyalgia is not a disease diagnosis; rather, it is a restatement in Latin/Greek of the symptoms. "Fibro" refers to connective tissue, "my" refers to the muscles, and "algia" means pain. However, in this case the pain is without obvious cause.

Six million Americans have been diagnosed with fibromyalgia syndrome [19]. The **Journal of the American Medical Association** estimates that it occurs in 11% of AIDS patients [20], suggesting a common link with immune dysfunction, or CFIDS.

Autoimmune diseases such as arthritis and lupus, or any type of chronic inflammatory condition or infection, may be related.

How is fibromyalgia diagnosed?

Fibromyalgia is difficult for medicine to diagnose, much less treat, because there is rarely any inflammation or visible evidence that anything is wrong. Allopathic treatments generally consist of painkilling (symptom-suppressing) medications. Fibromyalgia may easily be misdiagnosed as arthritis, lupus, multiple sclerosis, gout, and /or a variety of others conditions, and thus mistreated.

As mentioned, fibromyalgia is a description rather than a disease diagnosis, so if the description fits and you think you have it, you do. Symptoms may include the following, alone or in combination:

- *Aching muscles*
- *Aching joints*
- *An overall feeling of "everything hurts" - bones, muscles, organs, skin*
- *Skin hypersensitivity to stroking or touch, as with a fever*
- *Fatigue is often also associated with fibromyalgia*

What are some of the causes of fibromyalgia?

As is the case with many chronic illnesses, there are many possible causes of or contributors to fibromyalgia:

- Structural problems such as whiplash, concussion, TMJ/TMD or a poorly aligned jaw can contribute to fibromyalgia in some people.

- If the head is too far forward on the body, muscles can fire continuously to balance the jaw and head. Then the muscles throughout the body release lactic acid which can contribute to muscle pain and fatigue. If this condition remains untreated, the acidity can decalcify the long bones as calcium is released to buffer the acid, setting the stage for osteoporosis.

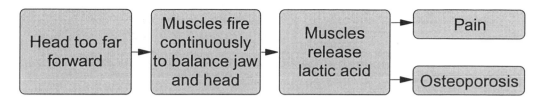

- Electrolyte (mineral) imbalance can cause muscle spasm and cramping, especially deficiencies of potassium, magnesium or calcium, or salt.

- Allergies such as nickel, foods, molds and airborne allergens can cause tightening of the meningeal mediated system, which can affect the head, neck and back.

- Microorganisms such as helicobacter, giardia or fungus can put out toxins, which can also cause tightening of the meningeal mediated system.

- A total body burden greater than one can handle can express itself as overall pain in those who are susceptible, just as the "weak link" of others may be headache or fatigue.

- Poor blood or lymph circulation, or clumping of blood (shown in Live Blood Analysis, which is discussed in the "A Visit To The Doctor" chapter). This reduces the oxygen to the muscles and tissues, causing aching similar to that experienced by runners who push themselves too far. This may be a cause if even moderate exercise brings on or worsens the pain.

- A blood pH that is too acidic may be a contributor [21]. This condition is similar to the aching caused by lactic acid buildup in the muscles of runners. Heavy metals and chemicals may be causing the acidity in the first place.

- The aching may be due to a heightened sensitivity to pain - nothing may actually change in the body to cause the pain, but the perception of it may be more acute. This is what happens with flu or fever - there are general body aches and even lightly stroking the skin may be uncomfortable. There may be a backache even though nothing is wrong with the back. Similar pain perception changes may occur with fibromyalgia.

- Disorders of the mitochondria, the power plants of the cell, can cause intolerance to exercise. An increase in pain or fatigue after even mild exercise could be related to mitochondrial disorders [16]. Although the existence of this problem and its cause should be evaluated professionally, a product called Mitochondrial Resuscitate by Metagenics contains nutrients which specifically support the mitochondrial system.

What can be done for fibromyalgia?
As with other chronic illnesses including those discussed in this chapter, reducing the total body burden can help eliminate the underlying cause. Keeping track of your activities, toxic exposure and diet and how they correlate with worsening or improvement in the pain can help to pinpoint

possible individual causes. Measures can then be taken to avoid the offending substances or activities:

1. *Structural work to realign head position properly on shoulders by moving neck vertebrae forward.*

2. *Balance jaw*

3. *Soft tissue work*

4. *Dental work, mercury and nickel removed from the mouth, and chelation to remove metals from the body.*

5. *Pathogenic microorganisms eliminated inside and out, and treating of other family members as well.*

6. *Allergy elimination and desensitization.*

Other remedies include:

- One source suggests avoiding acidic substances such as fried foods, wine, coffee, alcohol, tea, vinegar and excessive grains and meats [21]. Eat more alkaline foods, which include most vegetables. Don't limit your diet to vegetables, however, or nutritional imbalances will likely result. Use of the 40/30/30 dietary ratios of carbohydrates, protein and good oils should provide the proper balance for about 75% of us. The other 25% need more vegetables than protein.

- Localized application of heat with a hot-water bottle (an electric heating pad is not recommended due to harmful electromagnetic radiation), followed by the application of cold packs. This can improve circulation and relax the muscles.

- Structural work

- Massage or soft-tissue work

- Adequate sleep and rest. Discontinue use of sunglasses, which confuses day and night biorhythms.

- Supporters, especially potassium and calcium, GABA, melatonin or tyrosine

- Tai Chi type exercises consisting of a series of slow movements which develop use of fine motor skills, vs. gross motor skills. This both aids circulation and recruits muscle fibers.

- Fibroplex (Metagenics), malic acid and magnesium, balanced later with calcium

Capsaicin cream, derived from cayenne pepper, has been shown to alleviate some pain and tenderness in fibromyalgia patients. The 0.025% capsaicin cream applied to tender areas four times a day for four weeks produced significant improvement as compared to a placebo [22].

Electroacupuncture has shown some success in treating fibromyalgia [23]. The "Myers cocktail" of intravenous calcium, magnesium, B vitamins and vitamin C has also proven successful in the treatment of fibromyalgia [24].

Brain Fog

What is brain fog and what part does it play in Toxic Immune Syndrome?
Brain fog, sometimes called mind fog, has received less publicity than the other ailments covered in this chapter. However, it is included here because it is quite prevalent, especially with chronic fatigue or chemical sensitivity.

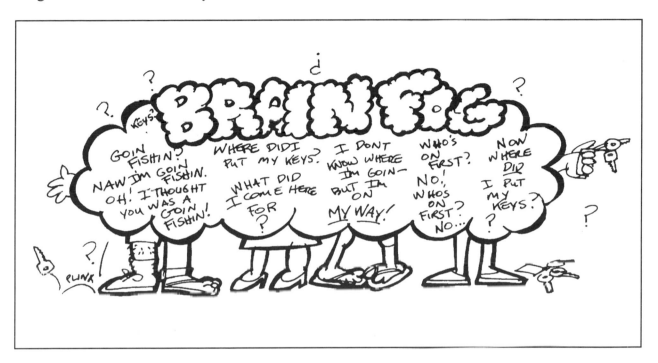

Brain fog, a condition in which the mind doesn't work as well as it used to, affects short term memory and can include the following - do any of them fit you?

- Trouble concentrating. It may be difficult to follow a book or television program. You may be halfway through a magazine article and realize that you don't know what it is about. You may be completely lost trying to follow a movie with a convoluted plot.

- Trouble remembering things like phone numbers, the last known location of the car keys, or why you went from one room to another, and yes, "where did I park my car in the mall parking lot!"

- A feeling of being spacey, foggy, out-of-it.

- Feeling disconnected from people or events around you.

- Coming up with a good answer to a question - several minutes after it's asked.

- Needing to be told the answer to your question several times.

- A feeling that your mind is not as clear as it used to be. If you are past the age of 40, you may be seized with a nagging fear that you are getting senile, or even developing Alzheimer's disease.

Why is brain fog not better known?
Brain fog is not as widely discussed as chronic fatigue or other illnesses. There may be several reasons for this:

- An individual may not be aware of the extent of their problem, since the mind being used to judge the degree of impairment may itself be impaired. This is like the person who, to others, is obviously drunk but insists that he is sober enough to drive - his impaired mind can't see its impairment.

- It may be mistaken for Attention Deficit Disorder (ADD) or other learning disabilities.

- There is a stigma in this society against having mental problems.

- Other people are not talking about it, so the person must be the only one with the problem.

In a not-unusual scenario, a patient goes to the doctor with a whole list of physical symptoms; brain fog is not even mentioned. Yet if an alert doctor asks whether you have the typical symptoms of brain fog (trouble concentrating or remembering, a spacey feeling), they often reply that, yes, that's exactly how they feel.

What are the causes of brain fog?
There are a number of causes of brain fog, several of which are related to the brain's use of oxygen. The brain needs more oxygen than anywhere else in the body, and a reduction in the oxygen getting to the brain can reduce the clarity of thinking.

- **Chemicals** such as petrochemicals (solvents, gasoline) can cause toxic effects to all body cells, including brain cells. This is true whether or not the person is hypersensitive to chemicals. Chemicals can also cause **meningeal mediated contractions**, which can reduce blood flow to the brain and central nervous system. Since blood carries oxygen, less oxygen can get to the brain. Most of the following causes can also involve meningeal mediated contraction.

- **Structural** problems, especially in the neck, can reduce blood flow to the brain as subluxations compress the blood vessels, especially those to the fourth ventricle of the brain. Whiplash and structural problems of the jaw and face may also contribute to brain fog for similar reasons.

- **Parasites, yeast and fungi** put out acetaldehyde as a byproduct of their life cycle. Acetaldehyde, which is chemically related to formaldehyde (embalming fluid), binds with oxygen in the body and brain. The brain will then get less oxygen. Yeast also takes blood sugar (glucose) needed by the cells, including brain cells, for proper function.

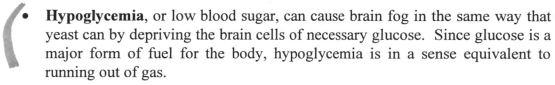

- **Hypoglycemia**, or low blood sugar, can cause brain fog in the same way that yeast can by depriving the brain cells of necessary glucose. Since glucose is a major form of fuel for the body, hypoglycemia is in a sense equivalent to running out of gas.

- **Allergies** can cause brain fog, possibly by causing brain swelling. The brain, if affected by an allergen, can't sneeze or develop a rash. Instead, the most common allergic reaction affecting the brain is swelling. Allergies, like chemicals, can also cause meningeal mediated contractions, reducing blood flow to the brain.

- **Hormones** can affect brain function and brain swelling. Women may notice that before their periods, when there may be water retention in other parts of the body, brain fog may be at its most severe, clearing dramatically around the fourth day of the period when the water weight is lost.

- **Mineral** deficiencies such as potassium can contribute to brain fog.

What can be done about brain fog?
As with other conditions, the first thing to do is identify, then remove and/or treat the cause.

Certain nutrients can help sharpen the mind:

- *Amino acids, especially glutamine, histidine, tyrosine, glutathione*
- *Phosphatidyl choline (MaxiCholine by Phillips Nutritionals) and lecithin*
- *B vitamins*
- *Ginseng*
- *Ginkgo biloba (Enzymatic Therapy)*
- *PCO Phytosome (PhytoPharmica)*
- *Magnesium, potassium*
- *Sun Chlorella*
- *ToxiCleanse (Metagenics)*

What Can Be Done?

All of these conditions, and other chronic conditions, are usually related to Toxic Immune Syndrome. It is important to identify the root cause(s) of the symptoms and treat them. The identification and treatment of these causes are the focus of *Surviving The Toxic Crisis*, in which are detailed the identification and methods of getting to the root cause, and how to eliminate and eradicate:

- *Chemicals, including organics, pesticides, cologne, drugs, and food additives*
- *Metals, especially dental mercury and nickel*
- *Electromagnetic radiation*
- *Structural problems such as whiplash and an unbalanced bite*
- *Emotional stresses*
- *Microorganisms*

In order to help you to better understand how the toxic suppressors have impacted your health today, it is important to have an understanding of how the human body operates at its optimum level and of the systems involved in maintaining your health. It is important to also understand how they are integrated and how a problem in one can have a profound affect on the state of your health overall.

This section of the book, How It All Works, will further your understanding of what happens at the cellular level and the importance of the immune system in maintaining your health and protecting you from the many assaults it must deal with in fighting to keep you healthy. You will begin to understand how important it is to be aware of what the toxic threats are to your health and how you can turn the tide and thrive in this toxic world. Knowledge is power.

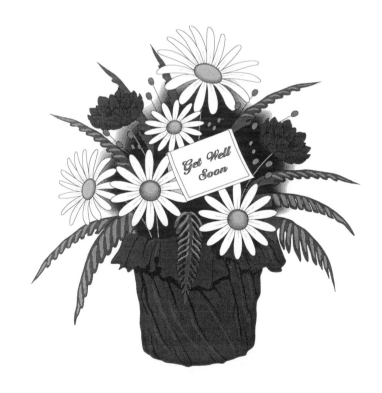

References and Resources

General

- Rogers, Sherry, *Tired or Toxic?*, Prestige Publishing, Syracuse NY, 1990.

Chronic Fatigue Syndrome

- Bell, David S., *The Doctor's Guide to Chronic Fatigue Syndrome*, Addison-Wesley Publishing Group, 1994.

- Berne, Katrina, *Running On Empty*, Hunter House, 1996.

- The Burton Goldberg Group, *Alternative Medicine: The Definitive Guide*, Future Medicine Publishing, Puyallup WA, 1994.
    "Chronic Fatigue Syndrome", pp. 616-624
    "Environmental Medicine", pp. 205-214

- Chaitow, Leon, *Post Viral Fatigue Syndrome*, Dents, London England, 1989.

- Collinge, William, *Recovering From Chronic Fatigue Syndrome*, The Body Press / Perigree Books, NY, 1993.

- Crook, William, *Chronic Fatigue Syndrome and the Yeast Connection*, Professional Books, 1992.

- Feide, Karyn, *Hope and Help for Chronic Fatigue Syndrome*, Fireside Books, NY, 1990.

- Friedberg, Fred, *Coping With CFS*, New Harbinger, 1995. *Offers practical coping strategies for living with CFS.*

- Hale, Mary and Chris Miller, *The CFS Cookbook*, Carol Publishing Group, 1994.

- Jacobs, Pamela D., *500 Tips For Coping With Chronic Illness*, Robert D. Reed Publishers, 1995.

- Johnson, Hillary, *Osler's Web*, Crown Books, 1996. *Chronological history of CFS research since 1984 and the medical and political implications.*

- Kenny, Timothy P., *Living With CFS: A Personal Story of the Struggle For Recovery*, Thunder's Mouth, 1994.

- Rosenbaum, Michael, and Murray Susser, *Solving The Puzzle of Chronic Fatigue Syndrome*, Life Sciences Press, Tacoma WA, 1992.

- Teitelbaum, Jacob, *From Fatigued to Fantastic!*, Deva Press, 1995.

- Vanderzalm, Lynn, *Finding Strength In Weakness*, Zondervan Publishing House, 1995. *Examines the impact of CFS on the family.*

- *The CFIDS Chronicle*, The CFIDS Association of America, Inc., PO Box 220398, Charlotte NC 28222-0398, phone 800-442-3437 or 704-365-2343. *This journal, published quarterly, combines first-person articles by those who have CFS or who have dealt with it or overcome it, articles about treatment, advocacy information, and other resources of interest.*

- **CFIDS Buyers Club**, 1187 Coast Village Road, #1-208, Santa Barbara CA 93108, phone 800-366-6056. *They publish a quarterly newsletter and catalog of supplements and products that could be of interest to those with CFS and chemical sensitivity.*

Chemical Sensitivity

- Rea, William J., *Chemical Sensitivity*, Volume I, Lewis Publishers, Boca Raton FL, 1992. *This book is very technical and is geared towards the scientist or physician.*

Allergy

- Astor, Stephen, *Hidden Food Allergies*, Avery Publishing Group, Garden City Park, NY, 1989.

- Buist, Robert, *Food Chemical Sensitivity*, Avery Publishing Group, Garden City Park, NY, 1988.

- Crook, William G., *Detecting Your Hidden Allergies*, Professional Books, Jackson TN, 1988.

- Gerrard, JW, *Food Allergies - New Perspectives*, Charles C. Thomas, Springfield IL, 1980.

- Mansfield, John, *Arthritis: The Allergy Connection*, Thorsons, San Francisco CA, 1990.

- Nambudripad, Devi, *Say Goodbye To Illness*, Delta Publishing Company, Buena Park CA, 1993.

- Nambudripad, Devi, *The NAET Guidebook*, Delta Publishing Company, Buena Park CA, 1994.

- Randolph, Theron G. and Ralph W. Moss, *An Alternative Approach to Allergies*, Bantam, NY, 1987.

- Rapp, Doris J., *Allergies and the Hyperactive Child*, Sovereign Books, NY, 1979.

- **National Allergy Supply, Inc.**, 4400 Georgia Highway 120, P.O. Box 1658, Duluth GA 30136. Phone 1-800-522-1448. *They sell products for reducing allergens in the home environment.*

SYSTEMS OF THE BODY

The Body Is A Team Sport

Seventeen reasons to read this chapter:

1. *Find out how the body systems are interrelated and can serve multiple purposes like parts of a motor home.*

2. *Are bones alive, and are they more than just the body's framework?*

3. *Are teeth bones, how are they connected to the rest of the body, and do they have a purpose besides chewing?*

4. *Why older people get stiff.*

5. *What causes pimples?*

6. *How can you make your hair fuller and your nails stronger?*

7. *What are the five senses and what else do they do besides the obvious?*

8. *What is a simple, safe, and effective substitute for a common, expensive heart drug?*

9. *What is the down side of breathing?*

10. *Why were we given an appendix?*

11. *Why must the bladder be emptied completely?*

12. *How is the reproductive system different from the other systems?*

13. *Is it true that we all start life the same gender?*

14. *What causes and relieves PMS?*

15. *Why do women have menstrual periods?*

16. *How can a hysterectomy cause problems?*

17. *Is there such a thing as female frigidity?*

Even though the immune system, discussed in its own chapter, is the most important system in the body and the key to the health of the entire body, the other body systems are also vital to life and well-being.

So what is a system anyway?

The term "system" refers to a set of interrelated parts within the body which work together to perform a basic function, or functions. All body systems are designed to work together, so it is not surprising that a problem in one system will affect the others. The body can be compared to a house, which has structural components such as wiring and plumbing. If one system doesn't work properly, the house will not function adequately and the needs of its inhabitants will not be met. For example, if the electricity to the house is out, your washing machine will not work even if the plumbing works perfectly.

Are the body systems interrelated?

Not all medical sources and textbooks break up the body systems in the exact same way. Some organs are classified as being part of more than one system. These organs can be considered to be "junction boxes" between the two systems. For example,

- *The pancreas produces both insulin (endocrine glandular system) and digestive enzymes (digestive system).*

- *The liver manufactures enzymes, aids in digestion and is part of the cleanup crew that filters out and metabolizes toxins.*

- *The lymph system is an important part of the immune system and has an equally important function in detoxifying and cleansing the body.*

Previously compared to a house, the body can also be compared to a well-designed camper or recreational vehicle, with many components doing double or triple duty - the table that turns into a bed, or the bench that provides storage.

An example of another type of junction box is the prostate gland in men, which has the blood, lymph, urinary, and reproductive systems running through it. A problem with the prostate gland can thus affect the entire body, with fatigue, anger, depression, difficulty urinating, urinary tract infection, swollen tired legs, bowel blockage, and resultant high blood pressure. This is somewhat like full-time PMS for males.

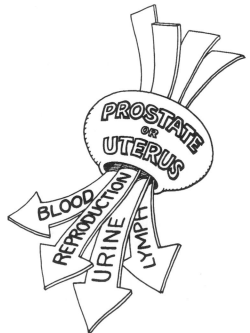

The important point here is the concept that no system stands on its own, nor can it be isolated for treatment. Another example of the concept of interconnectedness is how the liver, kidneys, lungs, skin, bowel, and lymph are each parts of different systems, yet they can all be considered parts of a system that cleanses the body of toxins.

Why is it important to understand the body systems?
It is important to have this basic knowledge of the structure and function of the parts of the body to facilitate understanding of much of the discussion in this book. Knowing, for example, that a certain chemical harms the liver or kidney is not very useful unless one understands why the liver or kidney is so important. This chapter also presents terms used frequently throughout this book and *Surviving The Toxic Crisis*.

Bones and Teeth

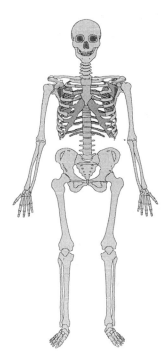

Are the bones more than just the body's framework?
The skeletal system consists of 206 bones. These bones range in size from the femur (thighbone) to the tiny bones in the ear. Bones form the framework of the body and serve as a means of attachment for the skeletal muscles. Without bones we would be like jellyfish. Along with the joints and muscles, bones allow movement. Yet bones do more than simply provide structure to the body.

Are bones alive?
The marrow, which is the soft living internal tissue in some bones, is involved in the production of red blood cells. Certain types of white cells such as the stem cells and mast cells which later differentiate to become part of the immune system also originate in the bone marrow. Leukemia, a cancer which results in uncontrolled production of white blood cells, can be treated with bone marrow transplants since healthy bone marrow makes healthy white blood cells which multiply as they should.

Bones act as storehouses for calcium and phosphorus, releasing these minerals to the blood as needed. This storing and releasing capability acts as a buffer if you have inflammation from alkalosis (high pH resulting from fermentation) or acidosis (low pH resulting from lactic acid buildup in the muscles). If too much calcium is taken from the long bones in the body for buffering or other purposes, one can develop long bone pain, hip and knee ailments, tennis elbow, bursitis, and eventually osteoarthritis and osteoporosis. Such ailments are best dealt with in the long run by treating the underlying systemic inflammation that is taking the calcium from the bones. Taking supplemental calcium seems like a logical solution, but the ingested calcium will go to buffer the inflammation. This may take the form of plaque in the arteries, which may eventually lead to arterial blockage. Solve the primary problem, then take calcium.

Although some people think of inert skeletons when they think of bones, bones are actually composed of living cells. They are one of the few parts of the body that can regenerate, leading to the knitting and repair of broken bones.

What are some bone-related problems?

Osteoporosis is a bone disease, usually showing up symptomatically after age 40, in which bone density is reduced and the person is more prone to fractures and height reduction. It affects about 20 million Americans [1]. 1.3 million people in the U.S. experience osteoporosis-related bone fractures annually [2], especially in the hip. An estimated 12-20% of older people with hip fractures die within the year [1]. Since 1920, a high protein intake has been correlated with calcium loss, which can lead to bone loss [3].

Does the skull do more than house the brain?

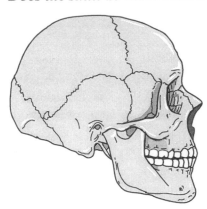

Popular belief is that the skull is merely an inert casing for the brain. Most people also believe that the sutures of the skull serve no purpose other than to allow the plates of the skull to move during birth to ease the infant's passage, and that these sutures serve no purpose after that.

This is not the case. The bony skull plates move when you chew and act as a pump for cerebrospinal fluid, which nourishes nerves all over the body. Spinal fluid should pump about twelve times per minute, but in sick people it may pump as little as 4-5 times per minute.

The expansion and contraction of the skull also increases blood flow to the pituitary gland in the brain, which regulates the function of other glands (endocrine glands) and hormone levels throughout the body [4]. The meningeal system, discussed in this chapter, can also be involved. Toxins can cause the meninges to inflame, causing the muscles to contract, which in turn restricts the motion of the skull plates as well as the positioning of the entire spinal column.

Birth injury, especially common in forceps deliveries, can compress these plates so fluid is not pumped properly. Techniques to relieve this misalignment and compression are described in the chapter on Structural Problems in *Surviving The Toxic Crisis*.

Most chronically ill people have had one or more suture-altering injuries or malformations:

- *Dental bridge crossing front teeth, blocking suture movement*
- *Concussion*
- *TMJ/TMD*
- *Whiplash*
- *Jammed facial bones, allowing uneven sutures*
- *Teeth make contact unevenly, turning the jaw*

Are teeth bones?

The teeth are sometimes considered to be part of the skeletal system. Like the bones, they are living structures with nerves and blood supply.

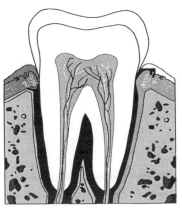

Calcium is pumped into and out of the tubules within the tooth when you eat. Dentin in the teeth is the buffer between the outside and the nerves. Drilling or problems with your collagen (which makes dentin), discussed in the following pages, may lead to dentin problems which result in tooth pain. This pain may be an early warning of other collagen problems in the body, such as ankylosing spondylitis, soft tissue problems, and arthritis.

Mercury from fillings, nickel from root canals, and bacteria from tooth abscesses and infections do not simply sit passively in the tooth or gum. These metals enter the system through lymph, blood, and bone to cause many chronic problems elsewhere in the body, such as the immune, circulatory, and collagen systems.

The teeth are linked to various other body systems through the meridians, or pathways, that traverse the body. Problems in or removal of the teeth can adversely affect the associated organs. These relationships are shown in this chart.

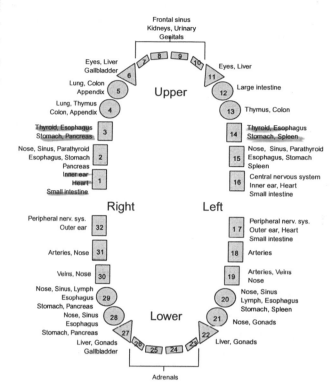

Skin

What system holds the body together? or: In a bag of bones, what is the bag?

The integumentary system consists of the skin, hair, nails, and the glands within the skin. The skin can be considered the largest organ in the body. Its primary role is one of protecting the organs from the outside environment. It is nearly waterproof, preventing both drying of tissues and over-absorption of water when immersed. The skin protects against outside agents such as most microbes, chemicals, UV radiation from the sun, and dust and pollutants. It conserves heat on exposure to cold and facilitates cooling and cleansing of the body through surface area exposure and sweating. The skin's pores can absorb toxic gaseous vapors, as well as substances such as chlorine from your shower water.

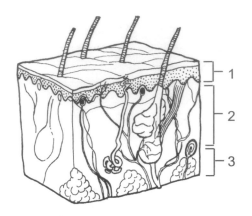

What is in the skin?

The skin consists of three layers: the epidermis (1), the dermis (2), and the subcutaneous tissue (3). The epidermis, or outer layer, which is scaly and dead, has no nerve endings. It is continually being sloughed off, sometimes visibly as in dandruff. The dermis lies between the subcutaneous tissue and the epidermis and contains nerves, blood capillaries, hair follicles, and tiny muscles. These muscles contract when cold to produce goose bumps. The same types of muscles cause animals to fluff up their fur for extra insulation, or a cat's fur to stand on end when it is threatened and takes a defensive stance.

What is collagen and why is it important?

Collagen is a substance that makes up 30% of the body's protein. It is the major structural component of the skin, as well as the ligaments, muscles, tendons, cartilage, bones, and teeth.

Some collagen is mineralized and hardens to form the bones and teeth, while the rest of it is not mineralized. Some toxins, such as fluoride, interfere with the proper synthesis of collagen leading to tooth and bone damage, skin wrinkling, and weakening of muscles and tendons [5]. Vitamin C helps in the building and cleansing of collagen.

Collagen and tendons perform a function like that of a suspension bridge. Picture the Golden Gate Bridge, with its cables rising into the air to help support the bridge. These cables allow the bridge to sway without harm, helping the bridge to withstand high winds and earthquakes. Collagen similarly allows the body much flexibility without harm.

CONNECTIVE TISSUE: Structure

COLLAGEN: **STRUCTURE**

1. The basic unit of collagen is a long protein chain assembled from amino acids.

long protein chain

2. Three chains combine to form a triple helix called a *tropocollagen* unit.

tropocollagen unit

3. Tropocollagen units are cross linked to form bundles or sheaves and then are connected end to end to form a *collagen microfibril*.

bundle — *collagen microfibril*

4. Microfibrils may be formed into parallel bundles in the case of tendon formation, or in sheets, like fibers forming paper, in the case of skin.

Tendons: microfibrils arranged in a parallel manner - high tensil strength.

Eye cornea: microfibrils laid perpendicularly- transparent.

Skin: microfibrils randomly arranged like fibers in paper.

© Chris Katke. Used with permission.

Why do older people get stiff?

In collagen diseases, fibers cross and toughen, accounting for much of the progressive stiffness felt as we grow older. These fibers also turn from white to gray with age. If a person is cremated, the ashes of a younger person are whiter while those of an older person are grayer. The difference lies in the cross-linking as the collagen ages.

Cross-linking of collagen (see above picture) causes rubber to harden and crack with age. Cross-linked arteries lose flexibility and can no longer pulse normally, leading to high blood pressure.

Cross-linking of collagen (see above picture) causes rubber to harden and crack with age. Cross-linked arteries lose flexibility and can no longer pulse normally, leading to high blood pressure.

Here's a test you can do to test yourself for flexibility. Pinch the skin of your hand. If the pinched portion returns to normal within a second or two, your collagen is normally flexible. If the skin stays pinched-looking for several seconds, your collagen has likely started to cross-link. A temporary cause of lack of skin flexibility is dehydration from too little water. Make sure you drink enough water daily; 64 ounces or eight 8-ounce glasses.

Why do some people sunburn easily?
Sebaceous oil glands lubricate the skin from the inside, serving as a barrier to water and water soluble substances, including some chemical toxins. This oil, along with good non-rancid oils and the B vitamin PABA, help protect the skin from the toxic far-UV rays of the sun. This explains why PABA is also an active ingredient in many sunscreens. A tendency to sunburn easily can be genetic, or it can be a warning sign of deficiency of oils and B vitamins, including PABA.

What causes pimples?
Pimples and acne are the result of blocking and inflammation of the sebaceous glands, whether caused by internal and/or external toxins. These toxins accumulate faster than the sebaceous oil can clear them out, resulting in visible inflammation. Acne usually develops from within, however, so topical acne treatments (applied to skin) are usually a waste of time. They are, in fact, worse than a waste of time, as some of them such as retinoic acid are toxic. Retinoic acid can lead to birth defects when used by pregnant women. Tetracycline, taken orally for acne, can kill and deplete the good bacteria in the intestinal system, leading to fungus and yeast infections. Fungus can double in number every 24 hours when not controlled by the protective bacteria, so it doesn't take long for runaway yeast overgrowth to develop. As your face gets clear from the tetracycline, your mind gets fuzzy from the fungus -- not a good tradeoff.

What purpose do sweat glands serve?
Sweat glands open onto the skin surface (eccrine) or are associated with hair follicles (apocrine). Apocrine sweat, especially from the armpits, can be malodorous or not, depending on bacterial or fungal growth. The odor can be managed naturally by bathing and staying healthy. It can also

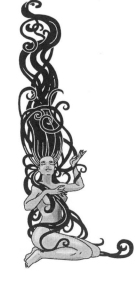

be masked artificially by deodorants and antiperspirants, many of which contain toxic drying aluminum. If deodorant is desired, magnesium is a non-toxic drying agent that is better than aluminum. Deodorants without aluminum are sometimes available in health food stores.

Sweat is one of the body's pathways for the elimination of chemical toxins, especially those that are volatile, or easily vaporized. These toxins, when excreted by the sweat glands, can also cause an unpleasant odor.

How can you make your hair fuller and your nails stronger?
Hair and nails, like the epidermis, are formed of a material called keratin, which is composed partly of silica, calcium, and the proteins in gelatin. Both hair and nails come from a living follicle, but hair and nails are dead and

nerveless. Products applied to the hair and nails to increase their health or "body" simply smooth down the scaly outer layer and improve the appearance. The surest way to have shiny hair, strong, healthy nails, and glowing skin is from within, through proper nutrition. Especially important are biotin and the rest of the B vitamins, and sufficient intake of calcium and essential non-rancid fatty acids. Silica and horsetail tea also contribute to strong, healthy hair and nails.

What can your nails tell about your health?
The fingernails provide clues to possible disorders throughout the body [6]:

- Thick nails   Poor circulation
- Brittle nails   Thyroid, kidney and circulation problems; nutritional deficiency
- Yellow nails   Internal disorders of any of several systems
- White nails   Liver or kidney disorders, anemia
- Bluish nails   Lung problems
- Ridges   Systemic infection

Muscles

How do muscles fit in?
The muscular system includes two types of muscle:

- Skeletal, also called striated or voluntary, which are attached to bones and cause movement. They are under our conscious control, and to a great extent determine our outward shape.

- Smooth, or involuntary, which form the muscle layers of hollow organs such as the stomach and heart and are not under our conscious control.

Nerve impulses control the movement of both types of muscle by causing the muscle cells to contract and expand in unison.

Carbohydrates, taken in as grains and roots, are broken down by the digestive system and stored in the muscle in the form of glycogen (stored cell sugar). They are then broken down to the simple sugar glucose to be released and burned by the muscle for energy. Muscle fatigue from exercise, as opposed to that from overall fatigue and weakness, can be due to a buildup of lactic acid and uric acid in the muscles, which in turn is caused by an oxygen deficit that builds up during certain types of exercise. These exercises include anaerobic weight lifting and aerobic exercise such as jogging which becomes anaerobic at the cellular level if you continue to jog after you've run out of breath.

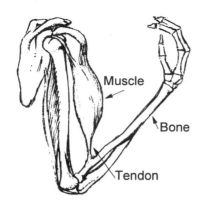

Muscle is composed of muscle cells surrounded by collagen, called the myofascia, which provides support and keeps the muscle from ripping. Towards the end of the muscle, there are fewer and fewer muscle cells until only collagen is left; this is called the tendon. The tendon collagen merges with the bone collagen. This muscle-tendon-bone bridge allows the muscle to move the bone for such activities as walking and lifting. This bridge can tear when abused, requiring major surgical repair.

Nervous System

What does the nervous system do?

The nervous system consists of the brain and spinal cord, which together make up the central nervous system (CNS), and the peripheral nerves which go to the organs and limbs. It is also considered by some to include the eyes and ears.

The nervous system is the communication system of the body, receiving information from the environment and both sending and receiving internal information. For example, an incoming message of "ouch" or "brrr" reaches the brain, which analyzes the information and sends out a message to the muscles. These respond by pulling away from the painful stimulus or by shivering. Shivering converts the thick blood triglycerides (fats) into energy to make heat to warm the body.

The peripheral nervous system controls the muscles while the autonomic portion of the nervous system controls many other body functions such as heartbeat and the peristaltic action that moves food through the digestive system. To remember the term "autonomic", think of "automatic", i.e. that part of the nervous system which works without conscious input.

The autonomic nervous system is divided into two parts, sympathetic and parasympathetic. The sympathetic portion is responsible for fight-or-flight stress reactions, which have survival value when one is confronted with danger. However, when stress is chronic, such as allergies, worry, or constant job deadlines, the fight-or-flight reaction can produce debilitating effects. Having the sympathetic part constantly "on" is like being in a continual fire drill with no food or sleep. The parasym-

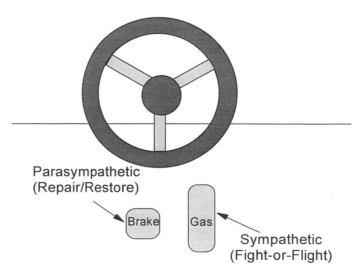

pathetic portion is responsible for counteracting the sympathetic response when danger is past, for digesting food, and for repairing and restoring body systems. The sympathetic part of the nervous system can be compared to the gas pedal of a car. The parasympathetic part of the nervous system can then be compared to the car's brake.

In another example of the gas pedal/brake effect which doesn't directly involve the nervous system, the pancreas stores sugar with insulin, and the adrenals release sugar with adrenaline. Like many other components of the body, adrenaline does more than one job.

What are the many functions of the brain?

The brain is the organ of thinking, learning, memory, emotions, and other functions that we think of as the mind. The brain is also the command post for the rest of the nervous system. Impulses from the brain travel down the spinal cord to the peripheral nerves. Nerve cells, or neurons, consist of an axon (tail), dendrite (head) and myelin, which is the protective fatty sheath around the axon.

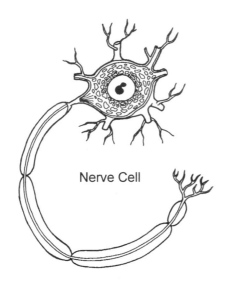

Nerve Cell

The myelin is believed to influence the speed of conduction of nerve impulses and amplify the impulses originating in the brain. Chemical solvents, whose purpose is to dissolve oils, can damage the fatty myelin and cause neurological symptoms and diseases such as multiple sclerosis (MS). They can also cause the dissipation of the nerve impulse which can result in slowing down of muscle response and shakiness.

How are nerve impulses conducted?

Nerve cells don't quite touch each other; the nerve impulse jumps across a gap called a synapse with the aid of chemicals called neurotransmitters. The faster the neurotransmitters fire, the faster the nerve impulse is relayed. Stimulant drugs such as cocaine, amphetamines, and caffeine stimulate the firing of neurotransmitters, while the low or crash that follows the high is the result of the premature depletion of the neurotransmitters.

There are at least fifty biochemical substances which are or can act as neurotransmitters. Some of these include [7]:

- Acetylcholine and catecholamines such as dopamine, epinephrine, (adrenaline), norepinephrine, and tyrosine. Choline, a B vitamin, is a necessary building block for these transmitters. A supplement called phosphatidyl choline (Phos-Chol) can improve mental alertness for this reason.

- Serotonin, responsible for a feeling of well-being and promoting restful sleep, is the neurotransmitter most influenced by drugs which affect the mind. The amino acid tryptophan, in conjunction with adequate levels of vitamin B-6 and niacin, is converted to serotonin in the brain. Warm milk, long used as a sleep aid, contains tryptophan, as does turkey.

- Gamma-aminobenzoic acid (GABA) is an amino acid which is a component of dietary protein. Other amino acids can also act as neurotransmitters in addition to having other functions.

- Some hormones such as estrogen, testosterone, and prostaglandins can act as neurotransmitters.

What are the five senses and what else do they do?

The five senses involve passing certain external information from the appropriate receptor to the brain. The senses and their receptor locations are:

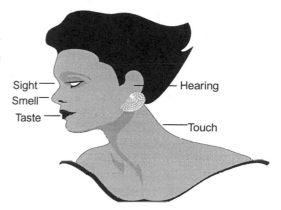

- *sight*   *eyes*
- *hearing*   *ears*
- *smell*   *nose*
- *taste*   *mouth*
- *touch*   *skin*

How can sunglasses contribute to cancer and arthritis?

As mentioned earlier, many parts of the body have more than one function. These receptor organs are no exception. The eyes see and also let in sunlight, stimulating the pineal and pituitary glands in the brain. These in turn produce the sleep promoting (and cancer fighting) hormone melatonin from serotonin and stimulate the adrenal glands to produce energy, explaining why we are awake during the day. Sunglasses and colored contact lenses worn during the day, artificial light that is missing certain frequencies, and bright light at night confuse this mechanism. This confusion provides one explanation of daytime tiredness and nighttime sleeplessness, although these can have many other causes. Different frequencies of light affect different parts of the body, and an imbalance of frequencies results in internal imbalance.

Albert Schweitzer observed arthritis and cancer among the African population who were free of such diseases just thirty years previously. Their diet and lifestyle had not changed in these intervening years. Western-style sunglasses, however, had become a coveted status symbol during this time. The sunglass-wearing natives subsequently developed Western diseases within one generation.

Shari was one of our patients who came in with recurring upper respiratory infections. She refrained from wearing her sunglasses for a year and a half and got well. She then put them on again for six months and got sick again. Finally, removing them for good after her doctor re-reminded her of their effect, she got well. It is interesting to note that sunlight sensitivity strongly correlates with signs of suppressed adrenal function or toxic depleted neurotransmitters.

Another patient, a woman in her mid thirties, developed health problems including chronic fatigue and pain when she started wearing colored contact lenses. These problems went away when she stopped using the lenses.

What keeps you from tilting when you walk?
The ears, along with the jaw, are the balancing system, or gyroscope, of the body, allowing us to walk upright over tilted terrain.

A malfunction of this inner ear balancing system can cause one to become dizzy, or to misalign (tilt) the head and neck and consequently the whole body, in order to compensate. Pain elsewhere in the body can result from this structural misalignment .

How can the other senses do double and triple duty?
The skin has protective and waste-releasing functions as well as transmitting the signals of touch and pain. The mouth is needed for speech and eating, and is also one of the main ways a baby explores its environment (sometimes picking up worms and parasites in the process).

How can your nose help you walk down Memory Lane?
The nose transmits not only smell, but the chemical that causes the smell also travels up the olfactory nerve in the nose to the brain. As an example of the interconnectedness of the brain, mind, and body, the inhalation of cologne can produce:

- An awareness of the smell of the cologne.

- A stimulation of the mind, if the smell reminds you of something such as cologne associated with an old lover. Feelings of anger or nostalgia can thus be induced. Of the five senses, smell can be the strongest memory inducer.

- A judgment of the smell as being pleasant, unpleasant, or too strong.

- An allergic or toxic reaction, as the cologne's chemicals themselves travel to the brain and get into the bloodstream.

Zinc, an essential mineral, is necessary for smell and taste sensors to function properly.

Meningeal System

What is meningitis and what system is involved?
A three-layered covering of tissue covers the brain and spinal cord for additional protection. This covering is the meningeal system. The meningeal system, or meninges, also acts as a shock absorber by providing a spring effect to counteract movement.

The neck and back should not be straight, but should have certain curves to optimize stability. The spine should be symmetrical, with the right and left halves mirror images of each other. If the head is habitually held forward, meninges tighten, the curves in the neck and low back flatten, and the spring effect is lost to a certain extent.

Whiplash injury can also tighten the meninges. The meninges also tend to tighten to stabilize misalignment of the spinal vertebrae. The resulting contracture only worsens the misalignment by subluxing the joint and pinching nerves. The effects of misalignment are discussed in the chapter on Structural Problems in *Surviving The Toxic Crisis*. Many structural problems develop in compensation for the meningeal system contracting.

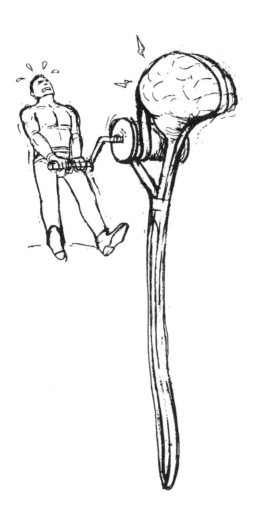

Allergy, chemical toxicity, electrical charges produced by metals in the mouth, and even emotional stress can cause meningeal inflammation, which in turn can lead to muscle contraction. An infectious inflammation of the meninges is called spinal meningitis. Meningitis can cause stiffness as the muscles and meninges contract in response to the inflammation.

Maybe you have played with a toy called Chinese handcuffs, in which an end is slipped over each of two fingers. Contrary to logic, the harder you pull, the tighter the ends get. The meningeal system is like that - the harder it is pulled, the more it compensates and the tighter it gets, so that contraction will cause further contraction in a downward spiral.

A form of treatment called meningeal release uses the same principle in reverse, in which a contracted spine is manually contracted even more by pulling the coccyx bone (tailbone) up and the head back. This allows the meninges to shorten like Chinese handcuffs and release. This principle is used by Dr. Lowell Ward, DC (Long Beach CA) in his Stressology work, tying the emotional to the meningeal system.

Another form of treatment called nasal specific involves inserting a special type of balloon into the nasal cavity, quickly filling it with air, and then releasing the air. The quick filling and release of the balloon facilitates meningeal release. This technique, used by Dr. Dean Howell, ND, (described in greater detail in the Structural chapter in *Surviving The Toxic Crisis*) changes the head pressure and releases it like a hydraulic system.

Circulatory System and Blood

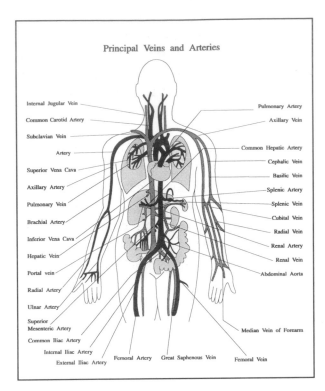

Principal Veins and Arteries

Internal Jugular Vein
Common Carotid Artery
Subclavian Vein
Artery
Superior Vena Cava
Axillary Artery
Pulmonary Vein
Brachial Artery
Inferior Vena Cava
Hepatic Vein
Portal vein
Radial Artery
Ulnar Artery
Superior
Mesenteric Artery
Common Iliac Artery
Internal Iliac Artery
External Iliac Artery
Femoral Artery
Great Saphenous Vein

Pulmonary Artery
Axillary Vein
Common Hepatic Artery
Cephalic Vein
Basilic Vein
Splenic Artery
Splenic Vein
Cubital Vein
Radial Vein
Renal Artery
Renal Vein
Abdominal Aorta
Median Vein of Forearm
Femoral Vein

What is included in the circulatory system?

The circulatory system, also called the cardio-vascular system, consists of the heart, the blood vessels, and the blood. These are analogous to a pump, a hose, and the water which goes through them.

Some sources consider the lymphatic system to be part of the circulatory system, part of the immune system, or a separate circulatory system. For the purposes of this book it is both part of the immune system and one of the cleansing/detoxification systems. It is discussed in detail in the chapter on the Immune System. Unlike the cardiovascular system, the lymph system has no self-powered pump. Rather, it has a bulb-type pump located in the upper abdomen. This pump relies on muscle contraction from deep gut breathing, walking, motion, and gravity for movement of lymph and waste from all directions towards the chest. An accumulation of toxins in the lymph system, caused by greater intake than elimination of toxins, will often cause immune suppression over a period of time.

The heart is located in the upper chest, between the lungs and slightly to the left.

The heart is a muscular organ about the size of a fist which acts to pump blood through the body. The heart consists of four chambers. The two atria (singular: atrium) are on top, and receive incoming blood from the veins. The two thicker-walled ventricles are on the bottom, and they send the blood out from the heart through the arteries.

The heart's pacemaker is electrical in nature and regulates the heartbeat in both speed and smoothness. Mineral imbalances, especially sodium, magnesium, calcium and potassium, can affect the smooth functioning of the heart. The adrenal glands and kidneys help to balance these electrolytes (minerals) as a priority even before the making of adrenaline. If the mineral potassium is deficient, the pulse can speed up,

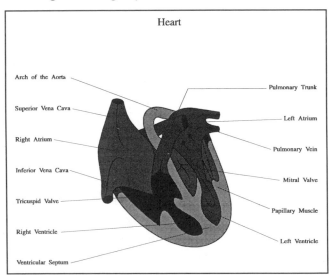

Heart

Arch of the Aorta
Superior Vena Cava
Right Atrium
Inferior Vena Cava
Tricuspid Valve
Right Ventricle
Ventricular Septum

Pulmonary Trunk
Left Atrium
Pulmonary Vein
Mitral Valve
Papillary Muscle
Left Ventricle

while a deficiency of sodium can cause the blood pressure to fall. A deficiency of magnesium can cause heart palpitations.

What else can go wrong with the cardiovascular system?

Cardiovascular problems are one of the leading causes of death in the U.S. Heart attacks cause over 550,000 deaths annually in the U.S. [8]. The medical cost of cardiovascular disease is in the U.S. is over $56 billion a year [9]. 500,000 people in the U.S. have a stroke every year, and there are currently over two million Americans disabled by stroke [10].

What drug is often erroneously taken because of a mineral deficiency?

Magnesium, as mentioned, is essential for a regular, even heartbeat. Calcium and magnesium compete for the same spaces on molecules in the body, so a high calcium/magnesium ratio can result in too little magnesium getting to where it is needed. The expensive allopathic drug Verapamil is a calcium channel blocker, which blocks calcium to allow magnesium to regulate the heart. This blocking of calcium over time can contribute to osteoporosis. Why not just supplement the diet with additional

> **Irregular heartbeat? The solution may be simpler than you think!**

magnesium? Verapamil is a moneymaker since it can be patented. Plainly, such is not the case with magnesium. Doctors may be well meaning, but they are influenced by pharmaceutical salespeople in their recommendations. On the other hand, some people just don't believe it can be that simple.

Cardiovascular activity can also be affected by electromagnetic and other radiation, electrical currents generated from dissimilar metals in the mouth, and a wide variety of toxins and deficiencies.

How is oxygen carried throughout the body?

The blood vessels consist of arteries and veins. The arteries carry oxygenated, bright red blood from the heart to the tissues in order to transfer oxygen to cells all over the body. The oxygen is picked up as the blood passes through the lungs. The veins return the darker deoxygenated blood back to the heart.

Sizes of blood vessels range from the aorta, which is the thickness of a thumb and is the main artery from the heart, to the capillaries, which are so small that blood cells can only pass through in single file. It is through the capillaries that oxygen passes from the blood to the tissues. If the blood vessel walls are narrowed due to fatty deposits made up of calcium, cholesterol, and triglycerides, blood pressure goes up, much the same as pinching a hose increases water pressure. Narrowed blood vessels and plugged capillaries also reduce the amount of oxygen getting to the cells, resulting in dying and ineffective cells with resultant fatigue.

Patients at Comprehensive Health Center are taught range of motion, tissue cleansing exercises which can clear both the capillaries and lymph vessels.

Try this!

Blood vessels have valves inside them allowing the blood to flow in only one direction. There is an interesting trick to locate or illustrate the valves in a vein. Take an arm with a large, prominent vein - yours or a friend's. Keep in mind that the blood flows from the hand up the arm to the heart. Press down on the vein at the wrist to keep new blood from flowing into the vein, then slide a finger up the vein towards the shoulder to push the blood along towards the heart.

Keeping the finger at the wrist to block new blood flow, release the finger that did the sliding. Blood will then back up to refill the vein - but only up to the valve. The vein is flattened from the finger at the wrist to the valve, and the visible place where the flattened and full spots meet is the location of the valve.

What is blood made of?

Blood consists of several components:

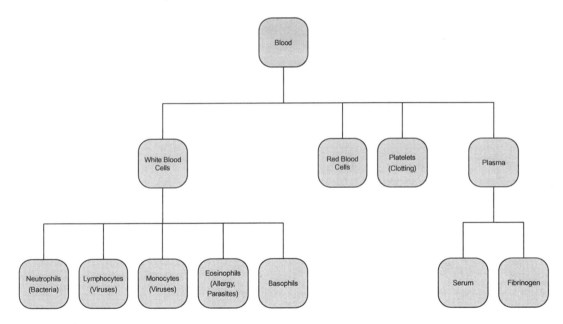

- **Red blood cells** carry oxygen to cells, tissues and organs. They are round disks which are concave in the center, and have an elastic membrane allowing them to bend to get through the smallest capillaries. They sometimes have to fold double to accomplish this. They look somewhat like a donut with a central membrane.

White blood cells of five different types are part of the body's defense against different types of infections:

- *Neutrophils*   *bacteria*
- *Lymphocytes*   *viruses*
- *Monocytes*   *viruses, some bacteria*
- *Eosinophils*   *parasites, allergy*

74

- *Basophils*   *function not yet fully understood*

An elevated count of one type of white cell (called a differential in a standard blood panel test) is normally an indication of the type of infection present. For example, an elevated lymphocyte count can indicate a viral infection, since the lymphocytes will multiply to better deal with viral invaders.

- **Platelets**, which are responsible for blood clotting. If the platelet count is too high, heart attack, stroke, and phlebitis (blood clots in veins) can result. A deficiency of vitamin K can lower the platelet count, possibly resulting in hemorrhage. Lowered vitamin K can contribute to suppression of the immune system.

- **Plasma**, the liquid part of the blood, consists of 90% water. The remainder is proteins, sugars, fats, vitamins, minerals, hormones, gases, metabolic waste products, and fibrinogen for clotting. Serum, part of plasma, is that part of the blood remaining after the blood clots. A laboratory uses a machine called a centrifuge to spin tubes of whole blood. The cells and heavier components form a thick dark plug at the bottom of the tube and the clear straw-colored liquid at the top is the plasma.

Respiratory System

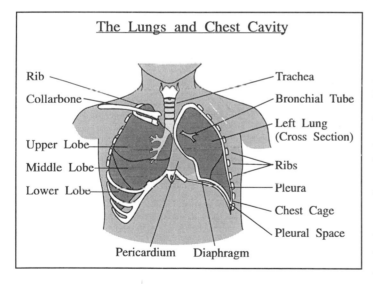

The Lungs and Chest Cavity

Rib
Collarbone
Upper Lobe
Middle Lobe
Lower Lobe
Trachea
Bronchial Tube
Left Lung (Cross Section)
Ribs
Pleura
Chest Cage
Pleural Space
Pericardium   Diaphragm

Why is breathing so important?
The respiratory system consists of the lungs and trachea. The important component of the air we breathe is oxygen. Taken in through the mouth and nose, it then goes through the trachea on into the lungs. Oxygen is necessary for the life of all of the body's cells.

The muscular motion of the diaphragm, located below the lungs, allows the lungs to expand to pull in oxygen and contract to release carbon dioxide. The alveoli, or tiny air sacs in the lungs, transfer the oxygen to the capillaries which surround them. Carbon dioxide, the primary exhaled metabolic waste product, is returned to the alveoli via the capillaries and then exhaled. About seven gallons of carbon dioxide is exhaled per day. Think about the fact that the body considers carbon dioxide to be a waste product the next time you drink a carbonated beverage (carbon dioxide produces the bubbles in soda).

> **Think about the fact that the body considers carbon dioxide to be a waste product the next time you drink a carbonated beverage.**

Why are some of us deficient in oxygen?
For a number of reasons, many of us do not breathe as deeply as we should to maximize energy-giving oxygen in the tissues.

- Think about the times you pass a diesel-fume belching truck or bus. You automatically breathe as shallowly as possible until the vehicle is past to minimize exposure to the fumes. This shallow breathing is done habitually to a lesser extent when air quality is poor.

- Stress can cause us to hold our breath.

- Exercise makes one breathe more deeply, so it follows that lack of exercise contributes to shallow breathing.

- People who are hard of hearing hold their breath when trying to listen.

- People who are sick or in pain tend to breathe more shallowly.

Many of us do not get enough oxygen for these reasons. It is helpful to consciously breathe as deeply as possible. Expand the abdomen visibly on the inhale, and push the breath out a little farther than usual on the exhale to remove more carbon dioxide. Breathe this way whenever you think of it, or set aside time for deep breathing on a regular basis. After a while, deeper breathing will become habitual. Deep breathing also massages the lymph collection points in the chest and the nearby organs towards the chest, promoting better function.

What is the down side of breathing?
Airborne toxins inhaled along with the oxygen can enter the bloodstream from the lungs or damage the lungs themselves. Cigarette smoke, for example, both damages the lungs and has systemic effects, which include zinc depletion due to heavy metals such as cadmium and nickel. Lowered zinc levels can adversely affect taste, smell, and appetite. When one stops smoking, appetite usually returns even without zinc supplementation, since the heavy metals from the smoke are no longer suppressing the zinc. Note: The eating disorders anorexia nervosa and bulimia can also lower zinc levels, which in turn can depress appetite in a vicious cycle.

Digestive System

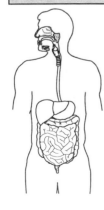

How are you like a donut?
In a sense, our bodies are like an elongated donut or a hose and the digestive system is the hole in the middle. In its simplest form, food enters the mouth and heads downward, nutrients are extracted and absorbed during the trip, and the waste products continue on to the end to be excreted from the body in the form of stools. Our digestive tract is considered by some to be outside of the body systems because it is not part of the inner workings of the closed blood system, and it runs through the body like a funnel, much like the donut hole in the donut.

Or think of a garden hose. The space both inside and outside of the hose walls is basically outside the plastic of the hose itself; in other words, they're both outside the interwoven plastic and fibers.

What are the parts of the digestive system?
The digestive system consists of, from top to bottom: mouth, esophagus, stomach, intestines (small and large, or duodenum, jejunum, ileum), rectum, and anus.

Accessory organs, those which aid in digestion but are not part of the digestive tube, secrete enzymes necessary for digestion. These organs and enzymes are discussed in more detail in the Digestion chapter. The accessory organs and associated enzymes include:

Organ	Enzyme	To digest
Pancreas	Amylase	Carbohydrates
Liver	Protease, Lipase	Protein, fat
Gallbladder	Bile	Fat; also stores enzymes

The salivary (parotid) glands in the mouth are sometimes also considered to be accessory glands. They secrete enzymes such as amylase that predigest starches. They also absorb certain toxins, especially when the tonsils have been removed. If overloaded with toxins, the parotid glands can become infected.

How is food digested?
The process of digestion involves the breaking down of food into particles (molecules) small enough to be absorbed and utilized by the body. Carbohydrates, proteins, and fats are macronutrients (macro means large), needed in larger quantities. They are broken down in different ways using the above enzymes. Vitamins and minerals are micronutrients (micro means small), needed in smaller amounts, and are also extracted from food during the digestive process.

Food does not simply fall through the digestive tract but is instead moved by peristaltic (flowing muscular) contractions which move like an inchworm moves. Food would move in the proper direction even if one is upside down or weightless in space. Peristalsis also serves the purpose of mixing the food together and with the beneficial bacteria in the intestines.

The mouth consists of tongue, teeth, palate, and salivary (parotid) glands. Saliva helps to predigest carbohydrates. The stomach holds the food for part of the digestive process. Gastric juice, or hydrochloric acid, is secreted into the stomach to soften proteins so they can be digested by enzymes. It is not uncommon for a person to have lower hydrochloric acid than is optimum due to stress or allergy. Stress and allergy keep the body in sympathetic fight-or-flight mode so that the parasympathetic mode, which is responsible for restoration of body functions, digestion, and manufacture of HCl, is suppressed. The result is that food is not completely digested and therefore not fully absorbed in usable form. Undigested food also sets up further allergic reactions as the immune system identifies the food as non-self.

Enzymes produced by the liver and pancreas empty into the small intestine to digest peptides (protein parts), starches, and fats. The small intestine itself also secretes enzymes which digest a variety of substances. The liver also produces bile, which digests fat and promotes the absorption of fat and the fat-soluble vitamins E, A, D, and K. Bile also helps in the excretion of certain toxic wastes such as mercury by adhering to them and carrying them out of the body.

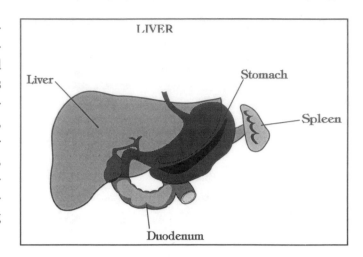

The liver, which at three pounds is the largest organ in the body, is located on the right side of the body above the waist. The liver makes enzymes which cause the many biochemical reactions in the body. It is assisted by the gallbladder in its digestion of fats. A poorly functioning gallbladder will cause a person to be intolerant of fats and oils.

The digestive system is discussed in more detail in its own chapter, Digestion, in the Supporters section.

Why do we need an appendix anyway?

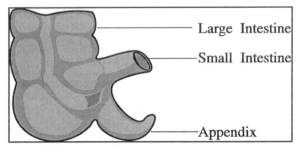

The appendix is located near the ileocecal valve of the small intestine. Although the appendix is considered by many doctors to be merely a vestigial remnant that can be removed without effect, it was put there for a reason. The appendix acts as a buffer to keep the pressure off the ileocecal valve. If the ileocecal valve is open, the appendix will collect toxins, functioning as a safety valve to keep these toxins from spreading through the digestive tract and being reabsorbed. Without the appendix as buffer, the poisons of the bowel can be absorbed back into the body by the small intestine.

What is the end of the digestive process?

The digestive process, including most nutrient absorption, is essentially completed in the small intestine. The large intestine, also called the colon or bowel, contains millions of beneficial bacteria which break down undigested food residues and combine these with unabsorbed digestive secretions, cell debris, and some metabolic byproducts to produce fecal matter, which is then excreted as stools. Bifidus, friendly bacteria which colonize in the colon, help make the B vitamin biotin which helps keep down the fungus population.

Urinary System

What happens when the blood is filtered through the kidneys?

The urinary system is responsible for waste collection and elimination, and for maintaining the water and electrolyte balance. The two kidneys, bean-shaped organs each the size of a small fist, are just above the waist. They maintain the relative constancy of the blood plasma and the acid-base balance. They also filter out waste products for elimination in the urine. The urine thus produced passes through the ureters into the bladder, which acts as a holding tank. Lower back pain can result if this system does not function properly, or if you are low in the mineral potassium.

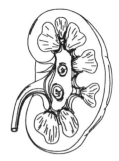

Kidney
(cross section)

When the bladder is full, sphincter muscles allow the urine to pass out of the body via the urethra. The urethra passes through the prostate gland, and then the penis, in the male. In the female, the urethra is shorter than in the male, about 1.5 inches, and its opening is just above - not in - the vagina.

Why must the bladder be emptied completely?

When urinating, the bladder should be emptied as completely as possible. This is accomplished by relaxing and taking enough time, and by squeezing the last bit of urine out. If this is not done, stale urine will remain in the bladder, bacteria will grow, and a bladder or urinary tract infection may result. In addition, the touching together of the sides of the bladder after completely voiding releases a natural antibiotic, and this signal might not occur if the bladder is not completely emptied. Infection may then grow unchecked.

When this doesn't happen properly, the lungs can act as a pseudo third kidney. In other words, when the kidneys aren't able to work optimally because of a problem with the bladder unable to perform its function because of an infectious process setting in, the lungs work like a backup system and start offloading some of the toxins from the blood, thereby giving the kidneys and bladder an opportunity to get back on track.

Endocrine System

Glands of the
Endocrine System

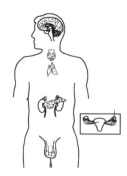

What is the endocrine glandular system?

The endocrine system consists of ductless glands which produce hormones and release them directly into the bloodstream. The blood then carries the hormones to their target organs to perform their function. The endocrine glands are listed and discussed here from top to bottom of the body. Like runners passing a baton, the endocrine glands work together, passing on information to each other.

What is the master gland of the body?

The pea sized **pituitary**, sometimes called the master gland, is located in the brain. It secretes growth hormone as well as a number of other hormones which regulate the activities of the other endocrine glands. Malfunctions of the other glands can often be traced to the pituitary's producing too much or not enough of these stimulating hormones. The pituitary has two parts: the anterior, which controls systems from the waist up, and the posterior, which controls systems from the waist down.

What gland helps keep us warm and regulate weight?

The **thyroid gland**, located in the neck, is responsible for the metabolic rate, i.e. the rate at which food is converted to energy. An overactive thyroid produces a thin, nervous bugged-eyed individual. An overactive but under-effective thyroid gland can cause a condition called Graves' disease. An underactive thyroid (hypothyroidism) produces mental retardation in children. In adults it can show up in sluggishness, overweight, retained fluid, and lowered body temperature. Thyroid underactivity can be related to adrenal underactivity and deficiencies of iodine, zinc, and copper. Hypothyroidism is common in chronic fatigue syndrome, discussed throughout the book. Thyroid problems can also lead to low adrenal function.

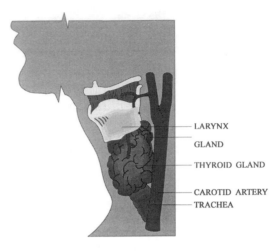

LARYNX
GLAND
THYROID GLAND
CAROTID ARTERY
TRACHEA

The level of the thyroid hormone T4, (not to be confused with the immune system's T4 cells), is most directly responsible for thyroid-caused nervousness or fatigue. T4 must be converted to T3, or triiodothyronine, in order for it to do its work. It is possible to have a high T4 level and a low T3 level, with fatigue and other symptoms associated with low thyroid levels. This is analogous to a car in which the engine is racing but the clutch is in. The car has energy but can go nowhere. The same is true of a person with high T4/ low T3. The clutch is lowered iodine.

Goiter, an advanced form of hypothyroidism due to iodine deficiency, used to be common in the Midwest, where natural salt levels are low. It is characterized by swollen thyroid glands which cause a visibly swollen neck, and symptoms of hypothyroidism.

What gland keeps your bones strong?

The four tiny **parathyroid glands**, with a combined weight of only 100 mg (1/280th of an ounce) are located next to and around the thyroid. Their primary function is to regulate calcium and phosphorus metabolism, and their primary action is on bone.

What gland functions as a brake?

The **pancreatic islet cells** produce insulin, which regulates glucose metabolism and its storage as glycogen. An inconsistent oversupply of insulin or an undersupply of adrenaline results in hypoglycemia, especially if a diet high in sugar is consumed. This causes attendant shakiness, headaches, mood swings, and sugar cravings. An undersupply of insulin results in the accumulation of glucose in the blood. This is called diabetes, which is sometimes considered to be an advanced case of hypoglycemia when it occurs in adulthood. Diabetes can be fatal if untreated, and is the third most common cause of death in adults.

One percent (1%) of the pancreas by weight produces hormones, while the remaining 99% produces digestive enzymes, yet both functions are equally important.

You may have seen or tasted spongy lamb or veal sweetbreads, sometimes sold in the meat section of the supermarket; the sweetbreads are the animal's pancreas.

What gland functions as a throttle?

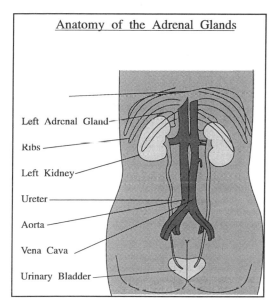

Anatomy of the Adrenal Glands

Left Adrenal Gland

Ribs

Left Kidney

Ureter

Aorta

Vena Cava

Urinary Bladder

The two **adrenal glands** lie just above the kidneys. They secrete adrenaline (also called epinephrine) for energy in the daytime, and noradrenaline (norepinephrine) at night which allows you to stay asleep. Adrenaline builds up all night, and releases energy for use during the day. The first rays of sunlight cause this adrenaline release. If you counteract this by sleeping late or by going back to sleep after waking, you may feel groggy all day.

Adrenaline is produced in reaction to stress, and is responsible for the "fight or flight" response involving the sympathetic nervous system. Norepinephrine (noradrenaline) constricts the blood vessels in response to shock. Anaphylactic shock is a severe allergic reaction in which the blood vessels close completely, the throat closes, and the body essentially shuts down. Epinephrine (the common name for adrenaline when used as a drug) is often administered to counteract norepinephrine in these cases and reverse anaphylactic shock. The adrenal cortex also secretes hormones called androgens, and controls progesterone which is involved in the sex drive.

The **gonads**, although they are endocrine glands which secrete hormones, are considered to be part of the reproductive system.

The endocrine system can be pictured using a baseball analogy: the pituitary is home plate, the thyroid and parathyroids are first base, the thymus is second base, the adrenals and pancreas are third base. In baseball, action at each of the four bases directly affects what happens at the next. Similarly, whatever happens to any endocrine system produces feedback affecting the other systems. For example, thyroxin (thyroid hormone) given orally does not stimulate the other glands as does naturally produced thyroxin since the thyroid is not working, thus affecting the whole endocrine system.

Reproductive System

How is the reproductive system different from the other systems?
The reproductive system, unlike the other systems, is not necessary for the physical existence of the individual, although it certainly adds to the person's vibrancy and enjoyment of life. Although its primary purpose is for procreation to insure survival of the species, associated hormones do help promote emotional balance.

Is it true that we all start life the same gender?
All embryos start out the same, gender-wise. In slightly over half of all embryos the hormone testosterone causes the reproductive organs to differentiate into male form. Virtually all organs and structures in the male are analogous to structures in the female:

Men		**Women**
male testes	↔	*female ovaries*
male scrotum	↔	*female vulva*
male penis	↔	*female clitoris*
male prostate	↔	*female uterus*
male foreskin	↔	*female clitoral hood*
male vas deferens	↔	*female fallopian tubes*

> **We are more alike than we may think - Nearly every part of the reproductive anatomy of one gender has its counterpart in the anatomy of the other.**

The female vulvae (plural of vulva, meaning vaginal lips) become the scrotum in the male. Vestiges of this are visible in the line, almost like a scar or suture line, that runs down the middle of the scrotum. This is where the would-be vulvae have fused during gestation. The ovaries-turned-testes drop down into this bag to be kept at a temperature a few degrees below body temperature. This lower temperature is necessary for sperm production. Some cases of male infertility can be traced to hot baths or tight jockey shorts for this reason. -- No, don't count on this as a birth control technique!

Why isn't early withdrawal an effective birth control technique?
The primary male sex organs are the penis and testicles (testes). The testes produce the hormone testosterone, which maintains the development and function of the male sex organs, and is responsible for much of the male's aggressiveness, motivation and sex drive in his early years. Testosterone production is highest around the age of 19.

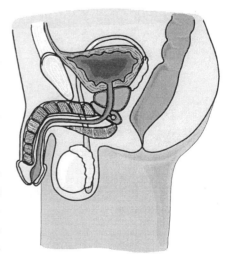

Sperm, the male sex cells which fertilize the ovum, are also manufactured in the testes. Sperm combines with secretions from the prostate and other glands to form semen which is released through the penis during ejaculation. Sperm are also released in small quantities prior to ejaculation along with lubricating secretions called seminal fluid, so therefore withdrawal is not an effective birth control technique.

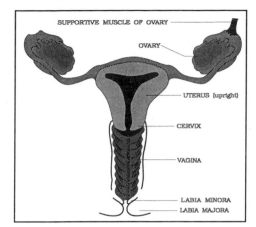

What are the female sex organs?

The primary female sex organs are the ovaries, uterus, and vagina. The ovaries produce the hormones estrogen and progesterone, which regulate the menstrual cycle. Estrogen protects a woman from losing her hair or being susceptible to heart attacks like men by preventing plaquing of calcium on the arterial walls. Estrogen also promotes the storage of calcium, which helps keep women comparatively calm during the childrearing years and provides protection from osteoporosis before menopause.

What causes and can relieve PMS?

Some women suffer from premenstrual syndrome (PMS). Bloating and pain can be caused by toxic buildup, and is alleviated when the toxins are released through menstruation. Anger, depression, and sugar and chocolate cravings can be due to low blood sugar, itself due in part to magnesium deficiency. Magnesium can counteract calcium's tendency to cause the body to hold onto sugar and will aid in releasing it into the blood, raising the blood sugar level back to normal. A raised calcium level can also contribute to cramps, and magnesium can help counteract this. A magnesium supplement equivalent to little more than the RDA recommendation which is usually one or two tablets, can often dramatically relieve cramps within a half hour.

> **Magnesium can dramatically relieve menstrual cramps within a half hour.**

Magnesium is found in chocolate, partially accounting for this common premenstrual craving, but chocolate contains refined sugar, caffeine and its chemical relative theobromine, along with unhealthy oils that will only tend to make matters worse. Vitamin B6 and healthy oils, particularly gamma-linolenic (GLA) oils such as evening primrose oil, borage oil, and black currant oil can also help relieve PMS symptoms.

Estrogen increases before the period, reducing blood sugar and increasing appetite. The buildup of progesterone after the period tends to reduce the appetite.

Why do women have menstrual periods?

The uterus prepares each month for possible impregnation, creating a cozy nest rich in blood vessels. Menstruation is the monthly elimination of this lining if there is no pregnancy, and healthy menstruation has a cleansing effect on the woman's system. If an ovum, or egg cell, is fertilized after release from the ovaries, the fertilized egg makes its home in the uterus for nine months. The resulting baby would then normally be delivered through the vaginal canal, barring medical complications.

A woman's monthly cycle provides a channel for the release of toxic buildup out of the system each month. With the onset of menopause this outlet is closed and the body then has to deal with this extra toxic burden. This may contribute to the difficult transition some women experience post-menopausally, trying to sweat out the toxins, while others make the transition without so much as a symptom, although I grant you this is more the exception than the rule.

What can be done for menstrual cramps?

Menstrual cramps regularly affect between 30% and 50% of women [11]. At least 10% of young women have cramps and other symptoms that are so severe as to interfere with their normal activities [12]. Several factors can increase the likelihood and severity of cramps, including:

- *The use of tampons*
- *IUD birth control devices*
- *Bladder infections*
- *Yeast infections*
- *Lack of exercise*
- *Poor posture*
- *Emotional stress*
- *Excessive salt*
- *Animal fats*
- *Allergy to dairy products, wheat, alcohol and sugar*

The following are useful in the treatment of cramps [13]:

- *GLA*
- *Biofeedback*
- *Wild yam*
- *Antifungals*
- *Soft tissue work*
- *Stretching exercises*
- *Vitamins B6, B3, C and E*
- *Calcium and magnesium, especially magnesium*
- *A number of herbs including cramp bark, ginger and valerian root*

How can a hysterectomy cause problems?

As mentioned early in this chapter, the prostate gland in men is related to the rest of the body, and its malfunction or removal can have negative system-wide effects. The uterus is the female analog of the prostate. Contrary to the apparent belief of some doctors, the uterus is not simply a "holding tank" useful only in pregnancy. Like the prostate, the uterus has functions throughout the body. Its malfunction or removal, like that of the prostate, can have system-wide effects, including fatigue, depression, and weight gain and sluggishness related to lowered thyroid function. These symptoms have been experienced by countless women who were advised to have a hysterectomy (uterus removal) based on minor ailments and the fact that they planned to have no more children.

More than 50% of women over age 65 have had hysterectomies. Many women are not informed prior to surgery about these common post-hysterectomy symptoms. In fact, they are often told by their doctors that the symptoms are all in their head. They aren't. Many doctors will prescribe hormones to relieve these symptoms, but hormone therapy can cause a whole new set of problems such as uterine and breast cancer.

A female patient in her late 40s experienced an avalanche of problems after her hysterectomy. By the time she came to the clinic, she suffered from major mood swings, weight gain, hot flashes, depression, and irritability. Oral hormones had been prescribed to relieve her symptoms but they only made things worse - she now had a major yeast infections on top of her other problems. Her system was finally rebalanced using Dong Quai, vitamin E and Remifemin (by Enzymatic Therapy), along with successfully eliminating the yeast overgrowth..

Is there such a thing as female frigidity?

The female analog for the penis is the clitoris, located above the vagina, and not the vagina itself. The vagina is actually quite insensitive. A three-inch-wide birth control diaphragm or a tampon can be in the vagina without being felt regardless of how the woman moves. Some women do not enjoy the deep penetration of intercourse. If this is the case, you are probably not frigid, physically abnormal, or emotionally stunted. The clitoris is analogous to the head of the penis, which is the most sensitive part of the man's anatomy. It follows that clitoral stimulation can provide the most pleasure for most women. Although intercourse will provide clitoral stimulation for many women, for others this type of stimulation is insufficient for full pleasure. By analogy, intercourse without additional stimulation for a woman can be compared to a man's having only the shaft of his penis stimulated without any contact with the head. While this may be pleasurable for a man, it may not be as fulfilling.

Much of sexual stimulation is between the ears, and mental and emotional stimulation and closeness with one's partner is often more important than technique.

Lubricating secretions are produced by glands which empty into the vagina in response to sexual arousal. Intercourse without arousal is thus likely to be dry, producing pain and discomfort.

Chlamydia and fungus infections such as an overgrowth of yeast cause secretions of a different type and are actually drying, causing painful intercourse and possible small tears in the mucous membrane of the vagina. This type of discomfort may be an indication that a previously undiscovered infection is present. When vaginal fungus is present, it is likely that you have a systemic fungus infection. Treating only the local infection will not remedy the underlying problem, and the local infection may keep coming back.

Women past menopause may also experience dryness as lowered estrogen levels produce lowered secretions. In this case good dietary oils will optimize hormone levels and may decrease the dryness. These oils are a good idea in any case.

What about men's prostate problems?

As mentioned previously, removal of the prostate can have aftereffects as drastic as those for women who have had a hysterectomy, and for similar reasons. As with most surgery, it is best to use less drastic measures whenever possible.

Saw palmetto berry is about three times more effective that the drug Proscar in relieving prostate symptoms, without the toxic side effects. These side effects include impotence, ejaculation problems, decreased sex drive and birth defects [14]. Yet the FDA has recommended that saw palmetto berry - but not Proscar, made by the pharmaceutical giant Merck - be removed from the market [15].

What Can You Do?

In addition to the oils mentioned previously, estrogen production in women is supported by Remifemin, Dong Quai, vitamin E, and soy protein. YamCon, extra strength, (Philips Nutritionals) and ProYam Cream supply a natural form of progesterone, and can help with female hormonal balance.

The rest of the body is supported by measures discussed throughout this book.

Summary

The body's systems are interrelated, and many of them have more than one function, in a masterpiece of efficient design. It is necessary to understand the body's systems in order to appreciate how toxic suppressors affect the body and to understand how to treat the associated problems.

References and Resources

General

- The Burton Goldberg Group, *Alternative Medicine: The Definitive Guide*, Future Medicine Publishing Inc., Puyallup WA, 1994. *The following chapters are pertinent to the Systems of the Body:*

    "Female Health", pp. 657-679

    "Male Health", pp. 733-743

    "Gallbladder Disorders", pp. 923-4

    "Hyperthyroidism", p. 934

    "Hypothyroidism", pp. 936-7

    "Urinary Problems", pp. 984-6

    "Heart Disease", pp. 711-724.

    "Hypertension", pp. 725-732,

    "Respiratory Conditions", pp. 813-826.

- Bevan, James, *Anatomy and Physiology*, Simon and Schuster, New York, 1978.

- *There are many other textbooks on human anatomy (structure) and physiology (function) which range in complexity from grade-school level to highly technical. Check your library.*

Skeletal System

- Appleton, Nancy, *Healthy Bones: What You Should Do About Osteoporosis*, Avery Publishing Group, Garden City Park, NY, 1991.

- Gaby, Alan R., *Preventing and Reversing Osteoporosis*, Prima Publishing, Rocklin CA.

Cardiovascular System

- Bennett, Charles, *Controlling High Blood Pressure Without Drugs*, Doubleday Books, NY, 1984.

- Carlson, Wade, *Hypertension and Your Diet*, Keats Publishing, New Canaan CT, 1990.

- Chaitow, Leon, *High Blood Pressure*, Thorsons, San Francisco CA, 1988.

- Charash, Bruce D., *Heart Myths*, Viking Penguin, NY, 1992.

- Cooper, Kenneth, *Overcoming Hypertension*, Bantam, NY, 1990.

- Gruberg, E.R. and S.A. Raymond, *Beyond Cholesterol: Vitamin B6, Arteriosclerosis and Your Heart*, St. Martin's Press, NY, 1981.

- Karpman, Harold L., *Preventing Silent Heart Disease*, Henry Holt and Co., NY, 1991.

- Kwiterovich, Peter, *The Johns Hopkins Complete Guide for Preventing and Reversing Heart Disease*, Prima Publishers, Rocklin CA, 1993.

- Ornish, Dean, *Dr. Dean Ornish's Program for Reversing Heard Disease*, Ballantine, NY, 1990.

- Ornish, Dean, *Stress, Diet and Your Heart*, Holt, Rinehart and Winston, NY, 1983.

- Piscatelli, Joseph C., *Choices for a Healthy Heart*, Workman Publishing, NY, 1987.

- Wallace, Louise M., *Coping With Angina*, Thorsons, UK, 1990.

- Whitaker, Julian, *Reversing Heart Disease*, Warner Books, NY, 1985.

Respiratory System

Gagnon, David and Amadea Morningstar, *Breathe Free*, Lotus Press, Willimot WI, 1990. *Nutritional and herbal treatments for respiratory problems.*

Gastrointestinal System

- Hoffman, Ronald, *Seven Weeks to a Healthy Stomach*, Pocket Books, NY, 1990.

- Perkin, Steven, *Gastrointestinal Health*, Harper Perennial, NY, 1992.

- Scala, James, *Eating Right For A Bad Gut*, Plume Books, NY, 1992.

Endocrine System

- Barnes, Broda O. and Lawrence Galton, *Hypothyroidism: The Unsuspected Illness*, Harper and Row, NY, 1976.

Reproductive System

- The Boston Women's Health Collective, *The New Our Bodies, Ourselves,* Simon and Schuster, NY, 1992.

- Chaitow, Leon, *Prostate Troubles*, Thorsons, UK, 1988.

- Ford, Gillian, *What's Wrong With My Hormones?*, Desmond Ford Publications, Newcastle CA, 1992.

- Lark, Susan M., *Dr. Susan Lark's The Menopause Self Help Book: A Woman's Guide to Feeling Wonderful the Second Half of Her Life*, Celestial Arts, Berkeley CA, 1990.

- Lark, Susan M., *Premenstrual Syndrome Self-Help Book: A Women's Guide*, Celestial Arts, Berkeley CA, revised 1993.

- Lark, Susan M., *Menstrual Cramps: A Self-Help Program*, Westchester Publishing Co., Los Altos CA, 1993.

- Ojeda, Linda, *Exclusively Female: A Nutrition Guide for Better Menstrual Health*, Borgo Press, San Bernardino CA, 1985.

- Stuart, F.H., *My Body, My Health: The Concerned Woman's Book of Gynecology*, Wiley and Sons, NY, 1979.

- Wolfe, Honora Lee, *Menopause: A Second Spring*, Blue Poppy Press, Boulder CO, 1990.

- Vliet, Elizabeth Lee, *Listening to Hormones: When They Speak, Your Body Changes*, M. Evans and Co., NY, 1995.

MEDICAL TERMINOLOGY AND WORD ROOTS

Medical terminology may seem terribly complex and multisyllabic, but a knowledge of basic Greek word roots will enable one to understand many, if not most, medical terms. These word roots refer to parts of the body and basic body conditions (inflammation, cancer, etc.). With these word roots, you will probably be able to figure out the meaning of most of the examples, even if you are unfamiliar with the word.

Body Part	Word Root	Examples
Skin	derm	epidermis, dermatology
Muscle	myo	myocardial, myositis
Bone	osteo	osteopath, osteoporosis
Kidney	nephr	nephritis, nephron
Liver	hepat	hepatitis, hepatic
Heart	cardio	cardiologist, pericardium
Lung	pulm	pulmonary
Gallbladder	chole	cholecystectomy
Uterus	hyster	hysterectomy
Vessel	vas	vascular, vas deferens
Nerve	neur	neuritis, neurotransmitter
Blood	hem	hematocrit, hemoglobin
Cell	cyte	lymphocyte, cytology, cytotoxic
Forming cell	blast	osteoblast, blastocyst
Spleen	splen	splenectomy
Urine	uria	anuria, hematuria
Milk	lact	lactation, lactose

Meaning	Word Root	Examples
Tumor	oma	carcinoma, myeloma
Condition of	osis	diverticulosis
Inflammation	itis	mastitis, meningitis
Over	hyper	hypertension, hyperthyroidism
Under	hypo	hypodermic, hypoglycemia
None, not	a, an	anuria, anosmia
Enzyme	ase	amylase, lactase
Sugar	ose	glucose, sucrose
Growth	trophy	hypertrophy, atrophy
Disease	path	cardiomyopathy, pathologist
Cutting	otomy	keratotomy
Removal	ectomy	appendectomy, hysterectomy
Study of	ology	biology, dermatology
Hard(ening)	scler	arteriosclerosis

The Cell

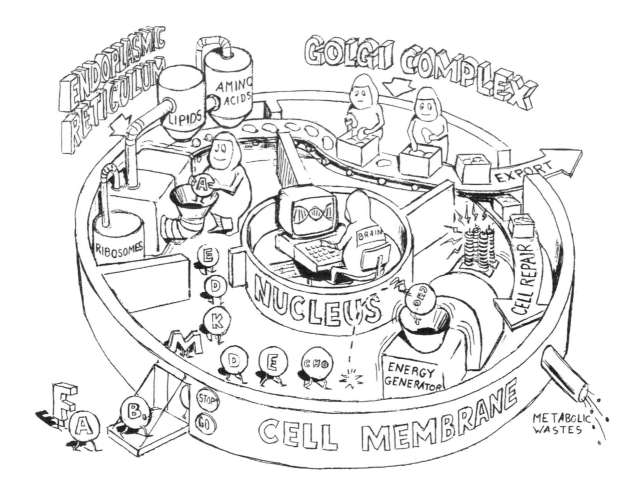

THE CELL

As The Cell Goes, So Goes Your Body

In this chapter you can learn:

- *Why cells are so important*
- *How a cell is like a factory*
- *What happens as we age*
- *Why women have more difficulty losing weight than men*
- *How the body's internal environment affects us*
- *Why cleansing the body is so important*
- *How the body deals with waste products, and how we can hinder or help this process*
- *Is cholesterol always the bad guy?*
- *Where we get our energy from*
- *What hormones are for*

Why are cells so important?

Billions of cells make up our bodies. Cells are the living units that form the structure of all of our tissues. Perhaps more importantly, each cell is a tiny self-contained factory that manufactures something needed for optimal function of the entire body. An understanding of the structure and function of cells is necessary in order to have a full appreciation of the workings of the body and the ways in which malfunction can occur.

How do the cells in your body resemble your body?

There is an amazing parallel between the functions of the different parts of the cell and the different parts of your body. These functions are illustrated here and described throughout the chapter.

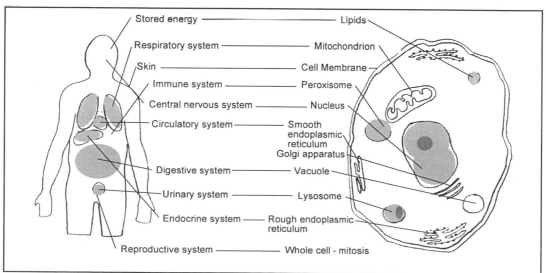

What's in a cell?

The cell is somewhat like a chicken egg, with a cell wall (the shell), a nucleus (like the yolk), and the cytoplasm (like the egg white). Other structures within the cell and their functions are shown in the stylized picture at the beginning of this chapter and discussed throughout this chapter.

Are all cells the same?

Yes and no. There are hundreds of different types of cells, each with a specialized function. However, all cells have certain structures and processes in common. Cells can be compared to manufacturing companies: as varied as the products they produce yet still having many things in common.

So the cell wall protects the cell like the shell protects an egg?

The cell wall surrounds the cell and performs the function of a security guard and chain link fence around a factory. In both cases (cell and factory) it keeps that which should be inside on the inside, and that which should be outside on the outside. Supplies - nutrients such as vitamins and amino acids - are delivered and taken into the cell in an orderly fashion, and wastes such as carbon dioxide are excreted.

The cell wall is very thin and is composed of a double layer of fat molecules sandwiched between two layers of protein. Cavities, and in some cases fingerlike projections called villi, increase the surface area of the cell wall to maximize absorption of nutrients and facilitate elimination of wastes.

Is cholesterol the bad guy portrayed by the media? -- Not always.

> **Cholesterol is not always the bad guy.**

Cholesterol is vital to the function of the cell and other body structures. It helps build and repair cellular membranes, in addition to other functions such as making hormones. In spite of its bad name it is so important for this purpose that the liver will manufacture cholesterol primarily from dietary sugar - and very little from fat as is commonly believed - as a backup system if insufficient cholesterol is ingested in the diet. The fatty bilayer of the cell walls require good oils for their integrity and maintenance. Insufficient good oil may result in cell walls that do not do their job properly. The remedy for this is outlined in the Oils and Fats chapter of the Supporters section.

Solvents such as acetone and benzene, which are made to dissolve fats and oils, can damage these cell membranes if taken into the body. This allows things such as toxins that do not belong in the cell to get in and do their damage. Carcinogens, which are chemicals that cause cancer, can then get in and damage the DNA of the cell (described in the next paragraphs), resulting in the possible eventual formation of a tumor.

Who's the brain of the whole operation?

In a corporation there is a governing body overseeing operations, making decisions, telling workers what to do, and hiring new workers when needed. The cell **nucleus**, which is the brain of the cell, performs these functions in the cell. The nucleus controls the characteristics of the cell and stores genetic information in the form of DNA for the duplication and creation of new cells.

The nucleus of the cell is like the brain of the body in its command functions. In fact, many parts of the cell mirror the functions of the body: the cell membrane is like the skin, the adrenal glands produce energy like the cell's mitochondria, and both the body and the cell have pathways for taking in nutrients and eliminating waste products. Testing techniques (see the chapter on A Visit To The Doctor) such as Live Blood Cell Analysis make use of these analogies to see what is happening in the body by observing cells.

How do we make new cells?

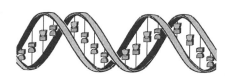

The nucleus, surrounded by its own membrane, is protected by its position in the center of the cell like an egg yolk in an egg. The nucleus is filled with a densely packed material called **chromatin**, which uncoils when the cell divides to form **chromosomes**. These chromosomes contain deoxyribonucleic acid (**DNA**) which encodes the genetic information necessary to recreate new cells just like itself. This allows us to replace cells as they die off or, in the case of the sex cells (ovum and sperm) to create a whole new individual.

DNA makes copies of itself using an enzyme called DNA transcriptase, similar to the process of making copies of a video tape. The DNA can be damaged, however, by many agents and toxins such as chemicals, radiation, and bad oils, and cause detrimental changes in the cells which are reproduced. You can get a picture of what happens by looking at the results of reproducing copies of a damaged video tape with blurred or missing sections of the tape. This error will be duplicated in further copies of that tape. In the body, the cells formed from this damaged genetic material, like a damaged tape, reproduces a genetically inferior copies and may not be able to do their job properly. They may even lose their identity entirely to become undifferentiated cancer cells.

What happens as we age?

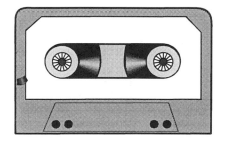

Making a copy of a cell from another cell's DNA is like making a copy of a tape from a master tape. Consider what happens when tape #2 is made from tape #1, then #3 is made from #2, etc.

Even using high quality tapes, the quality of the information on the tapes will degrade progressively with each successive copy. This is similar to what happens when we age. The quality of the original set of instructions becomes progressively poorer and is lost to an increasingly greater extent. Think about how much faster the information will degrade if poor quality tapes are used or if the tapes are exposed to heat and sunlight. When our cells are poorly nourished or exposed to toxins, our own cellular information degrades. As we age, we may feel as blurry as a tenth-generation tape.

The life of an average cell is about 120 days, although this varies somewhat by type of cell. This adds up to about three cycles a year or about 180 cellular life cycles in a lifetime of sixty years. That's a lot of potential cellular degradation.

How does the "egg white" of our cells help our bodies move?

Jelly-like **cytoplasm**, similar to the white of an egg, makes up the bulk of the cell, but it does more than simply take up space. Cytoplasm contains minerals which have important jobs to do. Potassium, a necessary mineral, is found inside the cell, while sodium is found on the outside; the sodium-potassium pump through the cell walls enables muscle movement. Magnesium, another essential mineral, has a number of functions, one of which is to move potassium by way of a biochemical pump into the blood to enable muscles to expand and contract. This is an example of how necessary minerals taken in from the diet can bring about their effects at the cellular level.

Where do we get our energy from?

The **mitochondria** are the power plants of the cell. They are sausage-shaped organelles (literally small organs, or cell parts) that contain a multiple-folded membrane. The folds create more surface area for increased absorption. Though all cells contain mitochondria, they are most abundant in active cells such as muscle fibers and spermatozoa. Mitochondria can be induced to increase in size and number to provide more energy through exercise, especially aerobic exercise such as running.

The cell takes in fuel in the form of amino acids from protein, glucose from carbohydrates, and fatty acids from good oils which themselves are broken down from the food we eat. This fuel is stored in the mitochondria as glycogen (stored blood sugar) and fat. Glycogen is short term energy storage. Everyone has on store about 1200 calories worth of stored energy, in the form of glycogen, which can be quickly transformed into a burst of energy when needed. (Fat is used for longer term storage.) Glycogen, reacting with oxygen, is released in the form of the biochemical adenosine triphosphate (ATP). ATP is a form of energy that the cell can use directly in protein manufacture, cell repair, and transport of minerals and other molecules.

Why do women have more difficulty losing weight than men?

There's a reason women have more difficulty losing weight than men.

On an average, the cells of men contain about 40% more mitochondria than those of women [1]. This is because women are made in such a way that they store food to nourish a potential pregnancy. Since mitochondria convert ingested calories to energy, it follows that people with more mitochondria (men) will burn more calories and deposit less of their food intake as fat. Women therefore gain weight more easily, and lose it with more difficulty than men.

The good news is that women can increase the number of mitochondria in their cells through a regular program of aerobic exercise such as walking or running. This will both provide more energy and burn off excess calories that you would otherwise end up wearing. You may never have to worry again about "a moment on the lips, a lifetime on the hips".

What are hormones for?

Hormones such as thyroxin from the thyroid gland or corticosteroids from the adrenal gland help regulate the speed of the cell's activity. Some hormones have a specific effect on only one type of cell, such as thyroid stimulating hormone (TSH) from the anterior pituitary gland, which tells the thyroid to make thyroxin. Other hormones affect one type of activity in all cells, such as the way insulin from the pancreatic islet cells affects carbohydrate metabolism.

What is the cell's packaging and shipping department?

The **Golgi bodies**, also called the Golgi complex, are the packaging plant of the cell. This is where materials made in the cell are collected for secretion. The Golgi bodies are stacks of thin, flat, saucer-shaped sacs, especially prominent in cells which secrete mucus and other glycoprotein solutions. Mucous membranes form a system which includes the lungs and digestive system. The IgA antibodies in the immune system and the mucus from the Golgi bodies work together to eliminate toxins from the body through the lungs, nasal passages, and digestive tract.

Irritation of the mucous membrane from smoking, infection, parasites, or allergy can cause mucus production that seems to be unrelated to the source. Intestinal parasites or food allergy can thus lead to a runny or congested nose or excessive throat clearing. The elimination of foreign material via mucus is one of your body's first detoxification steps.

Do you clear your throat a lot? Suspect parasites or food allergies.

Where is the manufacturing department?

The **endoplasmic reticulum** (ER) is an extension of the wall of the nucleus. The ER consists of large numbers of irregular folds throughout the cytoplasm (jelly-like material). Thousands of structures called ribosomes dot the outer surface of the ER.

These **ribosomes** are the sites where proteins are manufactured from protein components called amino acids, the building blocks of the body. Amino acids are like bricks in that they are put together to form polypeptides (poly = more than one, peptide = amino acid). So these proteins are assemblages of polypeptides, comparable to houses built brick by brick to form small or massive structures, depending on the blueprint. These specialized proteins can be used within the cell or are released as materials to manufacture enzymes, hormones, and other products.

What kinds of different cells are there?

The main purpose of a factory is to produce something that can be used by many segments of society in such a way that society as a whole appears to benefit. Factories produce many products, from cars to computers. Just as there are many thousands of possible consumer products, there are many thousands of specialized factories which use different types and combinations of raw materials and manufacturing processes.

Similarly, each cell is a specialized factory producing something needed by a part of the body for the benefit of the whole. Each of the hundreds of types of manufacturing cells exists for production purposes. Thus a thyroid cell produces thyroid hormone, a liver cell produces bile and hundreds of types of enzymes, a pancreatic cell produces digestive enzymes, an adrenal gland cell produces adrenaline, and stomach (parietal) cell produces hydrochloric acid.

Just as not all companies produce a tangible product, not all cells are manufacturing cells. Some cells, like some companies, provide services rather than goods. Nerve cells conduct biochemical/electrical impulses, like a power plant with transmission and distribution lines. Muscle cells expand and contract in unison to cause a biceps muscle on the arm to contract or the heart muscle to expand and contract. Bone and tooth cells have strong, rigid walls to form the skeleton, as well as to store and release calcium. Each type of cell works synergistically and symbiotically with the others to help make the body a better place in which to live.

How can you improve cell function?

In factory production, the final product can only be as good as the raw materials used. If inferior or insufficient raw materials are used, an inferior product will result - one which will not function optimally, or will break or wear out sooner. The raw materials for manufacturing cellular products and for the manufacture and upkeep of the cells themselves come from the nutrients we take into our bodies. Contrary to what some may think, these nutrients - amino acids, sugars, fatty acids, vitamins, and minerals - are all needed by every cell in the body. They are discussed in detail in the Supporters section. While nutrients don't heal in the strict sense of the word, a lack of quality nutrients can make you sick.

What environmental elements can affect the function of cells?

Factory workers cannot do their best in a poor working environment. If the temperature is too hot or too cold, the air stale, or the work atmosphere stressful, productivity will suffer. Similarly, the internal environment of the body must be optimal to ensure the best possible function. If there is too little oxygen, too hot or cold an internal temperature, body fluids too acid or alkaline, too many free radicals, or too much emotional or physical stress, cellular productivity will suffer.

If factory workers are spending much of their time repairing equipment, keeping employees from stealing (as fungus or parasites steal by cutting into the body's supplies), or dealing with inefficient transportation systems (like blocked arteries or anemia), this will also cut into productivity. Similarly, if the body is busy detoxifying solvents that break down cell membranes and trying to pry loose from the cells, metals that interfere with mineral absorption, it can't work very efficiently either.

Trash collection and disposal

Factories have garbage chutes and dumpsters, and hire companies to take away the trash on a regular basis. If this isn't done, garbage piles up, clutter in every room increases, the garbage chute clogs up, and the air becomes foul from rotting garbage. Each cell has ways to eliminate waste products such as carbon dioxide and ammonia through the cell wall, and the body as a whole has ways to eliminate waste altogether through the lungs, kidneys, the bowels, and the skin. These elimination or detoxification pathways can become saturated, clogged, or inefficient, with resulting harm to the system.

Why do painkillers make you constipated?

The painkilling drugs codeine, morphine, and related compounds which are found in preparations like Tylenol with codeine, Vicodan, and Demerol, slow down all body systems, including the elimination pathways, allowing toxins to build up in the body. This is similar to the way a New York City trash strike allows trash to pile up until the city is overloaded with garbage. The slowing down of the digestive system's elimination pathway often takes the form of constipation.

One of the purposes of this book and *Surviving The Toxic Crisis* is to pinpoint the many things which keep the body's cells from working optimally, and what can be done to correct the problems.

Remember: death starts in the cell, and as your cells go, so goes your whole body.

> As your cells go, so goes your whole body.

References and Resources

- Waterhouse, Debra, *Outsmarting the Female Fat Cell*, Hyperion, NY, 1993. *This book discusses the reasons, on a cellular level, why women have a harder time losing weight than men.*

- Stonehouse, Bernard, *The Way Your Body Works*, Crown Publishers, Inc., New York, 1974.

- Bevan, James, *Anatomy and Physiology*, Simon and Schuster, New York, 1978.

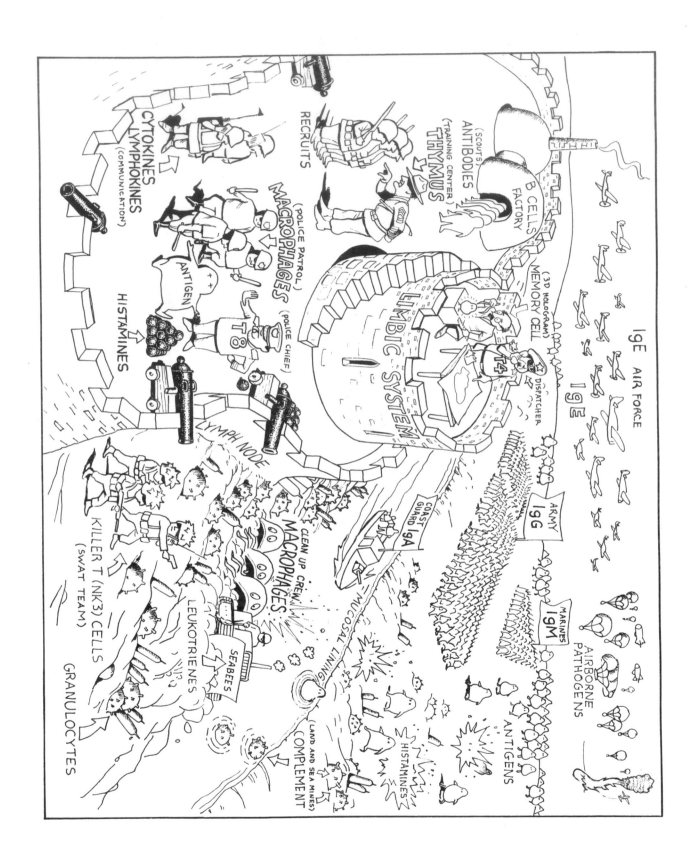

THE IMMUNE SYSTEM

In Defense of Your Defense

Twelve reasons to read this chapter:

1. *How is the immune system the most important system in the body?*

2. *What exactly is the immune system, and where is it located?*

3. *How does one develop a healthy immune system?*

4. *Are you what you eat?*

5. *How is the immune system like a country's defense system, and how does it work?*

6. *Why do my lymph glands need exercise?*

7. *How do antihistamine medications work, and are they a good idea?*

8. *Why do colds and some organ transplants last a week?*

9. *How can surgery adversely affect chronic disease?*

10. *How can your immune system attack you? or: Why does the body appear to attack itself?*

11. *Can the immune system be too efficient?*

12. *What are some symptoms of allergic reactions, including some you may not suspect?*

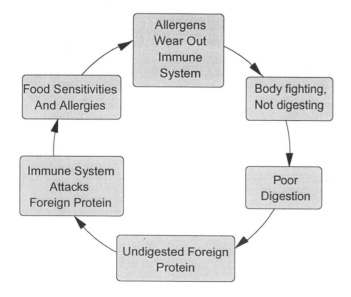

What is the most important system in the body?

The immune system, more than any other system in the body, is central to your health and well-being because it affects every other part of the body. The healthier your immune system is, the better your body can cope with the many toxic burdens it may encounter. Conversely, the fewer the toxic burdens, the more effectively your immune system will work. Allergens weaken the immune system, and a malfunctioning immune system in turn leads to allergies; a

99

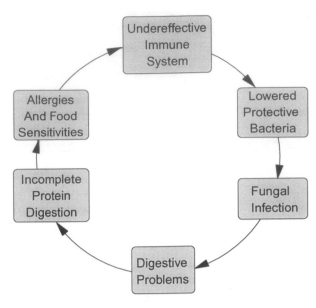

vicious cycle that can throw your health into a tailspin if the cycle is not stopped.

In a similar cyclic effect, a defective immune system can allow a fungal infection to take hold, which leads to digestive difficulties, which leads to allergies, which are a different type of defective immune response.

This syndrome, or collection of symptoms, is sometimes called Toxic Immune Syndrome (TIS).

What exactly is the immune system?

The immune system is the defense force against invaders from both outside and inside the body. These invaders can cause disease or death if not stopped. The importance of the immune system cannot be underestimated. A major focus of this entire book and of **Surviving The Toxic Crisis** is the immune system and how to improve its function by eliminating the toxic suppressors. The immune system is involved in all body systems and ties all the systems together.

How does one develop a healthy immune system?

Immune system health is dependent on three things:

- *Biochemical support (including nutrition)*
- *Genetic factors (heredity)*
- *Elimination of toxic suppressors*

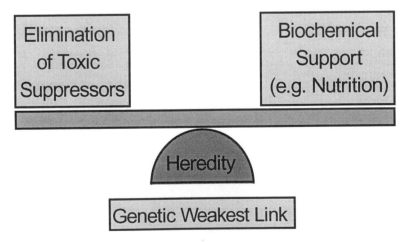

There are three ways you can win in developing a healthy immune system and having generally good health. Comparing your current health to an airplane needing to pull out of a tailspin or face imminent disaster, you can do a turnaround and reverse the downward descent of your health.

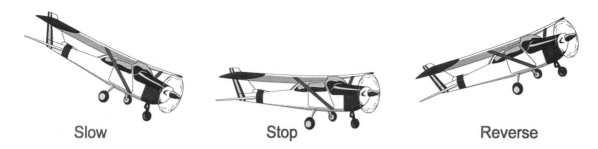

Slow   Stop   Reverse

Is it all in your genes?

The factor of heredity explains why some people can eat junk food or smoke and still lead long and healthy lives, while others follow all the rules and die early. Or why others have constant colds and infections and feel generally rundown year after year. Although your heredity cannot be changed, with today's technology, and by maximizing nutrition and other supporters and minimizing toxic burdens, you can make the most of the hand you've been dealt -- your genetic predisposition.

Are you what you eat?

Everything you eat will either strengthen or weaken your immune system, so nutrition is the key to its efficient function. However, there is more to nutrition than diet, as detailed in the Supporters section. Good foods are the tools which will provide necessary nutrients, and bad foods such as sugar and rancid oils are "negative nutrients", or toxins. If you go without food long enough, or limit yourself to toxic, nutrient deficient junk food, the body dies in stages beginning at the cellular level. For example, the mitochondria, the energy factories or generators of the cell, can lose the ability to make energy.

There is just no substitute for proper nutrition. Without it, all other measures have limited usefulness in restoring and maintaining immune system health. However, there is no guarantee that proper nutrition by itself will restore the immune system to health. Again, knowledge is power. And one of the purposes of this book is to provide knowledge that will empower you to maximize all the resources available to you to build and restore your immune system and your health!

Primary toxic suppressors such as metals, chemicals, and radiation can interfere with proper immune system function. Secondary microbiological suppressors such as fungi and bacteria which are fed by refined sugars in the diet can also damage the immune system. Primary toxic suppressors along with biochemical deficiencies can cause your immune system to be suppressed to the point that it is not working one hundred percent for you, and can open the door for opportunistic microorganisms to gain a foothold and undermine your health.

Toxic suppressors, or toxic burdens, such as chemicals, radiation, or parasites have the same effect on the immune system as a weighted backpack would have on a runner. Three pounds in the backpack would have no effect on the runner, 30 pounds would slow him down, 200 pounds would stop him, and 1000 pounds would crush and kill him regardless of his training or genetics.

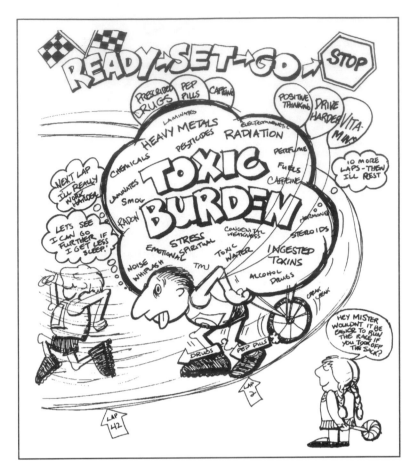

Although a healthy immune system, like a well-conditioned runner, can ignore a small burden - and in fact has systems to eliminate the small burdens - each toxic burden has an additive and cumulative effect on the immune system. The burdens pile up faster than the body can get rid of them. This makes the immune system less and less effective over time, with a concomitant increase in symptoms. This is like a boat filling up with water faster than you can bail it out.

You must take back responsibility for your health!

Chances are if you are reading this book you or someone you care about has a poorly functioning immune system, so some damage may have already been done. Fortunately, the body comes with self-repair systems that are activated with even a minimum of effort. Regardless of the state of your immune system, it is virtually guaranteed that any nutritional improvement and/or lowering of your toxic load will result in at least some improvement in immune system function. This improvement may or may not cause a noticeable decrease of symptoms, or the improvement may be very slow, but your body is still benefiting. Another way to look at it: if your symptoms or disease are slowing, stopping, or reversing, you are winning.

A generally healthy lifestyle, including good nutrition, low or no tobacco smoking or alcohol consumption, exercise, adequate sleep, and lowered stress levels has been correlated with higher natural killer cell (NK) activity, a positive indicator of a healthier immune system overall [1].

Just what is the immune system and where is it located?

Although no system works alone, the immune system, unlike the cardiovascular or digestive systems, cannot be isolated and pinpointed in a diagram of the human body. Because it is so important, and must react so quickly to invaders, its components and cells are found everywhere in the body. Like the defense system of a country or government, the immune system is set up to keep order and to recognize and attack enemies, to distinguish between friend and foe, self and non-self.

How is the immune system like a country's defense system?

The immune system is so similar to a country's defense system that direct parallels can be drawn between specific components of the defense system and those of the immune system. These are illustrated at the beginning of this chapter and described in greater detail in the chapter.

Immune Component	Defense Analog	Function
Macrophages	Police patrol	On-site attack
Helper T4	Dispatcher	Decide what to attack, send message
Suppressor T8	Police chief	Stop attack when over
Antigen	Enemy	Reason for attack
Histamines	Bullets	Used to fight and kill enemies
Granulocytes	Land mines	Empty shrapnel (granules) into enemy
Killer T (NK3) cell	SWAT team	Kill cancer and other deadly cells
Limbic system	Pentagon	Command post
Cytokines, lymphokines	Communication	Transmit information from one cell to another
Antibodies	Scouts	Recognize nonself, attack and signal others to attack
Lymph node	Fort	Protected place to mobilize forces from
IgA	Coast guard	Mucosal lining defense/shore patrol
IgE	Air Force	Fights airborne pathogens
IgM	Marines	Fierce early fighting, then leave
IgG	Army	Keep fighting
B cells	Arms factory	Make antibodies
Memory cell	3D Hologram	Remember shape of enemy for selective attack
Complement	Land and sea mines	Activated to explode and destroy
Leukotrienes	Seabees	Come in afterward and rebuild
Macrophages	Cleanup crew	Garbage collectors
Thymus	Training center	Training of new recruits

How does this defense system work?

The immune system is tremendously complex, and whole books have been written on the subject [2]. This complexity belies a simple explanation. The immune system is actually a series of nearly fail-safe systems and backup systems which work independently or together to varying degrees. Although this complexity hampers the simplicity of the explanation, it serves our body wonderfully well.

What happens when the enemy comes?

The appearance of an antigen, or foreign protein, is the signal for the immune system to swing into action. An antigen can be hostile (non-self, like a parasite) or friendly (self, food). An antigen can be a wolf in sheep's clothing, such as a bacteria or fungus infection which builds up so slowly that the immune system gets used to and accepts the invaders, like a Trojan horse. Conversely, an antigen can be a sheep in wolf's clothing, something that should be harmless but causes the immune system to react negatively to things such as food or even body parts. A seemingly inappropriate reaction to one's own body is called autoimmune disease, described later in this chapter.

Even before an antigen appears, however, lymphocytes, a type of white blood cell, are patrolling the bloodstream like police looking for anything that does not belong there. The body holds about one trillion lymphocytes, or about 3000 in every drop of blood. Over 800,000 of them are created and destroyed in the time it takes you to read this sentence [3].

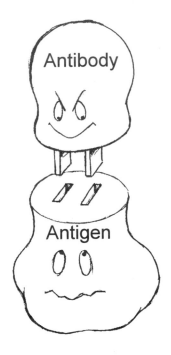

Every part of the immune system, except for granulocytes (described in the following pages), comes from or is related to lymphocytes. They transmit information to the plasma cells (precursors to more specialized cells), telling them what kind of antibodies to make. They travel through the lymph nodes and the thymus. They change into other types of cells such as killer T cells, helper T cells (called T4) or suppressor cells (called T8). The plasma cells that make antibodies were once lymphocytes [2]. Lymphocytes are themselves created from their precursors called lymphoid stem cells, which are undifferentiated (not a specific type of cell).

An antigen is a foreign substance (non-self) that incites an antibody's attack. An antigen can be a bacterium, a virus, a vaccine, a mutated cell, a pollen granule if one is sensitized to pollen (in which case it becomes an allergen), a transplanted organ, or a toxic metabolic byproduct such as acetaldehyde from alcohol.

Chemicals and metals can combine with body tissues to create non-self antigens, which the immune system then attacks. This can lead to autoimmune disease.

Each antigen has a marker on its surface, and each type of antigen has a different type of marker, like a fingerprint. There are, ideally, as many different antibodies as there are antigens, with each antibody specific to one type of antigen like a key to a lock.

An antibody is a protein substance in the blood stream that performs several functions. Antibodies both attack the invader themselves and, like scouts, signal other parts of the immune system to attack. Upon attacking, antibodies self-destruct. Like kamikaze pilots, they sacrifice themselves as they launch an all-out attach on the enemy attacking your body.

We are born with certain antibodies obtained from our mothers, and receive other valuable antibodies to antigens in the environment through the colostrum in mother's milk if we are breastfed as our Creator intended rather than artificially as with bottle feeding. Other antibodies are created through proper immune system response to infectious agents.

How does the lymphatic system fit into the defense system?

When an antigen (non-self) enters the system, a circulating lymphocyte picks off the antigen from the invader and carries the information to the nearest lymph node. Lymph nodes are located in the groin, armpits, neck, and near the major organ systems, as well as elsewhere in the body, and are the misnamed "swollen glands", which you can feel if you have an infection.

Lymph nodes are collection points in the lymph system, which also consists of tubes for transportation between nodes. The main collector lymph nodes are located in the chest. The wearing of the current fashion craze -- the "wonder bra", with its underwire construction, can constrict and block these lymph channels from properly draining from the feet to the chest, to the detriment of the body.

> **The wearing of an underwire bra can interfere with the immune system**

Underwire bras are not the only type to be implicated in immune-related health problems. It has been found that bras of any type, usually worn all day and sometimes even worn to bed at night, are associated with a 21-fold risk of breast cancer as compared to the risk of women who do not wear a bra at all [4,5]. Another study shows even higher numbers. In a study of 4700 women with and without breast cancer in five major U.S. cities, it was found that women who wear a bra more than 12 hours a day are *19 times* more likely to develop breast cancer than women who wear a bra less than 12 hours a day. Women who wear a bra to sleep in as well, or nearly 24 hours daily, have an incredible 113-fold breast cancer incidence [6]. The theory behind these statistics is that unnaturally compressing breast tissue, which is rich in lymph nodes, impairs lymph flow and causes toxins to accumulate in the breasts.

A patient in her mid 40s who wore an underwire bra complained of weight gain (edema, or toxic water weight), sluggishness and poor immune system function. She removed the underwire bra, raised the foot of her bed six inches (which helped lymph drainage), retired her sunglasses, and used an Alpine Air Cleaner. She then lost over 40 pounds and gained newfound energy.

The lymphatic vessels are more likely to be used when chronic conditions and infections are being dealt with. The lymph system also makes use of the vascular (blood vessel) system for transportation of its components in an acute, or emergency, situation. This is rather like having both air and ground transportation available for the armed forces depending on the urgency of a defense situation.

The lymph nodes are also collection points for toxins in the body, similar to how the military police would use the brig as a holding tank. The lymph system moves chemicals, metals, and other poisons to the lymph nodes until it can process or eliminate them. Not all toxins can be eliminated. For example, some clothing dyes and fat soluble food dyes collect in the lymph nodes and remain trapped there.

The immune system eliminates toxins because it recognizes the toxins combined with the body's protein-containing tissue as non-self. However, the immune system is not equipped to deal with non-antigenic (non-protein-containing) invaders by itself. So when the lymph nodes are full of these toxins, the lymph system is too clogged up to do its job effectively, which is one of the reasons that toxic overload contributes to immune system malfunction such as allergy and autoimmune disease.

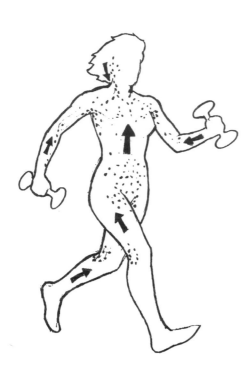

Why do my lymph glands need exercise?

Of our two circulatory systems, both have pumps. The heart is the pump for the cardiovascular system. But what type of pump does the other one, the lymph system, have? Toxins and infectious are released from the lymph nodes to be dealt with when the nodes are squeezed by the muscles as we exercise. We are designed in such a way that when we do even simple exercise like walking, most of the major lymph nodes are worked: the nodes in the groin, in the armpits, in the backs of the knees, at the shoulder blades, and in the neck are massaged when we move.

Deep breathing squeezes the lymph glands in the chest and upper abdomen. Chewing moves the head sutures, which stimulates the lymph nodes located in that area, as well as the movement of the spinal fluid. There is wisdom in the old adage - chew each mouthful of food thirty times.

All of these movements push toxins out through your pores as sweat and into the bloodstream for elimination, as well as the waste products lactic and uric acid which are byproducts of exercise.

If it is hard to bend and stretch, one possible cause may be lymph nodes which are full of toxins.

How is ammunition made and fired?

B-cells can be likened to the arms factories while the T-cells can be thought of as the SWAT team of the immune system. The outer part of each lymph node is filled with B-cell lymphocytes and the inner part is filled with T-cells, so called because they are formed in the bones and thymus respectively. When the lymphocyte bearing the antigen gets to the lymph node, it goes to either the B-cell area or the T-cell area based on its inner knowledge of what is needed to deal with this particular invader. If it touches B-cells, each B-cell becomes what is called a plasma cell which releases many thousands of antibodies to that particular non-self antigen. If it touches a T-cell, the T-cell changes to a killer T-cell which then leaves the node to attack the invader by itself.

How can you tell who's a cancer candidate?

These T-cells are sometimes called NK or NK3 cells, for Natural Killer. They form a sort of SWAT team for defense. They attack cancer cells like a homicide detective going after a serial killer. It can be said that most of us actually develop an early stage of cancer numerous times, but those of us with good immune function never know it because the NK3 cells

> The level of NK3 cells in the blood is a rough indicator of the chances of developing cancer.

take care of the problem long before symptoms develop. In fact, a look at the level of NK3 cells in the blood is a rough indication of the chances of a person's developing symptomatic cancer.

Granulocytes are white cells which have granular material in them that is visible under a microscope, in contrast to lymphocytes which are non-granular. They grab the invader and empty their histamine granules into the cell until it has been killed, like a wasp injecting its poison into the skin of its victim through its stinger.

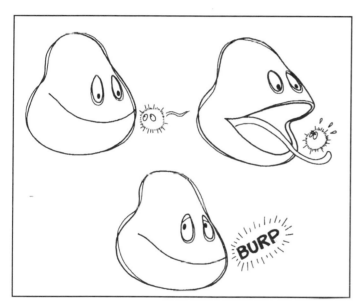

Antihistamine medications, which block histamine production and release, cause you to lose this part of your immune defense.

What are the garbage collectors of the immune system?

A macrophage is a larger, stronger white cell. Its name means "big eater", which describes its method of destruction. It engulfs the usually smaller invader and digests it by dissolving it with enzymes or swallowing it like some internal Pac-man. Macrophages are on site for small disturbances, like police patrolling the neighborhood or sentries on guard. They act as a combination of police and clean-up crew.

How are helper T-cells like a police dispatcher?

Helper cells, also called T4 (not to be confused with the thyroid component T4 - T stands for thymus here), decide what to attack, and convey this information to other immune system components. They perform the function of a police dispatcher. Low numbers of helper cells lead to poor immune function, as these immune system components can be aimlessly circulating around, totally unaware that they are needed. This is what happens in AIDS (Acquired Immune Deficiency Syndrome).

How are T8 cells like a police chief?

Suppressor cells are also called T8 cells. Their function is to keep the immune system from overreacting inappropriately. They act like a police chief or captain who keeps the police at a riot site from losing control. If the T8 count is too low, the immune system doesn't turn off and starts fighting everything, like a dazed punch-drunk boxer. The result is allergic reactions or autoimmune disease. Suppressors such as chemicals can be said to tire out the immune system so that it ends up like the arm-weary and ineffective boxer, swinging blindly at everything.

The ratio of T4 to T8 is more important than the actual count of either type of cell. A ratio of low T4/ high T8 is an indication of AIDS or other apparent immune system collapse. What actually happens in these cases is that the immune system is there and functional, but is nonresponsive. Low T8 is a sign of immune overactivity or allergic response, or in severe cases of the universal reactor. With low T8 counts, the immune system never turns off, while low T4 counts keep the immune system from turning on, leading to diseases such as cancer and pneumonia. The body, if its function is compromised by toxic suppressors, can tune out the T8 cells just as kids who are constantly nagged can tune out their parents by selective listening.

What part of the immune system is like land and sea mines that explode and destroy?

Another part of the immune system, besides the antibodies and white blood cells, is called the complement, which is manufactured in the liver and consists of nine individual proteins. These nine proteins help to minimize the chance of error, as each must be activated in sequence, within a tenth of a second, before the bacterium is destroyed. The complement essentially blows up and destroys the enemy like land and sea mines. Suppressed immune systems can be supported by a safe blood by-product called transfer factor, which contains complement.

What are the bullets used to fight and kill enemies?

Histamines are the bullets which are released to fight the antigens. They are also the components which cause the typical symptoms of colds and allergies: runny nose, wheezing, hives, itching and watery eyes, and to a certain extent a general sick feeling. Part of the sick, queasy feeling is due to the presence of alpha interferon, a substance which ignites the immune system's firing of histamines. Anaphylactic shock, the most severe and acute allergic reaction, is caused by a massive release of histamines and subsequent collapse of blood vessels and major body functions. Anaphylactic shock, also called anaphylaxis, can be fatal.

How do antihistamine medications work, and why should you sometimes not use them?

Antihistamine medications counteract the histamines, as their name implies, but they counteract the beneficial protective effects as well as the unpleasant symptoms. One danger of antihistamines is that a person with allergies who would otherwise identify and avoid the allergens will simply suppress the symptoms and live with the allergens. A person with, for example, an allergy to cats may take antihistamines (pills, inhalers) and continue to live with the cats. One day the body's reaction is stronger than the antihistamines can control, and a massive allergic reaction such as anaphylactic shock can come as a complete surprise. About 2000 people die annually from anaphylactic shock. In about half of the cases the victims are caught completely off guard, as they react to something that they did not realize was a problem. In the other half of the cases, the victims ignored milder allergic reactions, put their faith in drugs, pushed their luck, and lost the battle.

What are the fighting forces?

The body manufactures five types of antibodies, called immunoglobulins (Ig for short). These are called IgA, IgM, IgG, IgE, and IgD. They perform the functions of the armed services - Marines, Army, Air Force. These antibodies are not found in equal amounts in the body. Of the total serum immunoglobulin [7],

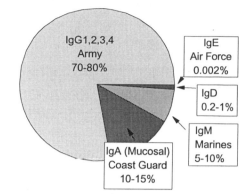

- *IgG (Army)*   is 70-80%
- *IgA (Coast Guard)*   is 10-15%
- *IgM (Marines)*   is 5-10%
- *IgD*   is 0.2-1%
- *IgE (Air Force)*   is 0.002%

IgA lines our mucous membranes and helps to keep out invaders. Like the Coast Guard or shore patrol on the alert for enemies invading by water, they stop them before they make it to land, IgA takes care of invaders before they penetrate the body. It is found primarily in secretions such as saliva, intestinal fluids, colostrum and breast milk, and tears. It causes toxins to be surrounded and carried out of the body by mucus. IgA problems usually show up as a disturbance in mucosal linings such as that in the stomach, which are analogous to the ocean shore line.

IgE are like the Air Force, dealing with airborne threats (inhalants). IgE, although present in extremely tiny amounts, is the immunoglobulin most involved in sometimes-fatal anaphylactic reactions. IgE deficiency can lead to inhalant allergies and vice versa.

IgM are like the Marine Corps. They are like assault troops that do the early fighting for about ten weeks, after which time they are inactive and leave the front to the IgG.

Why do colds and some organ transplants last a week?

IgG, found primarily in extracellular fluid, are like the Army, in that they take a while to mobilize (about seven days) but they fight steadily for as long as they are needed, taking over after the IgM launch their massive frontal attack. They stay on alert like a peace keeping force until the battle is won and peace is secured. The seven day wait accounts for the seven day duration of a cold, or the week before an organ transplant is rejected by the body (attacked by the immune system).

IgG is further subdivided into IgG1, 2, 3, and 4. Malfunctions of the IgG system, particularly IgG4, can lead to digestive sensitivities/allergies. The term allergy is sometimes used to refer to an inappropriate attack by the immune system in general. However, many allergists use the term allergy to refer only to an IgE mediated attack, and would therefore call a reaction to food a sensitivity rather than an allergy.

IgD has been shown to be present, but very little is understood about its function at this time.

What are the other parts of the immune system?

The spleen, located on the left side of the abdomen, is considered to be part of the immune system because it is made up largely of lymphoid tissue. It is used to make antibodies, as well as having non-immune system functions such as destroying old red blood cells. Tonsils and adenoids are lymphoid tissue as well. They filter out bacteria and drop them down through the esophagus into the stomach, where they are killed by the very acidic gastric juice.

The thymus is a flat, two-lobed organ lying in back of the sternum (breastbone). It manufactures lymphocytes and is especially active in childhood. Contrary to the beliefs of some doctors that the thymus is useful only in childhood, the thymus has an active function in adulthood.

It is believed that thumping on the thymus stimulates the immune system.

How can surgery adversely affect chronic disease?

There is so much redundancy and so many backup systems and buffers involved in the immune system that whole components can be removed or destroyed and other parts of the immune system will take over their function, at least in the short run. For example, the spleen can be surgically removed, the tonsils taken out, or the thymus destroyed by deliberate irradiation. This weakens the immune system, but it still works nearly as well as it is supposed to for short term purposes. However, the weakened immune system does not do as well with chronic long term problems. For example, when the spleen is removed, the liver takes over its function, but this overloads the liver with chronic symptoms worsening over time.

The main problem that arises when the immune system is interfered with is that, while backup systems work in the short run, the long term deficit can contribute to chronic disease.

A parable

The story is told of the championship frog that regularly outjumped the competition:

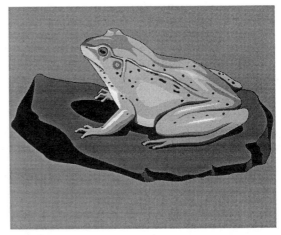

Day 1: The frog's owner said "Jump" and the frog jumped high and far. Alas, the competitors crept in one night and cut off one of the frog's legs.

Day 2: The next day the frog's owner said "Jump" and the frog still won. But that very night the competitors cut off the frog's other leg.

Day 3: The following day the owner said "Jump", and the frog just sat there. Everyone in the land concluded that the frog must be hard of hearing.

What does this parable have to do with the immune system?

Doctors removed the tonsils (lymph escape valve) of a hypothetical patient at age 8, the appendix (colon escape valve) at age 15, the spleen (blood cleaner) after an accident at age 25, the gallbladder (digestion and elimination of toxic waste) at age 35, and the lymph nodes under the arm during a mastectomy (breast removal for cancer) at age 42. When the patient developed severe chronic health problems by age 50, all the doctors in the land concluded that the problem was genetic. Like those who observed the frog, they reached an erroneous and misleading conclusion.

Such illness caused by medical intervention is so common that a word has been coined to describe the problem: **iatrogenic**, treatment caused damage, discussed in the "Treatment Caused Trauma" chapter at greater length.

What types of immune system malfunction are there?

An immune system that is functioning less than optimally can be either too aggressive or not aggressive enough towards internal or external antigens. Immune system malfunctions are of four basic types:

Immune System
Activity

	Overactive	Underactive
Internal	Autoimmune Disease	Cancer
External	Allergy	Infection

(left axis label: **Antigen Source**)

Nearly everyone who has any type of chronic problem has one or more of these types of malfunction. It is possible for the immune system to be both overactive (towards self) and undereffective (towards non-self), like an arm-weary boxer too tired lift his gloves, much less to punch.

How can your immune system attack you?

The immune system may be either overly aggressive in general, or may fail to distinguish between self and non-self -- between you and the bad guys. One's own tissues and systems come under attack. The resulting symptoms depend on the system being attacked. The immune system is set up to produce antibodies against a wide range of pathogens, or disease-causing organisms. It is also set up to *not* react against the molecules carried on the body's own cells.

Our immune system was designed to provide protection against foreign invaders, much the same way our country's defense systems are set to be on alert against dangers to its national security. Sophisticated military technology has developed heat-seeking missiles which go after anything "hot" picked up on radar. Added to this is a relatively new defense technology called holography, in which the shape of the enemy's planes, boats, and tanks is recorded holographically, as a three dimensional image. "Hits" are thus more accurately made than with heat-seeking missiles alone. An example of a hologram is the image on some credit cards. The missiles can now tell enemy from friend by comparing the object ahead with the holographic image.

This modern day technology is essentially the same as what the immune system has been doing for ages: telling friend from foe. The importance of this cannot be underestimated. Without the ability to tell friend from foe, soldiers can be killed by "friendly fire". Similarly, autoimmune disease can develop as the immune system which is supposed to protect and defend turns against its own system because of the confusion from incoming information, whereby it can no longer differentiate between self and non-self..

Why does the body attack itself?

This self-protective measure - telling self from non-self - can be disturbed by, among other things, chronic exposure to certain chemicals, metals, and types of radiation. When toxins go into and unite with soft tissue, the immune system attacks the soft tissue because the combination is recognized as non-self. For example, mercury from amalgam fillings may bind to tissues instead of the zinc that belongs there, causing a response leading to symptoms of arthritis.

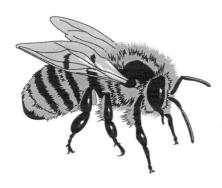

Autoimmune disease has sometimes been described as a body that has somehow gone crazy and started attacking itself. This does not just spontaneously happen. There is always a reason which makes sense to the immune system, even though the reason may not be apparent to us. For instance, suppose you were watching a person sit quietly in a chair, and she suddenly jumped up and started flailing around. It would look as though she had gone crazy, but her actions would make sense if you saw the bee that was buzzing around her head. Her actions make sense -- to her -- even if *you* don't see the bee.

Similarly, the actions of the immune system make sense whether or not they are understood by an observer. For example, people studying osteoarthritis, an autoimmune disease, have found blastocystis hominis, a parasite, in the joints. The immune system was attacking the parasite, not the joint tissue. Interestingly, a folk remedy for arthritis has been the wearing of copper bracelets. Since copper helps to kill parasites there may be some innate wisdom in the remedy. Some of the pharmaceutical companies which condemn such folk remedies as nonsense derive the basis for many of their drugs from these simple solutions.

Autoimmune disease is rarer in those who have a history of being breastfed, since the immune systems of breastfed babies have been programmed with additional instructions in how to behave properly.

What are some of the autoimmune diseases?

There are a number of autoimmune diseases. These include [8]:

- Lupus, or SLE, short for systemic lupus erythematosus. As the name implies, the whole system is affected, primarily the brain, kidneys, joints, skin and lungs. B cells go out of control and manufacture unusually large numbers of antibodies.

- Crohn's disease affects the intestines, causing diarrhea.

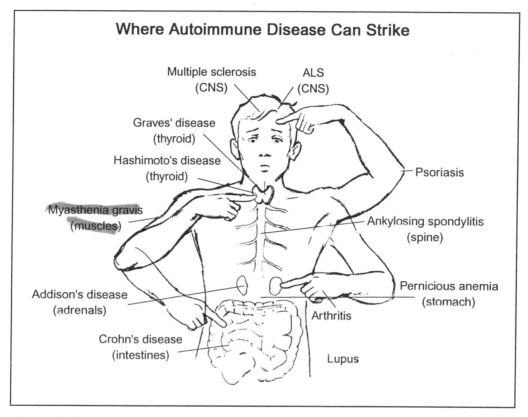

Where Autoimmune Disease Can Strike

Multiple sclerosis (CNS)

ALS (CNS)

Graves' disease (thyroid)

Hashimoto's disease (thyroid)

Myasthenia gravis (muscles)

Psoriasis

Ankylosing spondylitis (spine)

Pernicious anemia (stomach)

Addison's disease (adrenals)

Arthritis

Crohn's disease (intestines)

Lupus

- Graves' disease is a form of hyperthyroidism, causing bulging eyes and fatigue.

- Pernicious anemia affects stomach cells, leading to lack of absorption of vitamin B12.

- Addison's disease affects the adrenal gland.

- Psoriasis is an itchy, unsightly skin disease.

- Multiple sclerosis - The immune system turns against the central nervous system, breaking down the myelin sheath that protects the nerve cells.

- Rheumatoid arthritis - The tissues of the joints are attacked.

- Myasthenia gravis - The voluntary muscles are affected.

- Hashimoto's disease - The thyroid gland is destroyed by the immune system.

- Amyotrophic lateral sclerosis (ALS, or Lou Gehrig's disease) can be caused by mercury, root canals and nickel allergy, and parasites. The parasites are themselves secondary to mercury.

- Ankylosing spondylitis - the soft tissues of the head, neck, and spine are attacked, resulting in pain and stiffness. The klebsiella bacteria are often present in this disease.

How prevalent is autoimmune disease?

About 5% of adults in Europe and North America suffer from an autoimmune disease. Two-thirds of these are women [9].

What can cause autoimmune diseases?

These autoimmune disturbances, in which there is a breakdown in the ability of the immune system to distinguish between self and non-self, can be caused by:

- *A **pathogen** such as a bacteria, parasite, or virus, as described in some of the previous examples.*

- ***Chemicals** such as polycyclic aromatic hydrocarbons (PAH) and other solvents which break down cell membranes and mutate cells and blur the distinction between self and non-self.*

- ***Mercurials** - mercury can bind to soft tissue to form a combination identified as nonself, and can also open the door to parasites, fungus, chronic bacterial and viral infections.*

- *Many **drugs** can also bind with the body's tissues to incite an autoimmune reaction.*

- ***Allergy** / sensitivity such as sensitivity to nickel.*

- ***Electromagnetic fields**, discussed in the chapters on Electromagnetic Radiation in **Surviving The Toxic Crisis**.*

Can the immune system be too efficient?

A car alarm can be too sensitive, or too efficient, going off with the least provocation. The immune system can also be too sensitive, causing more harm than good.

Allergy is a hypersensitivity to an external (nonself) substance. The immune system goes into the cellular equivalent of a hysterical fit whenever something relatively harmless, such as pollen or eggs, enters the body. However, what seems like a random overreaction actually makes sense to the immune system, as is the case with autoimmune disease. The body is not doing wrong. We made a bad choice, and the body is doing the best it can to handle the situation.

Something which is toxic to everyone, such as mercury or pesticides, can also provoke an exaggerated reaction to even smaller amounts in some individuals than would affect most people. In either case, the reaction is akin to the entire National Guard being called out to deal with a neighborhood disturbance of the peace as if it were a major riot!.

Some chemicals, foods, and other substances can cause allergic reactions, either a hypersensitivity to that material when exposed to it in the future, or a predisposition to allergic reaction to other related or unrelated substances.

Allergy can be primary, an allergic response to the food or substance itself. Or allergy can also be secondary, a reaction to a byproduct. For example, fruit, grains, and refined sugar all turn to alcohol in the body. Allergy can be to the alcohol (the secondary product) or even to the acetaldehyde which is a breakdown product of the alcohol. Microorganisms in the body put out waste byproducts as a result of their life cycles to which some people become allergic. This is another example of secondary allergy or sensitivity.

Environmental illness (EI) is a type of multiple allergic response. A sufferer of EI, sometimes called a universal reactor in extreme cases, can be so sensitive that s/he cannot leave the house because of dangers in the outside environment. And sometimes it works the other way -- the afflicted person cannot remain in the house because of dangers in their own home environment.

What are some symptoms of allergic reactions?

There are a number of symptoms that can be caused by allergic reactions. Differences in symptoms and the degree of reactivity are determined by, among other factors, individual predisposition. The body system that is the target of the allergen is sometimes determined by the allergen and sometimes by the "weak link" in the individual. We need to look at genetic translators (weak link) vs. target systems (based on the chemical or allergen), since chemical toxins, like allergens, can produce symptoms based on either the person or the chemical itself.

- *For some people, the weakest part of their body can be their digestive system, the respiratory system, or the skin; this will have some bearing on the types of symptoms they develop.*

- *The type of toxin is another factor.*

- *Yet another is the method by which the toxin got into the body - inhaled through nasal passages, ingested through the mouth, or absorbed through skin contact.*

Are you allergic?

There are many possible allergic symptoms, including some that you or your doctor may not immediately attribute to allergy. Allergic symptoms and some possible causes include [10]:

- **Anaphylaxis**, which is an allergy-induced shock, and the most serious, can cause death due to high histamine release which can lead to throat closure and very low or loss of blood pressure.

- Urticaria, or **hives**, which combine visible skin swelling and intense itching is also caused by high histamine levels as a result of a systemic reaction or caustic chemicals.

- Rhinorrhea, or **nasal discharge**, sniffling and clogged sinuses can result from nickel in the teeth or microorganisms. Nasal polyps can also result from nickel exposure, particularly if the nickel is in the top four front teeth since they drain upwards towards the nose.

- **Head pressure and back stiffness** due to meningeal contraction from the allergic response are also possible.

- **Asthma**, which causes extreme difficulty in breathing, can come from inhalants to which one is allergic or from roundworms, which reside in the lungs and esophagus.

- **Digestive disturbances**, such as vomiting and diarrhea, can come from an allergic reaction. They can also be due to parasites such as giardia, helicobacter, fungi, or viruses.

- Contact **dermatitis**, which is a skin reaction to contact with certain chemicals and natural substances, including those in the air. Toxic byproducts of microorganisms and fungus can also cause dermatitis [11].

Are all allergic symptoms physical?

Allergy or sensitivity to a substance can cause mental or emotional impairment as well as physical symptoms. Brain fog is a fairly common symptom. For example, a person may be walking down the street, deep in conversation with a friend, and be exposed to diesel fumes or insecticide. The person can become instantly confused and lose track of the conversation in mid-sentence. A day-to-day lack of mental clarity can likewise be due to food, inhalant, or other allergy.

Mood swings and bursts of anger or tears are also sometimes attributable to allergy. For example, a person exposed to cologne from a passerby may feel disproportionately furious and violated, or suddenly want to burst into tears.

Panic attacks or agoraphobia (fear of leaving the home) may be brought on by allergy to substances in the environment. Hyperactivity and aggressiveness in children can be brought on by diet and can therefore be controlled by dietary modification.

Can anything be an allergen?

A list of possible allergens would be endless, as there are very few substances to which someone, somewhere, is not allergic. Foreign protein is almost always the antigen that causes the allergy. Nickel is one of the few exceptions, although nickel sensitivity is not IgE mediated and so is not considered a true allergy by some. This is strictly an academic distinction to anyone who has gone into life-threatening anaphylaxis from nickel.

Allergy can be compared to exhausted shell-shocked troops who flail around wildly, shooting at anything that moves. After doing this for a while, they become too fatigued to shoot at anything and just sit numbly by, no matter what happens. Similarly, allergy that continues long enough, such as untreated environmental illness, can eventually become immune suppression, in which the exhausted immune system no longer fights much of anything.

What happens when the immune system is not effective enough?
The immune system's purpose is to produce antibodies to outside invaders. Immune suppression causes the immune system to be less efficient at this than it should be. The result can be cancer, infection such as pneumonia, or AIDS.

What can cause immune suppression?
There are a number of causes for immune suppression which can work alone or together, including but not limited to:

- *Malnutrition*
- *Exposure to x-rays, microwaves, and other electromagnetic radiation*
- *Emotional or spiritual stress or lack of peace*
- *Structural problems and the effects of concussion or whiplash*
- *Removal of body parts or irradiation of the thymus*
- *Infectious diseases*
- *Treatment with or exposure to certain chemicals*
- *Toxic metals, including metal dental materials*
- *Lack of exposure to and stimulation of the eyes by beneficial UV rays due to wearing sunglasses or colored contact lenses*

What are the effects of immune suppression?
Immune suppression has two major effects:

- Cancer due to the lack of suppression of the growth of neoplasms (abnormal cells) or low NK3 cell counts

- Infection by bacteria or infestation by parasites due to insufficient fighting off of these pathogens. Fungus infections often precede the development of AIDS, as found in a study conducted by Walter Reed hospital (cited in **New England Journal of Medicine**, 1989).

Acquired immune deficiency syndrome (AIDS) is a system-wide and extreme form of immune suppression, in which both infections and cancers take over the body without resistance and eventually cause death. Immune suppression can be considered to be both the result and the cause of AIDS. The helper T cells, which are like the sentinels on guard whose responsibility it is to signal a warning of imminent danger, are disabled by AIDS.

Cancer - The immune system normally destroys the cell mutations that routinely occur in the body by recognizing them as nonself. If the immune system does not do this quickly and efficiently, the mutated cells encapsulate and then can multiply inside the capsule and form cancerous tumors. A weakened immune system that does not dispatch single mutated cells is certainly not up to dealing with large numbers of them [12].

Yeast infections, which gain a foothold when the immune system is weakened, are related to cancer, as both types of cells are fermenting cells. This means they are anaerobic, comparatively primitive cells that do better in conditions of lowered oxygen. By contrast, most body cells are respiratory, or oxygen using (also called aerobic).

If it ain't broke, don't fix it

An understanding of the immune system helps to explain symptoms of infection which, to many people, are signals that something is wrong. These symptoms are actually signs that the immune system is working properly. Lymph nodes near the area of infection - for example, the mandibular glands right under the jawbone that can be felt during a sore throat - swell and may be tender.

This swelling is a sign of the hard work taking place in the node as the antibodies gear up for battle. Redness and soreness around the site of an infected cut are also signs of the fight being waged locally. Pus is made up of large quantities of dead white blood cells, the allied and enemy soldiers killed in battle [13].

Some of the chemicals released from infectious processes signal the body to raise its temperature. This fever both increases the production and efficiency of the immune system components and provides a less hospitable environment for microbes. Just as fires in a riot-torn city will result in the calling out of the National Guard, fever is our internal fire that signals for reinforcements.

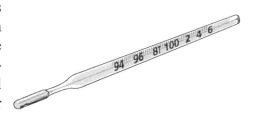

Fever can speed up the normal seven day wait for the immune system to reach peak fighting efficiency. For this reason, efforts to control these symptoms - aspirin for a fever, anti-inflammatory drugs, or an ice bag held against swollen, tender lymph nodes - will actually make the immune system work less effectively. An exception is a fever of 105 degrees or more, since such high temperatures can cause cellular or brain damage and should be controlled.

There is some speculation that childhood illnesses do more good than harm by stimulating the immune system so that it is stronger when needed. This can be likened to minor skirmishes which, like training exercises, prepare and train the troops so they will be able to fight the major battles when confronted by future enemies. It may be best to let these illnesses run their course.

What Can You Do?

Suggestions for immune system health are found throughout this book. Specific suggestions for boosting the immune system's effectiveness include:

- *First, remove suppressors*
- *Transfer factor*
- *c-AMP, gamma globulin*
- *Live cell, thymus*
- *Minerals - zinc, copper*
- *Herbs - echinacea, propolis, pau de arco*
- *Kyolic garlic*
- *Sun chlorella*
- *Vitamin C and A*
- *Sulfur based amino acids*
- *Lysine*

> **Your body knows what it's doing, and it does it best without interference for the most part.**

References and Resources

- Kellas, W. R., **Toxic Immune Syndrome Cookbook**, Comprehensive Health Centers, Encinitas CA, 2nd edition, 1995. *This book, written and edited by the co-authors of Thriving In A Toxic World and Surviving The Toxic Crisis, discusses the influence of food on the immune system and provides hundreds of hypoallergenic yeast-free recipes to maximize immune system support.*

- Berger, Stuart M., **Dr. Berger's Immune Power Diet**, New American Library, New York, 1985.

- The Burton Goldberg Group, "Allergies", pp. 510-520, **Alternative Medicine: The Definitive Guide**, Future Medicine Publishing Inc., Puyallup WA, 1994.

- Galland, Leo and Dian D. Buchman, **Superimmunity for Kids**, E.P.Dutton, NY, 1988.

- Glasser, Ronald J., **The Body is the Hero**, Random House, New York, 1976. *An excellent and interesting discussion of the immune system. Very readable.*

- Mansfield, John, **Arthritis: The Allergy Connection**, Thorsons, San Francisco CA, 1990.

- Mizel, Steven B. and Peter Jaret, **The Human Immune System**, Simon and Schuster Inc., New York, 1985.

- Null, Gary, **No More Allergies**, Villard Books, NY, 1992.

- Randolph, Theron G. and Ralph Moss, **An Alternative Approach To Allergies,** Harper Perennial, NY, 1990.

- Weiner, Michael A., **Maximum Immunity**, Houghton Mifflin Co., Boston MA, 1986.

CANCER

The Ultimate Parasite

Fifteen things in this chapter that can change your health and even save your life:

1. What are your chances of getting cancer, and why do they seem to keep going up?

2. What exactly is cancer, how does it start, and how does it kill?

3.-9. The following may be more prone to developing cancer:

Diabetics

People who wear sunglasses

People with yeast overgrowth

People with dietary deficiencies

People living in Northern states

Women on estrogen therapy

People whose immune systems are depressed

10. Are cancer tests a good idea?

11. What factors contribute to the development of cancer, and what can be done to avoid them?

12. Dietary fat (where fat soluble chemicals may be stored) has been implicated in the formation of some cancers (especially breast cancer).

13. What are the different types of cancer treatment, and their pros and cons?

14. Four major causes of the spread of cancer are cancer surgery, radiation, chemotherapy, and narcotics - the same as the list of the main treatments for cancer today.

15. The best treatment of cancer for a particular person may be a combination of orthodox and alternative treatments, decided on an individual basis.

Why is it so important to understand cancer?

One out of three people will get some kind of cancer during their lifetime, a rate that has been steadily increasing as we become more industrialized. 80% of these will die of their cancer eventually. Although the incidence of some cancers has declined, lung, skin, colon, and digestive system cancers -

> **By the year 2000 it is estimated that 1 out of 3 people will get cancer, and 80% of these will die of it.**

those caused by direct contact with toxins - are on the rise. There is a better than even chance you will be affected by cancer either directly (yourself) or indirectly (someone you know).

Cancer is the second leading cause of death in the U.S., accounting for 10% of the total health care cost [1]. About 1,040,000 new cancers are diagnosed each year, and it is estimated that 30% of Americans will develop some form of cancer [2]. It is estimated that 75-80% of all human cancers are induced by environmental factors, about 30-40% by diet [3]. The National Academy of Sciences puts that figure even higher, saying that 60% of all cancers in women and 40% of all cancers in men are related to nutritional and dietary factors [4]

What are the most common types of cancer?

The most common types of cancer in 1993 and the number of incidents, as reported by the American Cancer Society [5], are:

Cancer Type	Women	Men
Breast	182,000	*
Prostate	-------	165,000
Lung	70,000	100,000
Colon and Rectum	75,000	77,000
Uterus	44,500	------
Bladder	13,300	39,000
Lymphoma	22,400	28,500
Ovary	22,000	------
Oral	*	20,300
Skin Melanoma	15,000	17,000
Kidney	*	16,800
Pancreas	14,200	*
Leukemia	12,600	16,700
Stomach	*	14,800

(*) means that this is not in the top ten for this gender so figures are unavailable.

Everyone has heard of cancer, but what exactly is it?

The body is composed of cells. Normal cells have several things in common:

- *They are differentiated from each other - a kidney cell, a heart cell, a bone cell, and a skin cell are all different.*

- *They have specialized function - to carry oxygen, build bone, or filter wastes.*

- *In an adult, they reproduce in an orderly fashion and at a rate sufficient to replace dying cells of that type.*

- *Most cells (blood cells are an exception) do not travel within the body.*

Cancer cells differ from normal cells in all four ways. Cancer cells grow rapidly without stopping to form undifferentiated, disordered, nonfunctional cell clumps which can grow to weigh several pounds. In addition, cancer cells, unlike normal cells, can invade neighboring tissue and travel elsewhere in the body. These cells then crowd out normal cells, taking their supplies. As the normal cells starve and die, more cancer cells take their place.

Many people look at cancer as a disease which develops locally, in the form of a lump or tumor. The disease is then thought to spread systemically to other parts of the body if untreated. There is growing evidence that cancer is instead a systemic disease which forms a tumor if the immune system is not strong enough to deal with the first systemic stages of the disease, or unable to access the abnormal cells. The lump is then a symptom of cancer rather than the cancer itself, just as a herpes blister is a symptom of what is actually a systemic herpes infection.

We all get cancer many times during our lifetime, cancer being defined here as the growth of mutated cells. The immune system usually keeps these under control, so whether you actually develop the recognizable disease of cancer depends on the state of your immune system.

> **We all get cancer many times during our lives.**

What terms and concepts are necessary to understand cancer?

Some terms will be found in nearly any discussion of cancer, including this one. Some of these terms and their definitions are:

- **Tumor** - a growth of cells that forms a mass which does not belong in the body. Most cancers are tumors, but not all tumors are cancer.

- **Malignant** - referring to a cancer that can spread to other parts of the body, with the potential for fatal results if not stopped.

- **Metastasis** - the spreading of cancer cells to other parts of the body. The cells enter the bloodstream and travel to a new location like dandelion seeds blown by the wind to a new patch of soil.

- **Carcinogen** (noun), **carcinogenic** (adj.) - a substance which, in combination with other factors as described later in this chapter and in the chapter on Carcinogens in *Surviving The Toxic Crisis*, can cause cancer.

- **Oncology** - the study of cancer, or the medical specialty that attempts to treat cancer.

Why would the body have a mechanism that allows uncontrolled cell growth?

Rapid growth of relatively undifferentiated cells occurs in the first two months of fetal development as a necessary part of the gestation process. Primitive trophoblast cells are responsible for enormous fetal growth from day 1 to day 55-60. If the fetus continued to grow at the same rate throughout the pregnancy, it could be about the size of the Empire State Building at birth! [6]

At about day 56-60, the pancreas starts working, secreting an enzyme called chymotrypsin. Trophoblast cells are negatively charged and have a protein coating protecting them from your immune system's white blood cell attack, otherwise the mother's immune system would do away with the newly formed life before it had a chance to develop. Chymotrypsin destroys the protein coating and trophoblast cells die. Normal fetal growth then continues. After birth, trophoblast cells are produced only accidentally, and are essentially cancer cells. These cells, if unchecked by the NK3 cells of the immune system (your personal SWAT team), can kill you.

A rare form of cancer can occur when the fetal pancreas fails to form. Runaway trophoblast development will kill both the mother and fetus within 5-6 weeks if untreated by removal of the fetus.

The placenta, which nourishes the fetus, also stops growing at about day 56 due to the effect of the fetal pancreas. Both the fetus and the placenta share some characteristics with tumor growth, and pancreatic enzymes are the key to stopping fetal and placental growth when appropriate. It logically follows that a healthy well-functioning pancreas may be an element that stops or slows tumor or cancer growth. Giardia and fungus can decrease the effective functioning of the pancreas, and treatment for these conditions can raise pancreatic function back to optimal levels.

Can other conditions predispose one to cancer?
Diabetics are more prone to cancer than the general population, and an understanding of diabetes and of the above paragraphs explains why. In diabetes, the pancreas does not function properly, or at all, so that there is insufficient chymotrypsin enzyme produced. Trophoblast/cancer cells are therefore able to develop and spread unchecked, since the immune system can't attack them until the protein coating is removed.

Lifestyles of the rich and famous
Pancreatic and liver cancer, the types of cancer that killed actor Michael Landon, have some of the highest cancer fatality rates. This is probably because the cancer is damaging the function of the organ which could possibly stem its growth.

Michael Landon, as well as actress Lee Remick who also died of liver/pancreatic cancer, may have been victims of "Hollywood Mouth". The importance of a perfect smile in Hollywood leads many people in the entertainment industry to get enamel and porcelain caps and crowns which presents the image of a flashing white smile with perfectly formed teeth. However, underneath all the gleaming white bridgework lurks the toxic silver / nickel metal which provides the base upon which the porcelain is built. As discussed in the chapter on Nickel and Root Canals in *Surviving The Toxic Crisis*, nickel damages the RNA (duplicating system) of the cell and is a known carcinogen.

Non-stars can have similar problems. A 26-year-old nurse had dental braces with a loose bit of nickel-containing stainless steel wire that kept poking and irritating the inside of her mouth. Her orthodontist said not to worry about it, that it was no big deal and that it happens to most patients. She developed cancer right where the wire was poking her and essentially injecting nickel, a growth that was half the size of her head when she finally came to a clinic. She died two weeks later. She waited too long to search for root causes -- too little too late, sadly enough.

Doctors at the clinic studied this case so they were prepared when a similar case came in. This man in his early 40s, a Rolfing bodyworker and writer, came to the clinic with a baseball-sized tumor in his jaw, similarly caused by metal dental work. The doctors had him remove the dental metals and he got metal-removing glutathione injections. The cancer shrunk to the size of a pimple, and was still gone five years later.

How can cancer kill a person?

There are several mechanisms by which cancer can kill:

- By replacing normal functioning cells until the organ no longer works.

- By causing a general weakening of the body, called cachexia, until the systems fail.

- By blocking a major blood vessel, nerve pathway, or air passage

- By exerting pressure on the skull or brain.

- By damaging the immune system so the body cannot fight off other diseases. These other diseases, such as pneumonia, may kill before the cancer gets a chance to.

How does cancer start?

In the nucleus, or center, of a cell there is a nucleic acid called deoxyribonucleic acid, or DNA. The DNA contains up to 50,000 genes, which together form a blueprint enabling the cell to function and reproduce itself like copying a tape. Some of these genes, called oncogenes, have specialized functions of cell division, growth, and repair. These oncogenes in particular are targets of carcinogens.

When the DNA is exposed to a physical assault (such as radiation) or chemical insult, it can become permanently altered, or mutated, and these mutations are passed down to succeeding generations of cells. When oncogenes affecting growth are attacked, cell growth can spin out of control. Chemicals that cause these changes are known as carcinogens.

Oncogenes are supported by vitamin A, beta carotene, and other nutrients.

How does cancer progress?

As is the case with most chronic illness, cancer develops by way of a multi-step process, and decades can elapse between the initial DNA damage and the formation of a tumor. Still more time can pass before symptoms develop. Exposure to carcinogens is a chronic process; rarely is it a one-time event that can cause cancer 40 years later. An exception may be the actor John Wayne, who died of cancer. He was exposed to the radiation from an atomic bomb test blast while filming in Nevada.

It is unknown whether there were other factors contributing to his development of cancer. However, he was not the only actor who had been exposed to the same environment who later developed cancer. Susan Hayward, a well known star during the 40's and 50's and a contemporary of John Wayne, also died of cancer. Sadly enough, one of her last movies was about a woman who was dying of cancer. It was called *I Want To Live*.

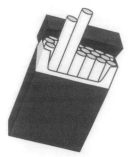

The amount of a chemical, its toxicity, and the duration of exposure play a part in the likelihood of developing cancer. For example, the chance of a smoker developing lung cancer depends on both the number of cigarettes smoked per day and the number of years that the person smokes. The tar, nickel, and some other compounds in cigarettes are carcinogens, and cadmium, a metal element found in cigarettes, suppresses the immune system thus allowing the cancer to gain a foothold.

Cells are of two basic types: respiratory and fermentative. Respiratory, or aerobic, cells require oxygen for energy, and do not function as well when the oxygen supply is compromised. Fermentative cells, so called because they ferment sugar for energy, are the more primitive type, and are characterized by their preference for an anaerobic environment. Anaerobic means without air or oxygen. Cancer cells, like yeast cells, are fermentative; they need fifteen times less oxygen than normal cells. It follows that a well-oxygenated body, provided by supplying clean air and breathing deeply and efficiently, will produce healthier body cells and retard the development of fermentative cancer cells. Aerobic (oxygen using) exercise such as jogging also helps oxygenate the body.

Patients with both AIDS and cancer have been treated with oxygen/ozone therapies, dioxychlor and hydrogen peroxide, which are all sources of activated oxygen. Several of these patients got well or at least had much less pain.

Once a tumor forms, the body attempts to control it by forming an encapsulating wall around it made of somatic (normal body) cells which would not otherwise be there. A cancerous tumor is a combination of malignant cells and nonmalignant encapsulating cells.

Not all cancers are encapsulated. Some cancers such as glioma (brain cancer) have no clearly defined boundaries but instead send tendrils into surrounding tissue.

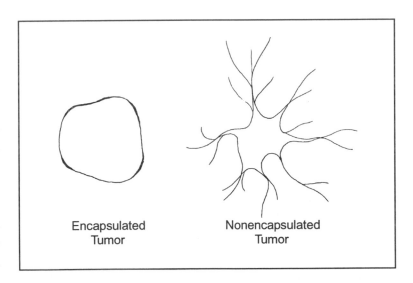

Encapsulated Tumor

Nonencapsulated Tumor

Can yeast turn into cancer?
Both yeast cells and cancer cells, as mentioned, are fermentative. Although yeast does not turn into cancer, the conditions which promote yeast growth also favor cancer development. An uncontrolled yeast overgrowth can therefore signal an increased cancer risk.

Are cancer tests a good idea?
When most doctors suspect cancer, the first thing they will often do is take x-rays or conduct other imaging tests. These are not always harmless, as described in the chapter on Electromag-

netic Radiation in *Surviving The Toxic Crisis*. The next thing they might do is take a biopsy, which is the removal of a small piece of tissue from the suspect mass. A knife or needle is necessarily used to pierce the tumor, which cuts through the encapsulation and can release malignant cells into the bloodstream.

Ironically, biopsy is often done just before surgery, or when cancer is virtually certain to be present, for legal reasons, as protection in a potential lawsuit. An event dreaded by most cancer surgeons is the accidental cutting of an encapsulated cancer, yet this is exactly what a biopsy does by design.

What factors contribute to cancer?

There are some factors which will not in themselves cause cancer, but can make cells more susceptible to the effects of carcinogens:

- **Heredity** - A weakness in certain oncogenes can be inherited. Breast cancer, for example, is more likely in the daughter of a woman with the disease. However, both heredity and microbiology, as well as toxicology such as nickel passed through the placenta, may be responsible for this relationship. Microorganisms which can be passed from mother to daughter put off toxic waste byproducts, and these and other toxins can contribute to cancer development. Beta carotene and other carotenoids, or vitamin A precursors, help soften the effect of a genetic tendency to cancer.

- **Immune system deficiencies** - There are many cell mutations that do not develop into cancer because a healthy immune system's NK3 cells recognize these mutated cells as invaders and destroy them before they can duplicate themselves. If the immune system is severely depressed, as with AIDS, certain cancers such as Kaposi's sarcoma (which is otherwise rare) can develop and spread quickly.

- **Vitamin and dietary deficiencies** - Cell walls, which form a barrier which protects the nucleus from chemical and infectious invaders, are made up of carbohydrates, protein, and fats. Dietary deficiencies can cause cell walls to become defective or weak. Smokers, for example, are at higher risk for lung cancer if they are deficient in vitamin A or beta-carotene. Adequate amounts of vitamins and minerals, as discussed in the Supporters section, also strengthen the immune system.

- **Hormones** - Excess sex hormones can cause a higher incidence of reproductive organ cancers, and female breast cancer has been linked to estrogen replacement therapy. There is some disagreement about the role of estrogen in certain cancers. Some believe that, while estrogen promotes the growth of pre-existing reproductive system cancers, natural estrogen may actually prevent their formation in the first place.

Dietary fat has been implicated in the formation of some cancers, especially breast cancer. It is likely that PCBs (polychlorinated biphenyls, a type of plastic) and other fat soluble chemicals stored in both dietary fat and breast and body fat are at least partially to blame, rather than the fat itself. Tissues of women with breast cancer had PCBs and certain pesticides at levels 50-60% higher than in women without breast cancer [7].

Animal fat has been consistently associated with higher cancer rates [8], especially cancers of the breast, colon, rectum, uterus, prostate and kidney [9]. Partially hydrogenated oils, commonly found in processed foods, are a major contributor to the carcinogenic effects of fats [10]. Experimentation with mice suggests that fat is a promoter working to increase the carcinogenicity of toxins rather than a carcinogen in itself [9]. The connection between animal fat and cancer may be due to the ingested toxins that concentrate in the fat of animals rather than to any quality inherent in fat itself.

Saturated (solid), heated, or rancid trans fats, the bad kind, can contribute to the formation of cancer. Beneficial cis oils, especially flax oil, have been found by Dr. Johanna Budwig of Germany and others to help clear cancer cells. Six to nine tablespoons, or about a half cup per day, is the usual amount used in

> **Healthy dietary oils can help clear cancer cells from the body.**

cases of cancer. However, fish oils may be even better, as flax oil contains omega-6 oils which stimulate the productions of arachidonic acid, an inflammation promoter and thus a cancer feeder. More information on oils is found in the chapter on Oils and Fats.

What are some other causes of cancer?

- Stress is the greatest single factor linked to recurring cancer, according to Dr. Carl Simonton [11].

- Obesity is a factor linked to cancer, especially in women. Overweight women are more likely to develop cancer of the uterine lining and do more poorly with breast cancer. Higher levels of fat usually correlate with higher levels of estrogen, which can worsen many female cancers. Obesity in women can also contribute to cervical, uterine and gallbladder cancer. Obesity in men may contribute to colon and rectal cancer [12].

- About 75% of breast cancers may be caused by exposure to ionizing radiation, primarily medical and dental x-rays [13].

What are some dietary factors contributing to cancer?
Dietary sugar is believed to increase cancer growth, possibly canceling out the protective effects of fiber [14,15]. Other dietary risk factors are too much iron [16], and nitrates in preserved meats and prolonged cooking of meats at high temperatures [17]. Caffeine intake (over 3 cups of coffee per day) is associated with higher cancer rates [18]; it can damage cellular DNA and interfere with its repair [19,20].

Alcohol intake, including and even especially beer, is also linked to higher cancer rates [21-23].

The risk of fatal cancer among Seventh-Day Adventist males is 53% that of white males in general of comparable age. The risk for Seventh-Day Adventist females is 68% that of white females in general [24]. Another study shows that incidence of cancer of all types is 30% to 40% lower among Seventh-Day Adventists [25]. The Seventh-Day Adventists are a religious group whose adherents follow a vegetarian diet and avoid alcohol, tobacco and caffeine. Since there is otherwise little or no difference between the Seventh-Day Adventists and the general population, except for their widely known healthy dietary practices, this could be the key factor responsible for halving the cancer death rate [26,27].

What can be done to avoid cancer?
There are two basic steps needed to minimize formation and growth of cancer cells:

- Avoid carcinogens such as cigarettes, nickel (from dental work, especially stainless steel posts, silver backed caps, crowns, and root canals), benzene (from gasoline and cleaners), and PCBs (from burning plastics). There are over 500 known carcinogens.

- Strengthen the cell walls and the immune system through diet.

In other words, avoid the enemy, lock your doors, and keep your weapons handy.

Dietary suggestions include:

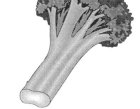

- Eating more good oils (cold or expeller-pressed) and less hydrogenated or heated oils and saturated fats

- Eating more orange and yellow vegetables such as carrots which are high in beta carotene.

- Cutting meat, animal byproducts, and dairy foods down or out to minimize ingestion of arachidonic acid which can promote fast growing cells, like cancer cells.

- Reducing or eliminating canned and preserved foods to maximize nutrition and minimize preservatives which are possibly carcinogenic.

- Eliminating or reducing sugar, including fruits and juices. Sugar ferments and feeds fermentative cancer cells.

- Eating cruciferous vegetables such as broccoli, cauliflower, and Brussels sprouts. They have been getting a lot of press lately as having protective properties against cancer.

- Sun Chlorella, Kyolic garlic.

How can avoiding sunglasses reduce cancer risk?

Another way to reduce your chances of getting cancer is, surprisingly, to get enough sunlight. While severe sunburns will increase the chances of getting skin cancer later in life, there is mounting evidence that moderate sun exposure to skin and eyes has a protective effect against internal cancers and even skin cancer. Albert Schweitzer found that African natives who wore sunglasses, a recent local status symbol, had a much higher incidence of cancer thirty years after starting to wear sunglasses, even without any other diet or lifestyle change.

A patient in her mid 40s who always wore sunglasses developed breast cancer. She stopped wearing sunglasses and was supported (versus "treated") with oxidative therapy, shark cartilage, flax oil, herbs, glutathione and other therapies. Her cancer is now gone.

The amount of sunlight considered to be enough varies greatly by skin type, as well as by geographical area and times of day and year. In general, the lighter the skin, the less sunlight that is needed. Even a slight sunburn means you have gotten too much sun.

How does geography influence your chances of developing cancer?

The overall cancer rate is highest in Alaska where residents spent most of their time indoors, and lowest in tropical Hawaii; sunlight exposure probably has a lot to do with this. Cancer rates are also higher in other northern states than in most southern states due to the lower sun exposure. (An exception may be Louisiana, where the eating of burnt Cajun food may increase the cancer risk there.)

Another factor in the difference in cancer rates may be the greater amount of clean outdoor air breathed by the average person in Hawaii, as compared with a cold climate such as Alaska where people are indoors breathing stale air most of the time. The abundance of fresh fruits and vegetables in Hawaii compared with the lack of fresh vegetables (fresh fruits and vegetables contain beneficial enzymes and more nutrients than canned produce) and the abundance of preserved meats (preservatives such as nitrites can be carcinogenic) in Alaska probably also contributes to the difference.

How can cancer be detected?

There are certain warning signs of different types of cancer. While these do not necessarily indicate cancer, they are indicators of a situation that may need to be checked [12].

Symptom	Type of cancer
Blood in urine, increased urinary frequency	Bladder, kidney
Lumps, thickening in breast	Breast
Bleeding between periods, unusual periods	Cervix, uterus, endometrial
Blood in stool, change in bowel habits	Colon
Cough or hoarseness	Throat, larynx
Paleness, fatigue, easy bruising, weight loss	Leukemia
Cough, bloody sputum, chest pain	Lung
Chronic ulcer in mouth	Mouth
Trouble urinating, pelvic pain	Prostate

Odd-looking mole, wart or ulceration	Skin
Indigestion and pain after eating	Stomach
Lumps, enlargement or thickening of scrotum	Testicular

How can cancer be detected noninvasively?

A blood test called AMAS, or Anti-Malignin Antibody in Serum, has been developed by Dr. Samuel Bodoch for the detection of cancer. The accuracy rate is said to be 95%, or up to 99% if the test is repeated. AMAS can be used for routine cancer screening or for monitoring the progress of cancer treatment. It can also be used in differential diagnosis, where a suspicious lump or x-ray spot has been found and a biopsy has been recommended - the AMAS test can be used instead [28-32].

What kinds of cancer treatments can doctors offer?

There are four basic treatments offered by the orthodox medical establishment:

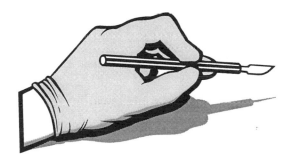

- *Surgery to remove the tumor.*
- *Radiation to shrink or kill remaining cancer cells at the tumor site.*
- *Chemotherapy (poison) to kill cancer cells in the bloodstream.*
- *Narcotic drugs and steroids for pain in the later stages of cancer.*

These treatments are used alone or in combination. They have a high failure (death) rate (would you believe 80%?) which is increasing as shown by these statistics: [33]

Death rate from cancer per 100,000 people total:

Year	Deaths
1900	64.0
1913	78.5
1950	139.8
1980	182.5
1985	191.7
1987	196.1
1988	198.6
1990	202.0

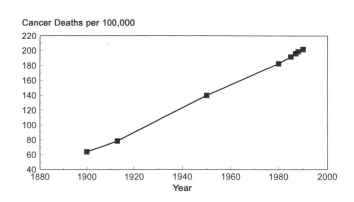

Obviously cancer death statistics are climbing despite supposed advances in treatment. Perhaps they are climbing **because** of these treatments (and perhaps in conjunction with the 500-plus carcinogens we are exposed to).

Looking at these figures in another perspective: 200 annual cancer deaths per 100,000 is equivalent to 1 in 500. Assuming a person has an 80-year lifespan, the chances of dying of cancer in those 80 years becomes 80 in 500, or about one in six.

How well do these treatments work?

As already mentioned, these treatments have an 80% failure rate in the long run. Four main causes of cancer spread and/or development are cancer surgery, radiation, chemotherapy, and narcotics. Hey, wait a minute - this list of cancer causes looks exactly like the list of orthodox cancer treatments!

The medical establishment seems to have little respect for what the body can accomplish. Rather than supporting the immune and detoxification systems so one's own body can work at eradicating the cancer, the doctors go after the cancer by treating it with the most toxic and potent drugs available to try to kill it. Unfortunately, since cancer cells are so like normal cells, anything toxic to cancer cells will also damage normal cells and body functions.

Along with mainstream medical focus on allopathic approaches to cancer treatment as being the only approach they have confidence in when facing a killer like cancer, there is the aspect of orthodox cancer therapies being enormously more profitable to the practitioner than nutritional supplements or lifestyle modification. And there is the additional component of human nature that often doesn't take well to making necessarily critical lifestyle changes that involve patient responsibility.

Western medicine's therapies are certainly not without value. The best treatment for a particular person may be some combination of orthodox and supportive treatments. Ultimately the choice of treatment is something that must be decided on an individual basis.

Even mainstream medicine is starting to realize that something needs to change in the so-called war against cancer. Two doctors from the Harvard School of Public Health have called for a shift in research, from just strictly cancer treatment to the aspect of prevention, as reported in the conservative *New England Journal of Medicine* [34].

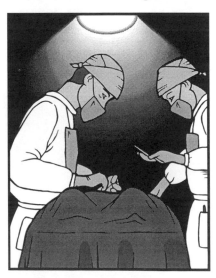

How effective is surgery?

Surgery, as is the case of biopsy, can open up the encapsulation around the tumor and spread cancer cells through the body (metastasize). It is also very stressful to the body, and immune function will likely suffer.

On the other hand, especially if the cancer is not cut into, it may be better to surgically remove all or even part of the tumor so the immune system will have a smaller, more manageable cancer to deal with. This would only be the case with a tumor that is not encapsulated such as a glioma or astrocytoma (brain cancers), or with multiple encapsulated tumors where only some of them are removed. Removing part but not all of an encapsulated tumor is still not a good idea.

Then what about radiation?

Radiation is normally used to shrink a tumor that is pressing on vital pathways like nerves and blood vessels. It is rarely used as a primary therapy to kill the cancer.

Radiation (photons of energy) affects the DNA of the cell, causing mutations to normal cells even as it kills some of the cancer cells. Radiation induces free radical damage. Free radicals are atoms with unpaired electrons. Electrons on atoms like to be in pairs, so the free radicals will grab an electron from the first atom they encounter. The new atom, now missing an electron, becomes a free radical itself, and the cycle continues. The effect is like a billiard ball hitting the other balls; the balls in motion then hit still other balls and so on.

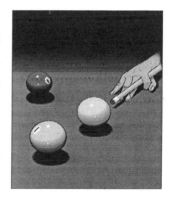

Those who give radiation treatments sometimes point out that the beam of x-radiation is aimed precisely through a tiny hole in a lead shield to pinpoint the tumor. Picture the billiards table just described, and then picture the white ball aimed at the others through a hole just larger than itself. It goes through the hole and even though it enters in one spot, balls fly all over the place just as before. This is the case also with free radical inducing radiation aimed through a tiny hole. It does not pinpoint the tumor any more than a white billiard ball aimed through a hole will affect only one ball on a crowded table.

Radiation can reduce tumor size in the short run, at least in the case of slow growing tumors, but it will make fast growing tumors grow even more rapidly because of its immune suppressive effects. When a tumor is irradiated, somatic (encapsulating body) cells are destroyed, reducing total mass and giving the impression that something is being accomplished. Malignant cells, the ones which are supposed to be destroyed, are radioresistant since they are tough primitive fermentative cells. Destroying the somatic cells around a tumor actually causes the cancer to spread, and cancer recurrence rates after radiation treatment are dismayingly high.

At best only 10% of people, once they get radiation treatment, end up living. Immune, detoxification, and lymph systems shut down once irradiated, and in this regard radiation is even worse than chemotherapy poisoning.

Does chemotherapy work?

Chemotherapy is the administration of powerful, toxic drugs which are intended to kill cancer cells. They are usually given by intravenous infusion, but are sometimes given orally. Typically they are given over a period of time rather than in a single large dose. Since the drugs are intended to kill fast-growing unwanted cells such as cancer cells, they also kill fast-growing wanted cells such as hair follicles. Hair loss is a common side effect for this reason. Chemotherapy drugs will also severely depress the immune system at a time when a strong immune system is most crucially needed.

Free radical processes, which in themselves can lead to cancer, may be set into motion by chemotherapy. These processes may also be behind some of its toxic side effects. Antioxidants may decrease free radical damage to healthy tissues from chemotherapy, resulting in reduced side effects [35].

Intense nausea and vomiting are common side effects of chemotherapy treatment. The body correctly recognizes the chemotherapeutic agent as being a poison that is harming the body, and does its best to expel it.

Chemotherapy drugs have been shown to *cause* cancer!

A pharmacist in New York described his experience working in a hospital preparing these drugs for cancer patients. He had to wear a "moon suit" complete with face mask, goggles, and gloves to do this. This was to protect him from the dangerous effects of the drugs he was working with - the same drugs that would be put into the veins of cancer patients. What was the main danger of these drugs? Brace yourself for a bit of irony here - the drugs are extremely carcinogenic. Without protection, he would run the risk of getting the very disease that the drugs were supposed to cure. These drugs are toxic to the cancer in the short run, but can be toxic to the body in the long run. Kill or be killed by chemotherapy - the race is on.

What about pain control measures?

Narcotic drugs such as morphine and codeine are often given to patients to control the pain often accompanying advanced cancer. Unlike surgery, radiation, and chemotherapy, narcotics are not intended to cure the cancer but are intended only for symptom relief. Narcotics block the pain signals, but also slow down all body systems - heart rate, respiration (breathing), detoxification and elimination, and others. Too large a dose of narcotics depresses heart rate and respiration to such a great extent that these functions may stop altogether, resulting in death.

Narcotics can not only cause constipation of the bowel, but can cause a sort of constipation, or blockage, of the detoxification systems as well. Since detoxification and elimination pathways are slowed down, toxins can build up in the body and cause their own damage. Narcotic drugs also have a strong depressant effect on the immune system, which is the last thing you want if you are fighting cancer.

Prednisone is a cortisone-like anti-inflammatory drug frequently given to control cancer pain. It is often given as part of a one-size-fits-all medical protocol whether or not pain is a problem. Such drugs are powerful immune suppressants by design. Inflammation is a sign that the immune system is working as it should, and a drug to suppress this mechanism also suppresses the immune system as a whole. That's its job - to reduce symptoms by turning down the immune system's responses.

One patient, a dentist in his early 40s, had lung and lymph cancer from exposure to job-related mercury and formaldehyde. His doctors treated him with prednisone, which suppressed his immune system which he so badly needed, even though he had no pain. When he questioned why he was on prednisone, he was taken off of it. Unfortunately, by this time his immune system was so badly suppressed that he couldn't recover. He started having pain from the cancer and was put on narcotic drugs, which further slowed his detoxification systems. He didn't survive.

So what kinds of treatments work?

Shark cartilage has been shown to have some effectiveness in the treatment of fast growing cancers. It suppresses angiogenesis, the formation of blood vessels that nourish the tumor, in effect cutting off its supply lines. Without a blood supply bringing food for the cancer, the tumor begins to die of malnourishment and ingest itself. Shark cartilage is most effective on heavily vascularized (many blood vessels) solid tumors such as those of the breast, cervix, prostate, and pancreas [36]. Several clinical trials have shown that shark cartilage has led to complete or partial remissions of cancer [37-39].

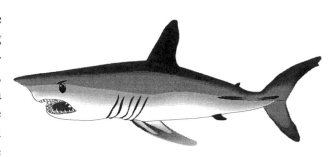

Alternative / supportive cancer clinics exist, although you may have to go outside this country for treatment specific to cancer. These clinics have some general procedures similar to those of alternative clinics within the United States. These procedures boost general health by means that work with the body rather than against it. Detoxification, chelation of free radical inducing metals, nutrition, herbs, and immune system support are some of the common alternative therapies.

Over 50% of the people diagnosed as having cancer by mainstream medicine go on to try alternative treatments. Either mainstream treatments do not work for them, or they are aware of the high risks and low benefits of the cut/burn/poison approach.

What about combining the two types of treatments?

Sometimes a combination of aggressive allopathic treatments, which may be necessary for a fast-growing cancer, and supportive therapies is the most effective course of treatment. There are several examples of patients who did well on the combination of treatments, or who followed toxic treatments with support so their bodies could heal from both the cancer and the treatment.

One patient in her 40s had chemotherapy, which brought her red blood cell count down. Nutrition therapy kept her strong enough to continue chemotherapy.

Another cancer patient in her 50s went through chemotherapy, which lowered her white blood cell count to the point where she kept getting secondary infections like pneumonia. She got well using a combination of conventional and supportive therapies such as zinc, vitamin A, echinacea, lymph drainage, SSKI, and the protective bacteria Megadophilus and Kyodophilus.

An ABC News study done around 1992 said that treating cancer with chemotherapy and surgery combined with dietary and other support was the best way to go, and had the greatest chance of success.

What are some other supportive (vs. suppressive) treatments?
Treatments fall into four categories:

- **Finding** and removing carcinogens. Also in this category is the removal of other toxins which would burden an immune system that should otherwise put most of its energy into fighting the cancer. Some of these toxins include nickel (from dental work), benzene (in gasoline), cigarette smoke, and electromagnetic and microwave radiation from some household appliances.

Amazingly, many doctors treat cancer without investigating and eliminating any possible contributing causes, although there are over 500 known carcinogens. Killing the cancer without finding the cause is like putting out an arson fire without looking for or finding the arsonist.

> **Amazingly, many doctors treat cancer without finding out and eliminating the cause**

- **Supporting** the immune system. These treatments include:

  - Hoxsey herbs for immune stimulation

  - Adaptogens, thymus, and PCM-4, which contains thymus for immune support and the antioxidant ginseng

  - Vaccine made from your tumor and injected back into your body to stimulate your immune system to make antibodies to fight the tumor

  - Material from your tumor can be injected into pregnant cows or goats, and antibodies will be made and secreted in the colostrum (first milk).

  - Transfer factor, the cellular communication system of healthy people or animals. There has been a 13% incidence of response in the treatment of renal (kidney) cancer with transfer factor [40].

  - Monoclonal antibodies have produced partial remission in 1 of 9 renal cancer patients. Immune RNA has been associated with a 14% incidence of response. Interferons have helped 10-20% of patients [40].

  - Vitamins A, B6, C, and beta-carotene [41]

  - Cruciferous vegetables such as broccoli and cauliflower [42]

  - Gaston Naessens' formula 714X, consisting of nitrogen-rich camphor and organic salts. Cancer cells use a tremendous amount of nitrogen, which they withdraw from the immune system, reducing the immune system's effectiveness. 714X floods the body with nitrogen so the cancer does not deplete the immune system of this element [43-45]. Former U.S. Congressman Berkley Bedell attributes his recovery from prostate cancer to 714X [44,46].

- **Cleansing** the body's cells. These include:
  - Hoxsey herbs
  - Glutathione, usually injectable but sometimes oral
  - Detoxifying sulfur based amino acids
  - DMSA, DMPS, or other chelation to pull out metals

- **Killing** the tumor, either directly or by making the environment inhospitable for tumor growth. These include:

  - Hydrogen peroxide, ozone, and dioxychlor oxygenate blood.

  - Chondriana and other microorganisms can attack cancer.

  - Cancer requires a low oxygen environment. A hyperbaric oxygen chamber, which oxygenates blood, works on the same principle.

  - Shark cartilage stops angiogenesis, the blood vessel supply to the tumor, as discussed earlier in this chapter.

  - Macrobiotic diet - eliminating meat reduces arachidonic acid, which then reduces the inflammatory prostaglandin E2.

  - Omega-3 fish oils and flax oil also lower arachidonic acid by raising prostaglandin E1, which is antagonistic to E2.

  - The Rife microscope and generator can put off frequencies which are toxic to cancer cells. A 60 year old woman kept her cancer under control using a Rife frequency generator.

  - Parasites such as entamoeba histolytica, which are known to cause cancer, should be killed or controlled as described in the Parasites and Protozoa chapters in *Surviving The Toxic Crisis*.

  - Antineoplastons are polypeptides (short-chain amino acids) that inhibit cancer cell growth and can even reprogram cancer cells to behave more like the normal cells that were their precursors [47,48]. Over 2000 patients have been treated with antineoplastons, and most have achieved partial or complete remission of their cancers [47]. A 1977 study found that 86% of advanced cancer patients given antineoplastons improved [49]. Phase II clinical trials were done from 1988-1990 on patients with advanced astrocytoma, a highly malignant cancer. These patients had had poor results from conventional treatments - their tumors kept growing - yet most of them improved rapidly within six weeks on antineoplastons and 80% had remission or stabilization of their tumors [47]. Antineoplastons are not only much more effective than conventional therapies but do not have as much of the dangerous and unpleasant side effects [50].

  - Hydrazine sulfate is a chemical that can reverse cachexia, the malnourishment and wasting away that characterizes and even kills many cancer patients. This was shown in double-blind studies, in which nearly 50% of patients with any type of cancer showed improvement in their cachexia. Hydrazine sulfate has also been shown to shrink tumors and even cause them to disappear [51-54].

- Laetrile, also known as amygdalin or vitamin B17, was first discovered in 1924. It has been shown to stimulate antibodies against spontaneous breast tumors in mice, resulting in complete tumor regression in 76% of the mice [55]. For best results, it should be used with proteolytic enzymes, vitamin A and a healthful diet with nutrient supplementation [56].

The key to success in cancer treatment is catching it early enough.

The key to success in cancer treatment is catching it early enough.

How effective is nutrition in the prevention and treatment of cancer?

Nutrition plays a major part in the body's effective prevention of and healing from cancer. In one study, cancer patients were divided into two groups - those with and those without nutritional support (special diet and supplements). Both groups otherwise had similar standard oncology (cancer treatment) care. The results were impressive - the patients in the control (unsupplemented) group lived an average of less than six months. Of the 98 patients in the supplemented group, 19 lived an average of ten months, 47 lived an average of six years, and 32 lived an average of ten years, with many still alive at the end of the eleven year study [57]. This is pretty convincing evidence of the value of diet and nutrition in cancer treatment, especially considering that oncologists are happy to find a drug that extends the lives of cancer patients by even three months.

Dietary recommendations for cancer are geared towards building up the immune system. Antioxidants prevent free radical damage that promotes cancer growth.

A totally meat-free diet is often recommended. Many cancer patients have had good results with a macrobiotic diet [58,59]. The macrobiotic diet has been shown to improve cancer survival rates [60]. A macrobiotic diet, even if not followed perfectly, has increased the one-year survival rate for pancreatic cancer from 10% to 52%. With prostate cancer the median survival time was increased from 72 months (6 years) to 228 months (19 years) [61].

Animal protein increases the level of estrogen, and many tumors rely on estrogen for growth. Animal products are also a source of inflammatory prostaglandin E2 producing arachidonic acid. Especially avoid smoked, pickled, or processed meats, which contain carcinogenic nitrosamines. Low fat diets are recommended in much of the literature, but many researchers did not differentiate between protective oils and harmful oils and fats, which are discussed in the Oils and Fats chapter. Animal fats, saturated fats, and heated oils (as with fried foods) should be avoided.

Vegetables, fruits and fiber all correlate with a higher survival rate in cancer patients. In a study of 675 lung cancer patients, lifespan after diagnosis was correlated with the amount of vegetables consumed, with an 18 month average for non-vegetable eaters and a 33 month average - almost twice as long - for vegetable eaters. Women showed a greater difference than men [57].

Cancer-fighting foods include [62]:

- *broccoli*
- *cabbage*
- *walnuts*
- *parsley*
- *garlic*

- *cauliflower*
- *cantaloupe*
- *fatty fish*
- *soybeans*
- *cucumbers*

- *carrots and other yellow vegetables*
- *legumes (peas, lentils)*
- *flaxseed and flaxseed oil*
- *citrus fruit*

Which nutrients are most useful in the prevention and/or treatment of cancer?
Many nutrients are useful for this purpose [63].

- The **antioxidant vitamins A, E and C**, as well as the vitamin A precursor beta-carotene and the mineral selenium, have been shown to have both preventive and treatment properties against cancer [64]. The amounts recommended for cancer prevention are : Vitamin E 200-800 IU; Vitamin A 12,500 IU; Vitamin C 1000 mg; selenium 50-200 mcg. [65]. A study of 30,000 rural Chinese showed that daily doses of beta-carotene, vitamin E and selenium reduced cancer deaths by 13% [66].

- **Beta carotene**, the vitamin A precursor, is found in yellow and leafy green vegetables and is protective against all cancers [67], especially cervical cancer [68] and lung cancer [69].

- **Vitamin B6** protects against cervical cancer [70].

- **Vitamin C** has both an immune-boosting and a protective role [71].

- **Vitamin E** can help protect against bowel cancer, and can counteract carcinogens found in smog [71].

- **Selenium** can protect against cancer by contributing to the formation of the enzyme glutathione, which helps eliminate carcinogens and other toxins [72].

- **Folic acid** helps protect against cervical cancer [73].

- **Calcium** helps protect against bone cancer [74].

- **Iodine** helps protect against breast cancer and is needed for the growth and repair of all tissues [75].

- **Zinc**, which targets the prostate and is depleted in semen, helps protect against prostate cancer [76].

- **Fiber** helps in the removal of potentially carcinogenic toxins from the digestive tract, and is especially protective against colon cancer. 20-30 grams of fiber per day is recommended from a variety of sources (different grains, vegetables) to get the different types of fiber [77].

What other nutrition based approaches have been shown to work?
The Gerson Therapy, which involves the use of diet (mostly fresh juices and supplements) and detoxification (including frequent coffee enemas), has been linked to many cancer cures including that of metastasized malignant melanoma, one of the deadliest cancers [78-87].

Other nutritional substances that have proven useful are garlic and the Maitake mushroom.

Garlic has been shown to inhibit colon cancer [88,89]. One or more servings of garlic per week was associated with a 35-50% decrease in the risk of developing colon cancer [90]. The best form of garlic is the raw natural form, but deodorized garlic supplements such as Kyolic may be best to insure a regular daily intake [91].

The Maitake mushroom (pronounced my-tah-key) has been found to have significant anti-tumor activity. it works not by killing cancer cells directly, but by stimulating the activities of immune competent cells so they will then fight cancer cells [92-94].

Science or political science? - some comments
Politics, greed, and personal interest masquerading as science can be called political science. Real science is predictable and reproducible, whether or not the observed results are understood or anyone profits.

It is illegal in some states for anyone other than an oncologist (MD) to treat cancer. The only approved treatments are surgery, radiation, and chemotherapy - otherwise known as "cut, burn, and poison". These have an 80% failure rate, i.e. are only 20% successful in the long run. This limited list of approved treatments sounds like restraint of trade as well as interference in freedom of choice in health care.

The orthodox medical establishment, like any bureaucracy in power, often criticizes alternative treatments because they keep the patient from getting "real" help such as drugs, surgery, and radiation. Ironically, these dangerous and ineffective orthodox treatments may buy the patient just enough time so that s/he does not seek treatment that will really help in the long run.

A true story
A 19 year old was diagnosed by a urologist with testicular and colon cancer. This urologist proceeded to surgically remove a testicle and told him that he would need full surgery and chemotherapy for the colon cancer. The patient then went to a comprehensive/integrated clinic and made a decision to change his diet to a meat-free one, eliminating inflammation-promoting arachidonic acid. This, along with other supportive therapies, helped his body eliminate his cancer, the disappearance of which was verified by an oncologist.

The urologist, meanwhile, was so upset at losing control of the patient that he reported the clinic to the California state medical board fraud division, telling them that the clinic was treating cancer without drugs, radiation or surgery, which is against the law, under, of all things, the Business Conduct Ethics Guidelines. The patient, who was thrilled at the outcome, had no complaint. The court case dragged on for several expensive years until the charges were finally dropped.

The deck is stacked against "alternative", i.e. effective, clinics - if they are charged with fraud, and if judgment rules against them, they must, by new law, pay *all* court costs, including those of the prosecution. Meanwhile, slanderous information is leaked to the media without giving the clinic a chance for rebuttal. The pressure is heavy to settle out of court, or in other words admit wrongdoing and guilt, whether guilty or not.

The doctors involved also face the threat of losing their medical licenses, or net worth. Being judged by a "board of peers" is like Jesus being judged by the Pharisees. These persecution tactics keep patients in a place where they have little recourse other than the "accepted" allowable and toxic treatments.

More comment

Lemmings are animals which are known for leaping en masse off cliffs to their deaths. If Big Business were in charge, they would build hospitals and mortuaries at the bottom of the cliff and await the victims. A government controlled by big business (such as ours) would build a fence leading the lemmings *to* the cliff. Socialism would build fences at the top of the cliff with the attitude that lemmings are too stupid to think for themselves and that the government should take care of everything. The free enterprise system would educate lemmings that cliffs are dangerous. The present medical establishment is Big Business. Supportive care, with its emphasis on personal responsibility and doing the least harm, is the free enterprise system.

If we don't defend free choice when we don't need it, it won't be there when we do.

References and Resources

General Information

- Airola, Paavo, *Cancer Causes, Prevention and Treatment: The Total Approach*, Health Plus Publishers, Phoenix AZ, 1972.

- The Burton Goldberg Group, *Alternative Medicine: The Definitive Guide*, Future Medicine Publishing, Puyallup WA, 1994, *especially the chapter on "Cancer", pp. 556-586. Pages 584-586 list many useful books and research and support groups, including resources for specific therapies.*

- Kaura, S.R., *Understanding and Preventing Cancer*, Health Press, Santa Fe NM, 1991.

- Levitt, Paul M. and Elissa S. Guralnick, *The Cancer Reference Book*, Facts on File Inc., New York, 2nd ed., 1983.

- Lynes, B., *The Healing of Cancer*, Marcus Books, Queensville, Ontario Canada, 1989.

- **International Association for Cancer Victors and Friends**, 7740 West Manchester Avenue, Suite 110, Playa del Rey CA 90293, phone 310-822-5032.

- **People Against Cancer**, P.O. Box 10, Otho Iowa 50569, phone 515-972-4444.

- **Cancer Control Society**, 2043 North Berendo Street, Los Angeles CA 90027, phone 213-663-7801.

Prevention

- Dreher, Henry, *The Complete Guide to Cancer Prevention*, Harper and Row, NY, 1988.

- Dreher, Henry, *Your Defense Against Cancer*, Harper and Row, NY, 1988.

- Epstein, Samuel S and David Steinman, *New Hope: Everything You Wanted to Know About Breast Cancer Prevention But The Cancer Establishment Never Told You: A Guide For Dramatically Reducing Your Risk*, Macmillan Publishing Group, NY, 1993.

- Gofman, John W., *Preventing Breast Cancer: The Story of a Major, Proven, Preventable Cause of the Disease*, Committee for Nuclear Responsibility, San Francisco CA, 1995. *Discusses the connection between x-rays and breast cancer.*

- Tobe, John H., *How To Prevent and Gain Remission From Cancer*, Provoker Press, St. Catharine's, Ontario Canada, 1975. *Toxins that can contribute to cancer and natural methods that can help heal it.*

Questioning Conventional Therapies

- Brown, Raymond Keith, *AIDS, Cancer and the Medical Establishment*, Robert Speller and Sons Publishers, NY, 1986.

- Evans, Richard A., ***Making The Right Choice***, Avery Publishing Group, Garden City Park, NY, 1995. *Explores treatment options in cancer surgery. Provides a balanced discussion of the options available without a blanket condemnation of surgery.*

- Heimlich, Jane, ***What Your Doctor Won't Tell You***, HarperCollins Publishers, NY, 1990.

- Lerner, Michael, ***Choices in Healing: Integrating the Best of Conventional and Complementary Approaches to Cancer***, The MIT Press, Cambridge MA, 1994.

- Lynes, Barry, ***The Healing of Cancer***, Marcus Books, Randolph NJ, 1989. *Research by journalist into the suppression of alternative cancer therapies by the medical establishment.*

- Moss, Ralph W., ***Questioning Chemotherapy***, Equinox Press, Brooklyn NY, 1995.

- Moss, Ralph W., ***The Cancer Industry: Unraveling the Politics***, Paragon House, New York, 1989. *This book discusses the political and financial motives for promoting harmful therapies and suppressing useful ones.*

Alternative / Progressive Therapies, General

- Fink, John M., ***Third Opinion***, Avery Publishing Group, NY, 1992. *An international directory to alternative therapy centers for the treatment and prevention of cancer.*

- Glassman, Judith, ***The Cancer Survivors and How They Did It***, Dial Press, Garden City NY, 1983.

- Hirschberg, Caryle and Marc Ian Barasch, ***Remarkable Recovery***, G.P.Putman's Sons, NY, 1995. *Looks at survivors of cancer and other illnesses who were given a death sentence by their doctors. Discusses the many types of treatment, primarily "alternative", that the survivors credited with their recovery.*

- Leroi, Rita, ***An Anthroposophical Approach to Cancer***, Mercury Press, Spring Valley NY, 1982.

- Marchetti, Albert, ***Beating The Odds,*** Contemporary Books, Chicago IL, 1988. *Alternative treatments that have proven successful in treating cancer.*

- Moss, Ralph W., ***Cancer Therapy: The Independent Consumer's Guide to Non-Toxic Treatment and Prevention***, Equinox Press, NY, 1992. *Alternative therapies for cancer, including contact addresses.*

- Null, Gary, ***Gary Null's Complete Guide to Healing Your Body Naturally***, McGraw-Hill, NY, 1988.

- Walters, Richard, ***Options: The Alternative Cancer Therapy Book***, Avery Publishing Group, Garden City Park, NY, 1993.

- **Foundation for Advancement in Cancer Therapy**, P.O. Box 1242, Old Chelsea Station, New York NY 10113, phone 212-741-2790.

- **World Research Foundation**, 15300 Ventura Blvd., Suite 405, Sherman Oaks CA 91403, phone 818-907-5483. *Large research library of alternative medicine; provides computer search of specific health issues for a nominal fee.*

Macrobiotic Diet

- East West Foundation, *Cancer Free: 30 Who Triumphed Over Cancer*, Japan Publications, NY, 1991.

- Esko, Edward (ed.), *Doctors Look at Macrobiotics*, Japan Publications, NY, 1988.

- Jochems, Ruth, *Dr. Moerman's Anti-Cancer Diet: Holland's Revolutionary Nutritional Program for Combating Cancer*, Avery Publishing Group, Garden City Park, NY, 1990.

- Kushi, Aveline and Wendy Esko, *The Macrobiotic Cancer Prevention Cookbook*, Avery Publishing Group, Garden City Park, NY, 1987.

- Kushi, Michio, *The Book of Macrobiotics*, Harper and Row, NY, 1986. *This book decribes how to follow a macrobiotic program, although this is not specific to cancer.*

- Kushi, Michio, *The Cancer Prevention Diet: Michio Kushi's Nutritional Blueprint for the Prevention and Relief of Disease*, St. Martin's Press, NY, 1983.

- Kushi, Michio, *The Macrobiotic Approach to Cancer*, Avery Publishing Group, Garden City Park, NY, 1991.

- Kushi, Michio, *The Macrobiotic Way*, Avery Publishing Group, Garden City Park, NY, 1986.

- Kushi, Michio et al, *Cancer and Heart Disease: The Macrobiotic Approach to Degenerative Disorders*, Japan Publications, NY, 1985.

- Nussbaum, Elaine, *Recovery From Cancer*, Avery Publishing Group Inc., Garden City Park NY, 1992. *One woman's story of her healing using a macrobiotic diet.*

- Rogers, Sherry A., *You Are What You Ate*, Prestige Publishing, Syracuse NY, 1987. *Discusses macrobiotics.*

- Satillaro, Anthony J., *Recalled By Life*, Avon, NY, 1984. *A physician's story of how he healed prostate cancer using a macrobiotic diet.*

Gerson Therapy

- Bishop, Beata, *My Triumph Over Cancer*, Keats Publishing, New Canaan CT, 1986.

- Davison, Jaquie, *Cancer Winner*, Pacific Press, Pierce City MO, 1977. *One woman's story of her healing using Gerson therapy.*

- Gerson, Max, *A Cancer Therapy: Results of Fifty Cases*, Gerson Institute, Bonita CA, 5th ed., 1990. *Gerson therapy.*

- Haught, SJ, *Cancer? Think Curable! The Gerson Therapy*, Gerson Institute, Bonita CA, 1983.

- Tropp, Jack, *Cancer: A Healing Crisis*, Exposition Press, NY, 1980.

- **The Gerson Institute**, P.O. Box 430, Bonita CA 91908-0430. Phone 619-838-2256 to request information 24 hours a day; 619-585-7600 to speak to a Gerson Institute representative M-F 9-5 Pacific time. *The Gerson Institute promotes the Gerson therapy for cancer and other degenerative diseases.*

Gaston Naessens

- Bird, Christopher, *The Persecution and Trial of Gaston Naessens*, H.J. Kramer Inc., Tiburon CA, 1991. *The development of Gaston Naessens' formula 714X and the legal difficulties he faced in trying to help people with it.*

- **C.O.S.E., Inc.**, 5270 Fontaine, Rock Forest, Quebec, Canada J1N3B6, phone 819-564-7883. *Resource for Gaston Naessens' formula 714X.*

Hoxsey Therapy

- Hoxsey, Harold, *You Don't Have To Die*, Milestone Books, NY, 1956. *Hoxsey herbs and therapy.*

- **Bio-Medical Center**, P.O. Box 727, 615 General Ferreira, Colonia Juarez, Tijuana, Mexico 22000. Phone 011-52-66-84-9011. *Resource for Hoxsey Therapy.*

Shark Cartilage

- Duarte, Alex, *Jaws For Life: The Story of Shark Cartilage*, Duarte, Grass Valley CA, 1993.

- Lane, William I. and Linda Comac, *Sharks Don't Get Cancer*, Avery Publishing Group Inc., Garden City Park, NY, 1992. *Explores the development, testing and use of shark cartilage in cancer treatment.*

- **Hospital Ernesto Contreras**, Paseo Playas de Tijuana, No. 19, Tijuana, BC, Mexico. Phone 011-52-66-80-1850 or 800-262-0212 (California) or 800-523-8795 (rest of U.S.). *Resource for Laetrile and Shark Cartilage.*

Alternative / Progressive Therapies, Other

- McCabe, Ed, *Oxygen Therapies: A New Way of Approaching Disease*, Energy Publications, Morrisville NY, 1988.

- Wright, Jane Riddle, *Diagnosis: Cancer - Prognosis: Life*, Albright and Co. Huntsville AL, 1985. *Immuno-Augmentive Therapy.*

- **Burzynski Clinic**, 6221 Corporate Drive, Houston TX 77036, phone 713-777-8233. *Resource for Antineoplaston therapy.*

- **Syracuse Cancer Research Institute**, Presidential Plaza, 600 East Genesee Street, Syracuwe, NY 13202, phone 315-472-6616. *Resource for Hydrazine Sulfate*.

Nutritional Approaches

- Breuss, Rudolf, ***Breuss Cancer Cure***, Alive Books, Burnaby BC, 1995. *Advocates juice fasting.*

- Budwig, Johanna, ***Flax Oil as a True Aid Against Arthritis, Heart Infarction, Cancer and Other Diseases***, Apple Publishing, Vancouver BC, 1994.

- Germann, Donald R., ***The Anti-Cancer Diet***, Wyden Books, NY, 1977.

- Heinerman, John, ***Heinerman's Encyclopedia of Fruits, Vegetables, and Herbs***, Parker Publishing Co., West Nyack, NY, 1988. *Dietary suggestions in general and for cancer prevention and treatment.*

- Hunsberger, Eydie Mae and Chris Loeffler, ***How I Conquered Cancer Naturally***, Avery Publishing Group, Garden City Park, NY, 1992.

- Nixon, DW and JA Zanca, ***The Cancer Recovery Eating Plan***, Times Books, NY, 1994.

- Nolfi, Kristine, ***My Experiences With Living Foods: The Raw Food Treatment of Cancer and Other Diseases***, Health Research, Mokelumne Hill CA.

- Quillin, Patrick, ***Beating Cancer With Nutrition***, The Nutrition Times Press, Tulsa OK, 1994.

- Simone, Charles B., ***Cancer and Nutrition***, Avery Publishing Group, Garden City Park NJ, 1992. *Using nutrition for the prevention and treatment of cancer, and minimizing risk factors.*

- Wigmore, Ann, ***The Wheatgrass Book***, Avery Publishing Company, Garden City Park NY, 1985. *Wheatgrass therapy.*

- Wigmore, Ann, ***Be Your Own Doctor***, Avery Publishing Company, Garden City Park NY, 1982.

Herbs

- Biser, Loren, ***The Layman's Course on Killing Cancer***, University of Natural Healing, Charlottesville VA. *Herbal treatments for cancer based on the work of John Christopher, medical herbalist.*

- Heinerman, John, ***The Treatment of Cancer With Herbs***, BiWorld Publishers, Orem UT, 1984.

- Kloss, Jethro, ***Back To Eden***, Back To Eden Books Publishing Company, Loma Linda CA, 1988.

- Naiman, Ingrid and Susan Meares, *Cancer Salves and Suppositories*, Bodhisattva Trust, Santa Fe NM, 1992.

Mind / Body, Emotional Aspects

- LeShan, Lawrence, *Cancer As A Turning Point: A Handbook for People With Cancer, Their Families and Health Professionals*, Plume, NY, 1991.

- LeShan, Lawrence, *You Can Fight For Your Life: Emotional Factors in the Treatment of Cancer*, M. Evans and Co., NY, 1977.

- Locke, Steven and Douglas Colligan, *The Healer Within: The New Medicine of Mind and Body*, New American Library / Mentor, NY, 1987.

- Rossman, Martin L., *Healing Yourself: A Step-By-Step Program for Better Health Through Imagery*, Pocket Books, NY, 1987.

- Siegel, Bernie, *Peace, Love and Healing*, Harper and Row, NY, 1989.

- Siegel, Bernie, *Love, Medicine and Miracles*, Harper and Row, NY, 1986. *Both of these books describe Dr. Siegel's work with cancer patients utilizing the mind/body connection.*

- Simonton, O. Carl, Stephanie Matthews-Simonton and James Creighton, *Getting Well Again*, Bantam Books, NY, 1980.

- **Exceptional Cancer Patients**, 1302 Chapel Street, New Haven CT 06511, phone 203-865-8392. *This organization was founded by Dr. Bernie Siegel to help cancer patients utilize the mind/body connection for healing.*

TREATMENT-CAUSED-TRAUMA

Designer or Disposable Parts?

Have you had any of the following body parts removed? More importantly, are you contemplating any of the following surgeries for yourself or your child? This chapter may have health-changing information for you.

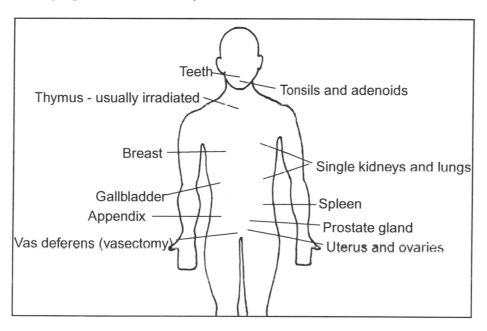

Twenty-one things in this chapter that can change your life:

1. How are nearly all of us suffering from treatment-caused trauma?

2. What are the strengths and weaknesses of our medical system?

3. Why would unnecessary surgical and other procedures be done?

4. What are some ways to weigh the pros and cons of a surgical procedure?

5. What organs are considered to be unnecessary, and are they really unnecessary?

6. What are these "unnecessary" organs, such as the tonsils, gallbladder, or appendix, good for?

7. What are some long term effects of the removal of these organs?

8. What are some simple, safe, and often effective alternatives to surgery?

9. What treatments, by dealing with the root cause, can help you avoid a tonsillectomy?

10. How can gallbladder removal cause colon cancer?

11. Is the uterus necessary once reproduction is not needed?

12. What are breasts good for besides attracting men and nursing babies?

13. *Are second kidneys and lungs "extra"?*
14. *Is the thymus needed in adulthood?*
15. *What is cosmetic surgery, and what are the risks?*
16. *Can removed fat be safely used elsewhere?*
17. *What about breast implants?*
18. *What are Hollywood teeth?*
19. *What happens when metal is placed in the body?*
20. *What damage can be done by scars?*
21. *Do vaccinations always help prevent disease? Can they be harmful?*

What is another name for treatment-caused trauma?
Iatrogenic damage is the term used to describe damage to the human body that is due to medical intervention. Some iatrogenic damage may be unavoidable when a life is being saved by heroic intervention. However, much of the damage can be averted by knowledgeable doctors and patients.

How prevalent is iatrogenic damage?
The following statistics were quoted in the *New England Journal of Medicine* [1]:

- 36% of patients on general medical services are suffering from diseases caused by medical intervention.

- Between 1981 and 1987, an estimated four million people died as a result of medical treatment. By contrast, 39,000 people died of AIDS and 47,000 people died in traffic accidents during the same period.

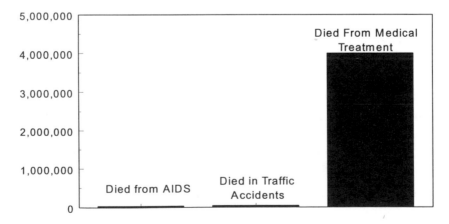

Deaths from Various Causes
Between 1981 and 1987

- There was a 300% increase in drug addiction from 1962 to 1988 as a direct result of medical prescriptions. Street-drug addiction increased by less than 30% during the same period.

Increase in Drug Addiction
Between 1962 and 1988
LBJ declared the U.S. the Great Society in 1965. Since then...

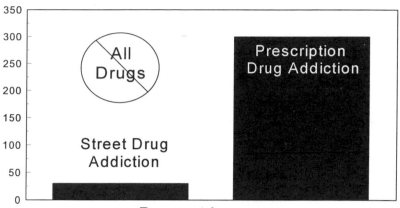

Percent Increase

- Every day 80% of the adults in the U.S. swallow a medically prescribed drug.

- According to the ***Johns Hopkins Medical Letter*** (March 1990), "Prescribed hospital drugs are so toxic they kill 130,000 Americans every year" [2].

What can cause iatrogenic damage?
Iatrogenic damage can be caused by:

- *Removal of organs*
- *Surgical scars*
- *Cosmetic surgery*
- *Mercury and metals in the mouth, root canals*
- *Vaccinations*
- *Antibiotics, anesthesia, and other drugs*
- *X-rays and other radiation*
- *Birth intervention can cause damage to both mother and baby*
- *Barium, iodine, and other dyes used in imaging testing such as a barium enema*

All of these are discussed in this chapter or in other chapters as referenced.

What are the strengths and weaknesses of our medical system?
Some of the best acute and trauma care in the world is found in this country. Some of the damage caused by medicine is minor compared to the benefits offered by our medical system.

There are a range of opinions concerning American medical care, ranging from blanket praise to blanket condemnation. In actuality, our medical system, like most systems, encompasses both the good and the bad.

- Many doctors feel that the good of the patient is foremost and practice medicine with this in mind.

- Some doctors mean well but are misinformed, and do not have the information needed to weigh the long-term risks of a procedure against its benefits.

- Many if not most doctors are over-specialized and don't know how to look at the whole patient.

- There are a few doctors who perform procedures for their own benefit, realizing that more surgery equals more money in their own pockets. Some of these end up on tabloid TV.

- Some doctors, particularly those who have recently graduated, may perform surgery of questionable necessity for the experience or in order to write and publish a journal article.

Western medicine, the type most often practiced in this country, can provide some of the best acute care in the world but as a tradeoff, is poorly equipped to provide care for chronic health problems and does little to avoid making an acute patient chronic.

Hospital care can be healthful or lifesaving for some people. Overall, however, statistics speak for themselves. If doctors and hospital personnel were to go on strike, available only for emergency treatment, the death rate might be expected to rise for the duration of the strike. However, analysis of the death rate during such strikes, gathered from several locations, showed a significant **decrease** in the death rate [3].

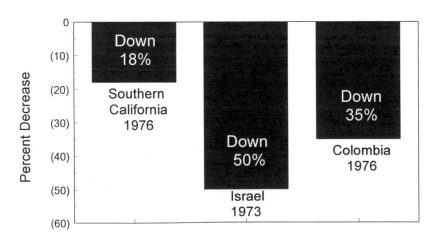

Decrease in Death Rate
During Hospital Strikes

On resumption of normal hospital and medical services, the death rate went back up to previous levels.

Infections contracted in the hospital, which, after all, is full of sick people, are so common that there is a medical term for such infections. Nosocomial infections are defined as those that one gets during a hospital visit or stay. Streptococcal bacterial infections are especially common.

Why is it important to know about trauma caused by medical intervention?
Reasons for surgery range from the life saving to the trivial. Patients, parents of potential patients, and doctors should have as much knowledge as possible of the risks of medical intervention in order to make an informed assessment of their options.

Our intent is not doctor-bashing or blanket condemnation of surgery but rather an attempt to provide information and balance. In many cases less-drastic measures discussed throughout this book and *Surviving The Toxic Crisis* should be tried first.

Why would unnecessary surgical and other procedures be done?
Western medicine is geared more towards treatment than prevention, and more towards acute short term results than long term effects. With this in mind, prevailing medical mentality tends to consider any part unnecessary whose removal does not cause death within a week or so. Organs whose function is not fully understood by the medical profession seem to be also considered to be unnecessary. However, removal of several of these "unnecessary" organs can cause a cumulative lifelong impediment to total health as the body's safety valves are removed.

By way of analogy, suppose you wanted to clean up your computer system, eliminating unnecessary files to make more storage space on your hard disk. You call up each file, notice that some appear to be written in gibberish rather than English, and conclude that since **you** don't understand the file it must not be necessary. You then delete these files. How well would your computer work when you are done? It would work about as well as your body would work after doctors removed everything whose function they didn't understand, or decided was no longer necessary, i.e., the appendix or gallbladder.

There is, especially since World War II, a great belief in science, which has become a god of sorts to many in medicine. Some people have sarcastically referred to the M.D. degree as meaning "Medical Deity". Some doctors in their arrogance believe they know better than God what belongs in a human body, and remove bits and pieces accordingly.

Unfortunately there are reasons for unnecessary surgery other than a misguided effort to do what is best for the patient. Some surgery is done for the money - a "walletectomy" - and some is done for the experience in an unusual procedure or to be able to write a medical journal article about it. As in all other professions, there are a certain percentage of doctors who have little or no feeling for other people, although this is especially reprehensible when the other people in question are their patients. One doctor overheard the following discussion in the hospital: A doctor had removed the appendix of a patient, which wasn't the original reason for the surgery. He said to the patient, "I got the appendix out just in time", then finished the sentence to his colleagues as they walked down the hall, "...just in time for lunch." They all laughed.

Patients sometimes feel that if a doctor goes in for exploratory surgery and doesn't remove anything, he hasn't actually done anything, adding to a doctor's pressure to remove something, anything, that might someday cause a problem, since he's already in there.

Drugs are often prescribed and taken in the belief that the drug, not the body, does the healing. Most drugs, in fact, cause harm to the body by giving it a foreign substance to detoxify and in some case deal with the long term or cumulative sided effects (i.e. Prednisone). All drugs have side effects, and many do more harm than good.

What are the dangers of surgery in general?

All surgery, even that which is comparatively minor, carries risks. These include:

- Dangers from anesthetic drugs, which, if improperly used, may cause just a bit too much unconsciousness. There is often a fine line between unconsciousness, coma, and death. In addition, anesthetic and other drugs lower immune system function, and infections after surgery are common partly for this reason.

- Another reason for infection is that the body is meant to be a closed system.

- Allergic reactions to anything used in the procedure, including anesthesia, drugs, and even latex operating gloves.

- Scars of any type can block the body's surface energy pathways.

- The root cause of the problem is usually not removed; for example, cancer often returns after removal of a tumor.

- Human error in technique or judgment.

Surgery, by suppressing symptoms, can keep the person from getting needed root-cause-oriented treatment. For example, a heart bypass operation can keep the patient from getting chelation (see the Metal Detoxification chapter in *Surviving The Toxic Crisis*), which is more effective because it cleans out *all* blood vessels. Ironically, critics of chelation - who may know little or nothing about it - contend that the opposite is true. So the patient is not informed at an earlier stage of the problem to take advantage of a procedure that could restore the health of the arteries so there would not be a need for expensive bypass surgery down the road. The real solution lies in understanding and stopping the cause of inflammation, and in using DMPS if the cause is heavy metals or chemicals, EDTA if not.

A female patient in her mid 30s went in for routine surgery, and a nerve was cut, resulting in the loss of use of muscles on the right side of her face. Also, a stainless steel jaw joint was put in, which caused a reaction that prevented the bone from healing. This finally caused so much allergic inflammation that surgeons removed her digestive tract. A progressive practitioner made the connection to a nickel allergy and the jaw joints were surgically removed. She tried to get compensation, but the company that made the joints had gone out of business because of the volume of related lawsuits.

What body parts and organs are considered to be unnecessary?

As mentioned, any organ whose removal does not cause immediate death is considered by some in medicine to be unnecessary. These body parts include, but are not limited to:

- *Tonsils and adenoids*
- *Single kidneys and lungs*
- *Uterus and ovaries*
- *Vas deferens (vasectomy)*
- *Teeth*
- *Thymus - usually irradiated*
- *Appendix*
- *Breast*
- *Prostate gland*
- *Spleen*
- *Gallbladder*

These are discussed on the following pages.

Why were tonsils removed?

The tonsils (also called palatine tonsils) and the adenoids (also called pharyngeal tonsils) are located in the throat and nasal cavity.

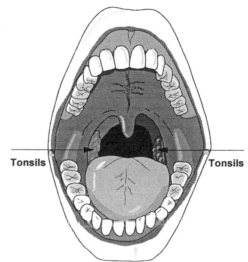

There are two of each, as well as two lingual tonsils at the base of the tongue. Tonsils were commonly removed in children, especially in the 1950s when respect for anything natural was at a low point. Even in 1992, tonsillectomy and adenoidectomy were the most common pediatric surgical procedures performed in the U.S. [4]. The usual indication for tonsil removal (tonsillectomy) was recurrent sore throats and redness and inflammation of the tonsils. The belief at the time was:

- The inflammation and soreness were due to infected tonsils.

- Since many in the medical profession didn't realize the residual problems resulting from their removal, tonsils were not deemed to be really necessary. Therefore, their removal was not considered to be a critical loss.

- Removal of the apparent source of inflammation, the tonsils, seemed to clear up the visible and immediate problem.

- There were no immediate and visible problems caused by tonsil removal.

These were all clear indications for a tonsillectomy. The fact that the procedure was simple and lucrative no doubt contributed to the prevalence of tonsillectomies. Sometimes tonsils which were not causing any trouble were removed for preventive reasons. Fortunately, tonsillectomies are now not nearly as widespread as they used to be.

Why can it be wrong to remove tonsils?

It is now known, although apparently not by all doctors, that tonsils have a purpose, and that removal of the tonsils usually does more harm than good.

The tonsils are part of the lymph system, which in turn is part of the immune system. Lymph tissue swells and sometimes becomes sore when a microbial or chemical invader or allergen is being attacked by large numbers of lymphocytes, which are white blood cells that destroy the invading microbes. Tonsil soreness is a sign that the good guys and the bad guys are slugging it out. Removal of the tonsils eliminates many of the good guys and destroys the battlefield, but the microbes are now free to do their damage elsewhere.

Tonsils are one of the escape valves used when the immune system is overwhelmed. The overflow of microbes are dropped into the stomach where they are killed by the hydrochloric acid in the stomach and then harmlessly excreted.

Much apparent tonsil inflammation is actually caused by an allergy, most often to milk, wheat, corn, or soy, or by a roundworm or giardial infestation. These possible causes should be investigated and ruled out before the body is permanently altered by surgery.

A ten-year-old boy had asthma all of his life. He was taken off milk, and his milk-allergy related asthma cleared up. Another asthmatic child, same age, was treated for roundworm and fungus and his asthma and attention deficit disorder (ADD) cleared. In both cases doctors wanted to remove the tonsils, which would have done nothing for the asthma and would have interfered with the body's optimal function for the rest of the patients' lives.

After a tonsillectomy is done, many of the sore throats are eliminated, but at a cost to the body for the rest of the person's life. The immune system has many redundancies and backup systems, but once a few of these are eliminated, the immune system is overloaded and its effectiveness is impaired.

In addition, the lungs and skin are the primary systems that the tonsils protect. Asthma and dermatitis (skin inflammation) can result later in life from tonsil removal. Overweight following surgery is a common complication of tonsillectomy in children [5]. This could be due to the body's retention of water to dilute toxins that would otherwise be removed by the lymph system, which includes the tonsils.

Having said all of this, there are legitimate reasons for tonsil removal. If tonsils are severely infected and more conservative treatments have been tried (such as removing allergens), tonsillectomy may be indicated.

One patient, a twenty-year-old male with asthma, reported that the asthma started after his tonsils were removed as a child. He was finally diagnosed with a milk allergy and his asthma got somewhat better. He could probably have regained his health if his tonsils could have been put back, but surgery is forever.

What is the appendix for?

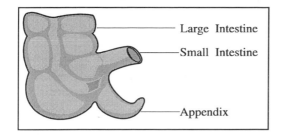

Large Intestine

Small Intestine

Appendix

The appendix is a wormlike appendage next to the ileocecal valve between the large and the small intestine. It acts as a buffer to keep the pressure off the ileocecal valve, and consequently keeps toxins in the large intestine from spreading back into the small intestine where nutrients and toxins are absorbed, and from where the toxins could spread throughout the body.

Are all appendectomies unnecessary?

Appendectomies are sometimes done when the appendix has ruptured or is about to rupture. In the case of rupture, toxins are explosively spread throughout the abdominal cavity and can cause infection, called peritonitis, and even death. In these cases an appendectomy can be life saving.

Some cases of appendicitis can be managed more conservatively by using antibiotics or herbal preparations. In these cases surgery is often not necessary, and the appendix heals on its own. Roundworms have been found in inflamed appendices (plural of appendix), and medication such as Vermox can often reduce the inflammation. Such cases should be closely monitored by a doctor.

The most unnecessary appendectomies are those which are done preventively. The doctor, opening the abdomen for an unrelated procedure, may suggest removing the appendix as long as he's already in there "just in case". This is not a good reason for appendix removal for anyone but the doctor's billing office. Removing any organ preventively is like hiring someone to clean your house, and they take your stereo with the excuse that it is cluttering up your living room.

An otherwise healthy twelve-year-old girl with appendicitis was treated for roundworm and bacteria. The appendicitis got better on its own, disproving the idea that surgery is always necessary for appendicitis. Within a month, her 40-year-old mother also developed appendicitis and had to have her appendix removed or it would have burst.

There are two morals to this story: The fact that both family members developed appendicitis at nearly the same time is a sign that the condition has a common infectious component. The second moral is the side-by-side illustration that there is a place for both mainstream or acute medicine (surgery) as well as integrated medicine (treating the infection/infestation). A wise doctor has knowledge of and access to both.

What is the gallbladder for?

The gallbladder stores bile, produced by the liver. Bile is released into the small intestine to aid in the digestion of fats and oils. A poorly functioning gallbladder may cause a person to be intolerant of fats and oils. Other early symptoms of gallbladder problems include pain between the shoulder blades, tight trapezius muscles, headaches, fatigue, and brain fog. Advanced symptoms include nausea and sharp pain on ingestion of oils and fats.

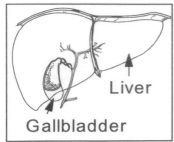

What causes gallbladder problems?

Many doctors do not look for the root cause of gallbladder problems. It is sufficient that the removal of the gallbladder eliminates the acute symptoms such as pain and gallstones, and they look no further. Many doctors now have adopted the view that gallstones are an indication of a diseased gallbladder and will only recommend surgery.

Giardia (an amoebic parasite), helicobacter pylori (a bacterium), and fungus, as well as mercury binding with bile sludge, are common causes of gallbladder problems. The common bile duct can become plugged by these organisms, as well as the sludge, causing symptoms. It is not necessary to remove the gallbladder in these cases. Just clean it out (Liver and Gallbladder Flush protocols are available from knowledgeable practitioners) and it will once again be able to perform its function. Some methods of eliminating the parasites are discussed in the Secondary Toxic Suppressors section in *Surviving The Toxic Crisis*.

It is not uncommon for patients to whom gallbladder surgery has been recommended to obtain relief from the liver/gallbladder flush. The flush is a combination of olive oil and lemon juice, and in conjunction with ultrasound to break up the stones, often flushes out the sludge as well as producing the passage of quantities of small to medium sized green gallstones. This is followed by the shrinkage of the gallbladder back to near-normal size. Surgery in many cases then may not be needed. An ultrasound procedure can determine if a patient would safely be able to do the flush, as it would reveal the presence of any large stones that might require surgical removal. Clinic patients are always advised to do an ultrasound before proceeding with a gallbladder flush.

Mercury fillings can set up an environment for the growth of giardia and other parasites. Removal of these fillings may be the first step in treating gallbladder problems.

What are some long term effects of gallbladder removal?

Oils are necessary for many body functions (see Oils and Fats chapter). Since the gallbladder is used in the digestion of oils, the lack of a gallbladder can cause oil deficiency problems, including lowered antioxidants and the fat soluble vitamins A and E, hormone imbalance, and chemical sensitivities.

There have been many scientific articles since the 1970s showing an increase in colon cancer among those who have had their gallbladder removed. The incidence of colon cancer is twice normal in women, and 40% more in men [6] when comparing colon cancer incidence between those without and those with gallbladders.

Gallbladder removal also caused colon cancer in mice in laboratory experiments. The postulated cause - the gallbladder stores bile which is released for digestion, and 6% of this bile goes to the colon. Bacteria in the colon interact with the bile to form carcinogens. When the gallbladder is gone, bile is released continuously, not just when fat is eaten, and more bile goes to the colon. Food in the colon increases transit time and gives the bacteria something else to do besides reacting with the bile.

If the gallbladder has already been removed, it is a good idea to eat frequent small meals which are high in fiber and low in fat. A predigested lecithin emulsified oil mixture for dressings and sauces is suggested to help break down oils for easier digestion. This oil mixture recipe is provided in the Oils and Fats chapter.

What does the prostate gland do?
The prostate gland, found only in men, provides seminal fluid which carries the sperm to their ultimate destination. It is believed by some that the prostate gland has no other use, and that it can therefore be removed without ill effect in any man who does not wish to reproduce.

What is the number one cancer in men?
Prostate problems, such as swelling, pain, and difficulty urinating, are common in older men. Prostate cancer is so common that it is the number one male cancer. Because of these symptoms, and because of the belief that the prostate is of no use to a man past his reproductive years, the prostate is often removed surgically.

Why is prostate surgery often inadvisable?
Sometimes prostate surgery is necessary, as in the case of prostate cancer. In other cases, removal of the prostate is not necessary and the risks of removal should be weighed against the benefits.

The prostate gland is one of the junction boxes of the body. The blood, lymph, urinary, and reproductive systems all run through it.

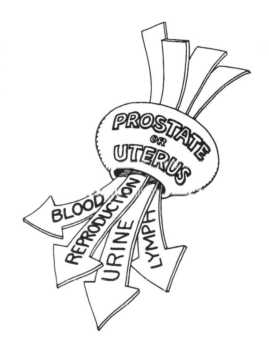

A prostate problem can affect the entire body, contributing to fatigue, anger, depression, mood swings, difficulty urinating and urinary tract infections, bowel blockage, swollen achy legs, and high blood pressure. It follows that the removal of the prostate can also have an effect on the rest of the body, sometimes in ways we do not fully understand.

There are 400,000 surgical operations to remove the prostate gland per year. The death rate from such surgery is as high as 1.8% [7]. The "freeze and remove" method, or heating to release the hardened fluids if caught at the prostatitis stage, are options. However, as of this writing, doctors, in some cases, are now taking a more cautious "wait and see" attitude because of the slow growing nature of the cancer.

Is vasectomy harmless?
Another common operation on the male reproductive system is vasectomy. This is the surgical cutting and tying of the vas deferens, the tube which carries sperm from the testes to be mixed

with semen. Vasectomy is undergone as a permanent birth control technique. The sperm are resorbed into the body rather than ejaculated.

There are risks to vasectomy which are now beginning to surface. In a study done at Harvard Medical School, 13,124 men who had vasectomies were compared to 12,392 men who didn't. The researchers found that the overall risk for prostate cancer was 56% higher in those men who had been vasectomized. By plotting the occurrence of prostate cancer over time, they found that vasectomized men had an 89% higher risk of prostate cancer after 20 years [8].

As many as two-thirds of vasectomized men develop antibodies to sperm following surgery [7]. The immune system encounters sperm where they don't belong, and gears up for attack against them. This immune response may weaken the immune system over time and may even lead to tumor growth.

Semen can be considered not just a reproductive fluid but also a detoxification, or waste, product of the body. Preventing its release is rather like being prevented from blowing your nose.

A patient who had a vasectomy in his 30s had cancer by his late 40s. Another vasectomy patient fathered a baby, evidence that the procedure doesn't always work. It is not uncommon to see men with lowered drive - both sex drive and overall ambition - as well as lowered immune function and weight gain after a vasectomy.

In an analogous procedure, women who have had their fallopian tubes tied as a sterilization procedure have also been known to gain weight after the procedure, especially below the waist. A 30 year old woman who had had three children gained little weight after the first two, but gained 80 pounds after the third child, after whose birth she had her tubes tied.

Is the uterus necessary once reproduction is not needed?
The prevailing belief among the medical establishment is that the uterus is simply a place to hold and nourish a developing baby. As such, it is often considered to be disposable once a woman has had all the children she wants or is able to have.

The uterus is often removed for the relief of menstrual problems, polyps (benign growths), or cancer. It is usually wise to remove a cancerous uterus, but other uterine problems can often be helped by less drastic measures.

Even the conservative *Journal of the American Medical Association* believes that 16-27% of hysterectomies are unnecessary. It is likely that even more hysterectomies than this could be prevented [9].

The uterus is the female analog of the prostate gland. Like the prostate, it is a junction box for several systems and therefore can be assumed to affect the entire body. Its removal, like the removal of the prostate gland, can also have effects throughout the system. It is not uncommon for a woman who has had a hysterectomy to ex-

> **Depressed or fatigued after a hysterectomy? It's not all in your head.**

perience depression, a symptom that many doctors attribute to purely psychological factors such as the feeling of losing one's femininity. Biological factors, such as blockage of other body systems as with prostate removal, are a more likely cause.

Menstruation is one way that a woman eliminates toxins. Removing the uterus ends menstruation and hence this cleansing pathway. Normally the onset of menopause also eliminates this cleansing pathway and a woman will have to deal with eliminating toxins in other ways. But having a hysterectomy may compound the intensity of the problem, and prematurely, if it occurs earlier than the normal onset of menopause. Synthetic hormone replacement therapy (HRT) taken to deal with the induced menopause may then replace the old anxiety about heart disease with a new one about developing cancer.

Why do women tend to gain weight and have other problems after a hysterectomy?
The ovaries produce the female hormones estrogen and progesterone. As part of the endocrine glandular system they affect and are affected by the other endocrine glands. They are sometimes removed in a procedure called an oophorectomy, which is often combined with hysterectomy. Reasons for ovary removal range from cancer to premenstrual syndrome (PMS). If one ovary is cancerous, the other is sometimes removed preventively. Other cancers such as breast cancer can be worsened by estrogen, and the ovaries are sometimes removed to halt estrogen production.

Bilateral oophorectomy (removal of both ovaries) brings about instant menopause, with cessation of menstruation, hot flashes in some women, and vaginal dryness. Depression, fatigue, and weight gain are common and are often wrongly attributed to psychological causes. Cats and dogs that have been spayed (uterus and ovaries removed) for birth control purposes often become overweight and sluggish just as do women, eliminating psychological factors from being considered a probable cause. Estrogen helps protect women from heart disease, and an increased risk of heart disease often results from oophorectomy.

Other problems related to hysterectomy include urination difficulties such as trouble voiding or incontinence. 15% of hysterectomy patients had gastrointestinal complications, and 21% had lymphedema, or water weight gain and puffiness [10]. In another study, premenopausal women who have had a hysterectomy without ovary removal had a significant loss of bone density, a precursor to osteoporosis, as compared with matched controls who had not had a hysterectomy [11].

Cesarean birth involves cutting the uterus open. Weight gain is common after the procedure, in part because lymph pathways have been cut and water is retained. One patient who did not have a previous weight problem gained 100 pounds after a Cesarean. She needed sclerotherapy - injection into the scar tissue - before balance was restored and she started losing the excess weight.

Can't estrogen be replaced?
Estrogen replacement in the form of pills or injections is not desirable because it is not the same in type or amount as that which is naturally produced. Synthetic estrogen is not the same as natural human estrogen.

Estrogen, when produced naturally by the body, is generally produced in exactly the amount needed via a mechanism which involves the other endocrine glands. Introducing a constant amount that is other than what the body would naturally produce can adversely affect the other endocrine glands and unbalance the amounts of the other hormones produced by these glands. The adrenal glands, which normally make a small amount of estrogen, are given the message that they no longer need to produce estrogen, and this can adversely affect their function.

Estrogen in pill form goes through the digestive tract, which estrogen is not designed to do. This can throw off digestion by creating a fungal environment.

Estrogen can promote the growth of certain cancers, especially reproductive system cancers such as those of the breast, ovary and cervix. The rate of fatal ovarian cancer in women who took estrogen was 40% higher compared to non-estrogen-using controls after 6-10 years of estrogen use, and 71% higher for those who took estrogen for 11 or more years [12].

The ovaries produce not only estrogen but also the hormone progesterone and even 1-2 mg/day of the male hormone testosterone. Hormone therapy usually replaces only the estrogen and occasionally the progesterone as well.

What are breasts there for?

Many people believe female breasts are only there to give definition to the female form which serves to attract the male, and only secondarily to fulfill the purpose of nursing babies. Actually, breasts contain lymph glands for detoxifying poisons, a vascular (blood) system, and milk glands which are actually specialized sweat glands. Sweat glands, like lymph glands, are important in detoxification. If a woman is toxic, the breasts get larger and sore. They function as overflow toxic depots. Breast soreness prior to menstruation is sometimes due in part to an accumulation of toxins. Some of these toxins are then eliminated through menstruation, easing the soreness.

Breast removal (mastectomy) is most often done when breast cancer is present. There has been no evidence that removal of the entire breast is any more effective in eliminating cancer than removing only the cancerous lump with a bit of surrounding tissue.

Are second kidneys and lungs "extra"?

There is no doubt among the medical profession that kidneys and lungs are necessary for life. However, the fact that we were given two of each leads some doctors to believe that one is an extra organ that can be removed if necessary, and the patient can still function adequately with just one. We were given two of each for a reason. The "extra" organ is a wonderful example of the body's backup systems, or fault tolerance. Because sometimes surgery is unavoidable and the patient is then grateful they still have viable function of the remaining organ. But is a far cry from the cavalier attitude that some take towards surgery.

Does the spleen have a use?

The spleen is one of the cleansing/detoxifying systems of the body. It has a large vascular (blood vessel) system for this purpose. Old blood cells are removed from circulation in the spleen, with some assistance from the liver. Because of the many blood vessels, life-threatening bleeding from the spleen is not uncommon after automobile accidents. Removal of the spleen is the usual remedy, but this surgery is not without its detrimental effects. Other body systems can take over the function of the spleen, but this can overload these other systems over time. As with your computer, if a system crashes it's comforting to have a backup.

Is the thymus needed in adulthood?
The thymus is larger in infancy and childhood and is usually small and shriveled in adulthood. This has led scientists to believe that the thymus outgrows its role after puberty. It used to be fashionable to irradiate (bombard with x-rays) the thymus gland if it was still large in a person's teens. The small shriveled form was thought to be the norm, and the thymus was essentially killed if it didn't conform to what doctors expected of it.

It is now known that the thymus, which makes infection-fighting B-cells, is an important part of the immune system. Its removal or destruction forces the rest of the immune system to take on its functions, and sometimes falter under stress.

What is cosmetic surgery?
Cosmetic surgery is that which is undertaken for the purpose of enhancing one's attractiveness. The primary benefit is psychological, although this benefit is not trivial. Reconstructive surgery is similar to cosmetic surgery in some respects, but it can have health benefits. An example is rebuilding a missing outer ear, which helps hearing as well as being more attractive. Cosmetic surgery, unlike reconstructive surgery, is defined as that which benefits only appearance, not function.

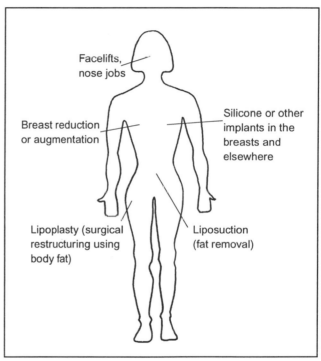

Some types of cosmetic surgery include but are not limited to these procedures in the box to the right.

What are the risks of cosmetic surgery?
Risks common to nearly all cosmetic surgery are those common to all surgery - risk of anesthetic reaction, allergy, scar interference, cutting through lymph and blood vessels, and a disappointing outcome. In the case of cosmetic surgery, the risks are higher compared with the benefits than is the case with other surgery. Knowledge of these risks is necessary in order to make an informed decision about such surgery.

A patient had cosmetic surgery all over her face with resulting poor lymph drainage throughout her body, since the scars restricted lymph drainage. She had immunological problems, chronic fatigue, mood swings and depression. The same woman had liposuction and lipoplasty (both described in the next paragraphs) and developed poor leg drainage, weight gain (edema) and auto-immune disease.

What is liposuction?

Liposuction, also called suction lipectomy, is becoming more common. The procedure involves suctioning local deposits of fat through a slit in the skin. Skill is needed to achieve smooth contouring. It is considered to be only minor surgery, as the body cavity is not entered and general anesthesia is rarely used.

Liposuction is normally recommended only for those of normal weight who have stubborn "saddlebags" or other local fat deposits. It is not intended for general fat removal over large areas. Local fat deposits, often called cellulite, are usually a mixture of fat, water, and toxic deposits. The ripply appearance of cellulite is due to lymph glands swollen with toxins and deposits of fat stored toxins under the skin. Dieting and exercise rarely has an effect on cellulite, since the cause is stored toxins and has nothing to do with calories. Detoxification procedures such as sauna or a detoxification diet can reduce the "cellulite" by removing the underlying cause, a far healthier approach.

The liposuction procedure involves cutting lymph and blood capillary tributaries, allowing toxic wastes to pool in the area. Infection sometimes results for this reason even if the procedure is done using sterile precautions. Since lymph glands are removed in the procedure, and the lymph glands are an important part of the immune system, their removal compromises the effectiveness of the immune system. Lymph glands are important in the storage of toxins. Removal of the lymph glands is like removing barrels which hold toxic waste without removing the source of the toxic waste.

Does liposuction work?

Apart from health effects of liposuction, long-term negative cosmetic effects of the procedure are not uncommon. In a questionnaire distributed to 1339 consecutive liposuction patients 5-8 years after the procedure, 19% reported asymmetry (both sides didn't match), 29% reported return of fat to the liposuction site, and 30% reported fat coming back elsewhere, almost as if in compensation. Overall weight gain and undesirable skin changes over the liposuction site were also common. The most problems were reported for liposuction of the buttocks [13]. Another study of 3511 procedures in 2009 patients reported similar results [14]. In a comparison of two liposuction techniques, syringe aspiration was associated with fewer short-term complications than pump aspiration [15].

Can removed fat be used elsewhere?

Lipoplasty (lipo- means fat) involves taking fat from the body and relocating it somewhere else. The usual desired destinations are the lips, cheeks, breasts, and buttocks. In the procedure, the removed fat is cleaned before it is injected where desired. Proponents of the procedure say that since the fat is your own, it is not a foreign substance and should not cause rejection or other undesirable reactions.

Fat which has been removed and cleaned is not the same as fat in its natural setting. Removed fat is no longer served by the vascular system, and becomes dead and rancid tissue which, despite its source, acts as foreign matter in the body. It can set up a long term infection in the body, and can lead to autoimmune reactions such as chronic fatigue and arthritis.

Injection of fat into the breasts has led to problems. The fat is either absorbed into the body, making for a short-lived result, or it hardens into a calcified (petrified) mass. Breast injections can interfere with a mammogram by either mimicking or concealing (or even causing) a malignancy.

What about breast implants?

Silicone breast implants have been in the news as their dangers are discovered to an increasing extent. Silicone has long been considered an inert (nonreactive) material, but long term problems are now surfacing.

About two million women have had silicone breast implants. About 80% of these are cosmetic, and 20% reconstructive after a mastectomy. The most common implant is a polyurethane coated membrane sac containing silicone gel. Both materials are reported to be cause for concern. Some of the problems caused by this material include [16]:

- *Liver damage*
- *Foreign body granulomas (noncancerous tumors)*
  in the breast and liver
- *Spleen and lymph node involvement*
- *Enlarged spleen*
- *Biliary cirrhosis (liver hardening)*
- *Autoimmune disorders*

Rheumatic disorders and lupus have also been linked to silicone implants [17].

Chronic fatigue syndrome, also an immune disorder, has been linked to these implants, as has overall pain (fibromyalgia) and multiple organ system abnormalities [18]. In a follow-up study of 50 consecutive silicone implant patients:

- 87% reported fatigue,
- 75% reported overall stiffness,
- 71% reported poor sleep, and
- 78% reported joint pain [19].

> **Chronic fatigue syndrome has been linked to breast implants.**

> **About *three-quarters* of silicone implant patients had adverse health effects that they attributed to the implants.**

In other words, about *three-quarters* of silicone implant patients had adverse health effects that they attributed to the implants. In another similar study, 103 of 142 patients had symptoms that they related to their implants. About half of these (52) reported improvement after implant removal [20], supporting a cause-effect relationship.

One patient with breast implants hit her breasts hard against the steering wheel during an automobile accident. The implants ruptured, driving the silicone into her body. The resulting immune suppression finally started resolving after she had the mercury fillings taken out of her teeth and had chelation to remove the metal from her body, which freed the detoxification pathways so they could finally start getting rid of the silicone.

Another patient, a 45 -year-old woman, had both breast implants and a Cesarean section birth. She gained weight below the waist and had to have her scars injected (sclerotherapy) to clear the pathways and relieve her symptoms. She then lost weight and reported an increase in energy.

What can be done about silicone implant related problems?

It is possible to regain your health after having silicone implants using a multi-modality approach [21]:

- Have the implants removed.

- Get counseling to deal with anger, sadness and guilt. Deal with the anger towards yourself, the medical profession, society's pressure to have a certain breast size, or a male partner who wanted you to look different than you did.

- Remove dental mercury and nickel, and then detoxify it from your body as through chelation. Mercury and silicone use similar detoxification pathways, and removing the mercury allows the body to concentrate on the silicone.

- Nutritional therapies to support the liver and kidneys in their detoxification role, e.g., Glutathione, Sun Chlorella, Kyolic garlic, and ToxiCleanse (by Metagenics)

- Cellulase and other enzymes to aid in the breakdown and removal of silicone

- Lymph massage and exercise helps the lymph system to dump toxins.

- Modified fasting.

- Colon cleansing through colonics or colemas.

What are Hollywood teeth?

Hollywood teeth is a name sometimes given to massive cosmetic mouth reconstruction. This involves root canals and caps, and large quantities of metals and foreign materials in the mouth. Actors Michael Landon and Lee Remick died of pancreatic and liver cancers which may have been related to their Hollywood smiles.

Most Americans have mercury fillings, nickel-containing root canals, and/or braces, contributing to toxic and allergic reactions and the equivalent of a battery in their mouths. Cancers of the breast, reproductive system, and lymph glands have been linked to root canals and nickel. Nickel is found in Root canal posts and silver-colored crowns. See the chapters on Mercury, Nickel and Root Canals, and The Battery Effect in *Surviving The Toxic Crisis* for more information.

A patient had wisdom teeth removed and had orthodontia (braces) in his teens. His low back and neck stiffened up and it was hard to bend over. He had pain throughout his body since his bite was so far off. He used to cramp so badly that he needed an analgesic wrap just to play football. The wisdom teeth, often considered to be unnecessary, are to stabilize the bite.

Where else can metal be placed in the body?

Stainless steel joints and pins of various types can be placed in the body to replace diseased or broken joints and bones. Stainless steel contains the toxic and allergenic metal nickel, a known carcinogen. Such bone replacements can lead to bone carcinoma (cancer) and a hollowing out of the bone after about ten years. Chronic inflammation can be set up next to the implant. This is especially common in jaw joint replacements. An additional problem with jaw joint replacements is the setting up of electrical currents by reaction with other metal in the mouth, causing pain and spasm. Metal elsewhere in the body can also react electrically with metal in the mouth.

What harm can surgical scars do?

Scars, surgical or otherwise, can block the meridians (pathways that acupuncturists use to change function and feeling) which run along the skin. This blockage can contribute to a wide variety of symptoms depending on which meridians have been cut. For example, a woman who has had a Cesarean delivery with the popular horizontal "bikini cut" often gains weight after the procedure, which is probably due to the cutting of three or four meridians as well as lymph channels.

A scar can act as a dam to block the flow of energy along the meridians. Sclerotherapy is a form of therapy that involves the injection of Lidocaine or homeopathic solutions along the scar, and, like punching holes in a dam to let water flow through, the energy flow can then be reestablished.

What about drugs?

Nearly all drugs are foreign substances to the body, and can cause undesirable side effects. These substances then need to be detoxified, adding to the burden of other toxins. Most drugs have deleterious (harmful) effects on the immune system, usually reducing immune system function.

Inappropriate use of antibiotics in childhood can cause more problems than such use solves. The immune system may need a sort of exercise in fighting minor and viral infections in order to strengthen it for larger battles. Antibiotics can rob the immune system of this exercise. In addition, microorganisms can become resistant to the antibiotics. Next time you're sick and don't use antibiotics, tell people this is your cancer prevention program. This will give you an opportunity to educate them about the indiscriminate use of antibiotics.

In a study of 56 volunteers with colds, aspirin and acetaminophen (Tylenol) caused increased nasal blockage and reduced virus fighting antibodies compared with an inert placebo [22].

These and many other drugs are discussed in the chapter on Drugs in *Surviving The Toxic Crisis*. Cancer drugs are discussed in the chapter on Cancer.

Can common testing procedures cause harm?

X-rays and other common testing procedures can be harmful. This is elaborated upon in the chapters on Electromagnetic Radiation in *Surviving The Toxic Crisis*, and the Cancer chapter.

Do vaccinations always help prevent disease?

Vaccinations stimulate the immune system to produce antibodies to a particular microbe, usually a virus. Vaccinations, also called immunizations, are usually given in infancy, childhood or before a trip to a Third World country. Weakened or dead viruses or bacteria are theoretically unable to cause disease but tell the immune system to be on the lookout for anything with that particular shape.

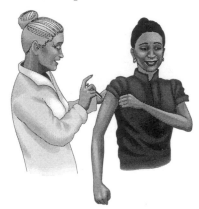

Many vaccinations cause a bit of fever and local soreness as the body prepares to fight a battle against the foreign material, but this is usually short-lived and not serious. Cases of serious illness and death, especially in children, have been reported as a direct result of vaccination. Cases have been reported of polio transmission to the father of a newly vaccinated infant [23], reactive arthritis after a flu shot [24], and potentially fatal anaphylactic shock after a hepatitis B vaccination [25]. These cases are rare, but one should be aware of the serious risks.

Vaccinations, like overuse of antibiotics, can prevent the immune system from getting the disease-fighting exercise it needs.

Another risk of vaccinations has recently surfaced. Women who were vaccinated for measles as children now have children with a higher rate of measles incidence in infancy, previously rare at this age. Vaccination produces lower levels of antibodies than are produced by fighting the actual disease. These lower antibody levels are passed on to their babies, who are now more susceptible to measles [26].

Vaccination has been linked to the development of autism [27].

Viral vaccines can depress cellular immunity [28,29]. A significant drop in T-helper lymphocytes was observed in healthy adults given routine tetanus vaccines; the effect on the immature immune systems of infants given the routine DPT shot (diphtheria-pertussis-tetanus) is likely even greater [30]. Children receiving the pertussis (whooping cough) vaccine were six times more likely to develop asthma than children not receiving the vaccine [31]. Japan has raised the age of pertussis vaccination to two years in 1975, with a resulting decline in crib death and infant spinal meningitis [32].

Vaccination has been found to be generally detrimental to the immune system [33], and is linked to Chronic Fatigue Syndrome in young adults [34].

A 60-year-old woman who had had a routine vaccination developed chronic fatigue and other health problems shortly after the vaccination.

Is vaccination linked to crib death?
Sudden infant death syndrome (SIDS) kills over 10,000 babies a year, and is the second largest cause of infant deaths in the U.S. In SIDS, an apparently healthy baby goes to sleep and simply doesn't wake up.

Dr. Viera Scheibner studied over 35,000 pages of medical papers dealing with vaccination and then wrote a book: *Vaccination, the Medical Assault on the Immune System*. She found that crib death, which has many possible causes, most commonly occurred soon after the common DPT (diphtheria-pertussis-tetanus) injection [35].

When childhood vaccination rates in Australia dropped by 50% after vaccination was made non-mandatory, SIDS cases also dropped by 50%. Japan moved the age of first vaccination up to two years (two months is the norm for first vaccination in the U.S.) in 1975, and since then crib death and infantile convulsions have virtually disappeared [36].

Can anything be done to reduce the risk and damage?
100 mg of vitamin C per day can reduce the risk of death caused by the DPT vaccination [37].

Summary

All organs of the body were put there for a purpose and have a use, and this purpose exists even if doctors don't understand what it is. Removal of any organ, surgical and other scars, and the implantation of anything in the body (metal joints, silicone, or vaccinations, among others) will interfere with the body's optimal function. However, there are sometimes legitimate and even life-saving indications for surgery. The understanding given in this chapter can help you weigh the pros and cons of surgery.

Summary Chart of "Unnecessary" Organs

Organ	Purpose	Potential Result of Removal
Gallbladder	Fat digester	Deficient hormones, allergy
Ovaries	Hormones	Mood swings, fungus
Appendix	Colon's buffer	Poisoning of intestinal tract
Spleen	Cleanse blood	Immune malfunction, allergy
Uterus/Prostate	Reproductive	Mood swings, fungus
Thymus	Immune function	Impaired immunity
Teeth	Pathways	Referred disease
Tonsils	Escape valve	Lung problems, asthma
Breast	Lymph storage	Immune dysfunction
Scars	Block pathways	Referred disease

References and Resources

General

- The Burton Goldberg Group, *Alternative Medicine: The Definitive Guide*, Future Medicine Publishing, Puyallup WA, 1994.

  Particular chapters of interest include:

  - *"Female Health", pp. 657-679, which discusses alternatives to hysterectomy and estrogen replacement therapy.*

  - *"Gallbladder Disorders", pp. 423-4, on non-surgical alternatives to gallbladder problems.*

  - *"Tonsillitis", pp. 982-3, on non-surgical alternatives to dealing with tonsillitis.*

- Berger, Stuart M., *What Your Doctor Didn't Learn in Medical School and What You Can Do About It*,. Avon Books, NY, 1989.

Vaccination

- Chaitow, Leon, *Vaccination and Immunization: Dangers, Delusions, and Alternatives*, Saffron Walden, UK, 1987.

- Coulter, Harris L, *Vaccination, Social Violence and Criminality: The Medical Assault on the American Brain*, North Atlantic Books, Berkeley CA, 1990.

- Coulter, Harris L. and Barbara Fisher, *A Shot in the Dark*, Avery Publishing Group, Garden City NY, 1991. *A well-referenced discussion of vaccination.*

- Kalokerinos, Archie, *Every Second Child*, Keats Publishing, New Canaan CT, 1981. *Discusses the dangers of vaccination.*

- Miller, Neil Z., *Vaccines - Are They Really Safe and Effective?*, New Atlantean Press, Santa Fe NM, 1992.

- Scheibner, Viera, *Vaccination*, Naturally Write, Australia, 1993. *Extensively referenced book documents the harm caused by vaccination.*

- **National Vaccine Information Center**, 512 West Maple Avenue, Suite 206, Vienna VA 22180, phone 703-938-0342.

TESTING METHODS AND BIAS

Protecting Ourselves From The Protectors

In this chapter you can learn:

- *What is a study?*
- *Is the conclusion necessarily correct?*
- *Why is it important to understand why a study is done?*
- *How are drugs tested?*
- *Does this testing and approval process protect us?*
- *Can studies be done incorrectly?*
- *Why do some study results appear to conflict?*
- *Is the double-blind placebo-controlled study the only accurate type?*
- *What is anecdotal evidence, and can it be valid?*
- *Is the FDA unbiased and looking out for our best interests?*
- *Are there other sources of bias in studies?*
- *To consider when evaluating studies or "public health" decisions: Is it science or "political science"?*

What is a study?

You will run into the term "study" in this book and maybe in other sources as well. The usual context for the term is "Studies show that..." or "A study done at the University of Whatever indicates that..." followed by particular results. Studies have shown that aspirin reduces heart attack risk, that vitamin C reduces cold symptoms, or that fish oils improve memory. What is meant by a "study"? Can all study results be believed?

A study is an experiment or series of experiments designed to test a hypothesis. A hypothesis is something which a research person or team would like to prove or disprove. The hypothesis is phrased as a statement or question, such as "Drug X cures headaches" or "Does drug X cure headaches?"

An experiment is then designed to prove or disprove the hypothesis. In its simplest form, an action is taken, the results are noted, and a conclusion related to the hypothesis is formed.

Is the conclusion necessarily correct?

The conclusion may or may not be correct. For example, a scientist forms the hypothesis "A rooster's crowing makes the sun come up." The scientist observes some roosters and makes note of the fact that the sun comes up after the roosters crow. These results are repeated after many days and many roosters. The scientist has proven his hypothesis, right? Obviously not. Designing a study properly is more complex than this, and an improperly designed study can result in conclusions which are not only incorrect but may be harmful.

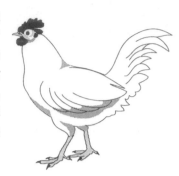

Why is it important to understand why a study is done?

Understanding the study process in general will help you to evaluate study results based on whether the study was done thoroughly and appropriately. This understanding will in turn allow you to know whether results can be believed, and to modify your behavior accordingly.

People without this understanding may take certain medications or expose themselves to toxins such as mercury or pesticides without realizing that safety claims may be based on poorly done or biased studies. Your health may be at stake here.

Many study results appear to contradict each other. Studies have shown, for example, that Vitamin C both does and does not relieve cold symptoms, and that aspirin both does and does not reduce heart attack risk. If you don't know which studies to believe, the information in this chapter can help you evaluate them.

A drug study is described here, but this process is used for the evaluation of many substances and procedures. In some cases, discussed later, this type of testing is not appropriate.

How are drugs tested?

You may have heard the terms "placebo" or "double-blind" used with respect to drug studies. What do these terms mean, and how is a drug study done?

Drug trials, also called clinical trials, go through several stages. These stages are mandated by the Food and Drug Association (FDA) to show that a drug is both safe and effective. The stages are listed here and discussed afterwards:

1. *Drug X is made.*
2. *A hypothesis is formed: Drug X will relieve headaches.*
3. *Drug X is tested on animals for safety.*
4. *Drug X is tested on animals for effectiveness where possible.*
5. *Drug X is tested on healthy human volunteers for safety.*
6. *Drug X is tested on volunteers with headaches for effectiveness.*
7. *Double-blind placebo-controlled studies are done on a small group.*
8. *These double blind studies are repeated on a larger group.*
9. *The hypothesis is proven: Drug X relieves headaches.*

> 10. *Further experiments refine the best dosage amounts and form.*
> 11. *Approval for marketing is given by the FDA (about $232,000,000 and ten years later).*

If Drug X does not pass at any stage - if it is toxic to animals or does not relieve headaches - then the study is discontinued.

Why are all of these stages necessary?
The necessity of these testing stages should become apparent as these stages are discussed.

Animal testing involves giving animals such as dogs different doses of Drug X and monitoring for toxicity. After the Thalidomide disaster in the 1960s, in which the sleep aid Thalidomide caused birth defects when taken by pregnant women, pregnant animals and their offspring have also been tested. After repeat testing, it was determined that dosages above a certain amount per pound of body weight are toxic, and those below this level are not.

Animals with the disease condition being tested for are given the drug when practical. Such testing is possible for cancer or some skin conditions, for example, but would clearly be useless for a subjective symptom such as headache. Results in this case would be impossible to measure and verify, so this step would be omitted in such cases.

Healthy human volunteers are then given dosages of Drug X below the amount, adjusted for body weight, found to be toxic in animals. If they have no short-term adverse effects, the drug is then tested for effectiveness.

How do the researchers know Drug X works?
At this stage volunteers with headaches are given Drug X. If the drug does not relieve headaches in a statistically significant number of the volunteers, the drug obviously does not work and the study is terminated.

If a significant number of patients report headache relief, this does not in itself mean that Drug X is responsible. There is an effect called the placebo (pronounced pluh-see-bo) effect. The mind can affect the body, and a certain number of people who take even an inert sugar pill will experience relief if they think they will. Further testing is necessary to eliminate interference from the placebo effect.

It is worth noting here that the placebo effect is generally considered to be only a nuisance factor that needs to be compensated for by further testing. The mind obviously has a powerful influence on the body or the placebo effect would not happen. The mind's placebo effect is so strong that not only subjective indicators (pain relief, for example) are affected, but objective observable indicators such as skin conditions and even cancer have been alleviated by a medically inert substance. There is the potential for this mind-body relationship to be harnessed rather than dismissed, and some progressive therapies utilize this relationship to improve health.

How do they know whether relief is actually due to the drug?
A double-blind placebo-controlled study is the next step. Several things are important here. Some people will get Drug X, and some people, called the controls, will get an inert substitute called a placebo, usually made of milk sugar (lactose). If significantly more people report relief from the drug than from the placebo, then the relief is considered to actually be due to the drug.

To eliminate the possibility of patient or researcher expectations biasing the results, precautions are taken. The active drug and the placebo pill look identical. Neither the patients nor the doctors / researchers administering the test know who is getting which type of pill, hence the name double-blind. The people who interpret the test results are told which patients, by number, have experienced relief, and they compare the results with the coded list of which patients (by number) were given the active drug.

A control group is nearly always necessary in any study. The control group is not subjected to the medication, toxin, or whatever is being tested so there will be some basis for comparison. In the case of Drug X, the trial is placebo-controlled; that is, those who get the placebo are the controls.

It is important that there be only one variable tested. A variable is, as the name suggests, the thing that is different between groups. Everything else should be the same. If, for example, everyone on the active drug were to make dietary changes while the control group does not, there would be more than one variable. It would then not be known which variable was most influential. A large patient population which is assigned active or placebo tablets randomly will tend to smooth out variables such as gender, age, or physical condition since people with different attributes are assigned fairly evenly to both groups.

Double-blind studies are very expensive. If the results done on a small group look promising, a larger trial is usually done to verify the results.

Other tests are done to refine dosage amount and form. These other tests include:

- *Tablets vs. capsules*
- *Immediate-release vs. timed-release*
- *Dosage amounts such as 75 mg vs. 100 mg*
- *Company's product vs. that of competitor*
- *Different formulations*

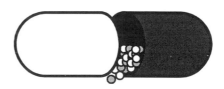

How is the drug then approved?
A New Drug Application (NDA) must be filed with the FDA, and the approval process can take up to seven years and cost millions of dollars (an average of $232 million per drug) in testing and other expenses. The drug must be proven safe, effective, and an improvement in some way over something already on the market. Many drugs are denied approval, and a small company which can only afford to develop one product at a time can go bankrupt if approval is denied.

The FDA can shorten the testing process at will. For example, the anti-anxiety drug Prozac, a serotonin reuptake inhibitor, was tested for less than seven **weeks** before approval, and long-term side effects were not monitored [1]. It is now recognized that Prozac's side effects can be quite serious and even fatal for the patient and those around him. Violent homicides in the news have been linked to the use of psychoactive drugs, including Prozac. Those who are taking Prozac are the long-term side effects "test subjects". Welcome to the world of drug testing -- you're saving the pharmaceutical companies a bundle of money!

How did it happen that Prozac was approved so quickly? It may or may not be coincidence that George Bush, who was the U.S. president when the drug was approved, used to be on the board of directors at Eli Lilly, the giant pharmaceutical company that manufactures Prozac.

Does this testing and approval process protect us?
It sounds as if the FDA's system should protect us, since the drug has been tested for both safety and effectiveness. This is not always the case, however. Many things can go wrong in even an FDA-approved study.

Safety is not an absolute. Nearly all drugs have the potential for side effects, long term toxicity, and allergic reactions. If drugs had to be proven absolutely safe, few if any drugs would be approved. Rather, the risk is assessed in relation to the benefit, and the risk-benefit ratio is determined subjectively by someone other than the patient who will actually be taking it. The danger in this lies in the fact that many people look to the government to protect them from harm, and blindly trust drugs that should not be trusted.

About half of all drugs that have been approved in the past are no longer on the market due to serious and sometimes fatal side effects. Since the testing process has not changed appreciably during this time, what does this say about the safety of drugs being approved today?

Many side effects of drugs and treatments do not show up for decades, and thus are not part of the approval process. This doesn't help those who may now have to deal with the residual side effects.

The FDA doesn't track problems with the drug by itself but does so through the drug company's own reports. Having drug companies monitor and report problems with their own products is rather like having the fox guard the henhouse.

So the FDA are the bad guys?
Although some questions have been raised regarding the FDA's motives, our intent is not FDA-bashing. A major purpose of this chapter - and this book - is to help the reader understand that blind trust in any agency, governmental or otherwise, giving up your own personal responsibility, is often not wise. The more knowledge you have, the more you can look out for your own best interests.

Can studies be done incorrectly?

There are many ways in which a study can be done incorrectly. Some studies have no controls, so there is nothing to compare the results to. Let's say that 45% of those taking Drug X experienced headache relief. Since it is quite possible that at least that many people could have their headaches go away without taking any medication, that 45% figure really says nothing about the efficacy of Drug X. A clinical study without controls, with rare exceptions, is a poorly designed study and the results are invalid.

Another problem is using a particular population for testing and extrapolating the results to the general population without further testing. Several large studies of middle-aged men with high blood pressure and heart problems showed that these men benefited from certain medications or dietary changes. Those who did the study erroneously figured that since nobody wanted heart problems, the recommendations fit everybody else, even women who tend to have *low* blood pressure.

Although the drug Valium is prescribed in much greater quantities for women than for men, the drug studies were done on men. Many studies are done only on men, with the reasoning that women have hormonal cycles which might confuse the results. In addition, women of childbearing age are routinely excluded from studies due to possible fetal risk. This exclusion of women from much of the testing makes no practical sense in light of the fact that women, with their hormonal cycles and potential for pregnancy, take at least half of all medication sold or prescribed.

Another problem in many studies lies in the choice of placebo, usually lactose, or milk sugar. Many people are allergic to lactose, and sugar of any sort can feed a fungus infection, so the placebo is not really inert as it should be in a valid study. Therefore worsening of symptoms in the placebo group may be due in part to the lactose rather than to the lack of the active drug.

A study may be poorly designed and give erroneous results. For example, a well-publicized study done in Finland in 1994 involved the administration of very low doses of the antioxidant vitamins A and E to long-time smokers to determine any protective effect. Not surprisingly, none was found, since the vitamin dosages were too low and given for too short a time to have any appreciable effect on people whose bodies were damaged by decades of smoking.

Why do some study results appear to conflict?

Sometimes a study which appears to have only one variable actually has two or more. A study done in the U.S. showed that low doses of aspirin prevented heart attacks in men. A similar study in Europe demonstrated that aspirin had no such effect. A closer look at the U.S. study showed that aspirin buffered with magnesium was used, on the erroneous assumption that magnesium was an inert (non-active) ingredient. The Europeans used plain aspirin without magnesium. The U.S. study therefore had two variables, aspirin and magnesium, and the favorable results likely caused by magnesium were wrongly attributed to aspirin. This shows that:

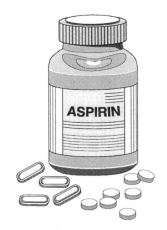

- *Studies with more than one variable are nearly useless.*

- *It is possible to have more than one variable without realizing it.*

- *Improperly done studies often account for conflicting results of two or more studies which are superficially similar.*

Another reason that some studies appear to conflict lies in the choice of test population. If one heart study looks at men and another looks at both men and women, or if one looks at healthy volunteers while another studies those with heart disease, the different studies may well reach different conclusions about what slows down heart disease. The results may not be incorrect; it is the interpretation of them which may be the problem.

Some studies look at too small a population sample and come up with biased results. For example, if you looked at a random sample of ten people, and eight of them were blondes, you might conclude incorrectly that 80% of the total population are blondes. Counting the number of blondes in a random sample of 500 people would yield results more applicable to the general population.

Is the double-blind placebo-controlled study the only accurate type?

Many critics of supportive health practices base their criticism on the fact that no FDA-approved clinical trials have been done. However, it is often not possible to test a treatment this way. Consider psychoanalysis, generally accepted as being a valid treatment for many psychological problems. To do a "proper" clinical trial of psychoanalysis, it would be necessary to give half of the patients real psychoanalysis and the other half fake psychoanalysis, with neither the doctor nor the patient knowing which was which. This would clearly be impossible to do. Other therapies which are highly individualized such as homeopathy, or for which there would be no meaningful placebo such as chiropractic, could likewise not be tested appropriately with a double-blind placebo-controlled study.

Double-blind studies are Western in thought, and concrete, and are usually inappropriate for evaluating Eastern or energy medicine. Using the wrong type of test for evaluation is like checking a car's electrical system to find out why it is leaking oil. If an EKG (heart rhythm test) does not detect a broken bone, this does not mean that the EKG does not work, it means that the wrong type of test is being used. Similarly, the standard clinical trial is the wrong type of test for evaluating many supportive therapies.

> **The standard clinical trial is the wrong type of test for evaluating many supportive therapies.**

What is anecdotal evidence?

Critics of alternative therapies often scornfully point out that only anecdotal evidence of the therapy's efficacy is available. An anecdote is a story, and anecdotal evidence is the report from one, a few, or many people that they experienced relief from a treatment.

Can anecdotal evidence be valid?

Consider the following statements:

- My uncle's secretary reported that she felt less fatigued after having her mercury fillings removed.

- 93% of 3000 people who filled out an anonymous questionnaire, with the results audited by an independent survey firm, reported a marked lessening of fatigue on removal of their mercury fillings.

The second statement is clearly more reliable and more applicable to the general population, yet critics of anecdotal evidence often would not distinguish between the two statements. However, such a survey is certainly valid evidence that the treatment, in this case mercury filling removal, is one which could clearly benefit a large majority of the population.

Many of those who claim that anecdotal evidence is invalid possibly have a protected interest or an ax to grind. They may want to refute any reason given for using supportive treatments. Scoffing at anecdotal evidence even when standard clinical testing is inappropriate provides a convenient smoke screen to hide behind.

Is the FDA unbiased?

The weight of evidence makes it appear as if, to an increasing degree, the FDA reflects the interests of the financially and politically powerful pharmaceutical companies rather than those of the consumer. However, more recently the FDA seems to be giving the pharmaceutical industry a hard time as well. There seem to be plans afoot to restrict our right to use nutritional supplements by redefining a drug as anything which has a health benefit, rather than a substance which can be harmful. In fact, a new law, which went into effect July 1994, sharply restricts health claims which can be made for supplements, with threats of jail and fines used as incentives to compliance.

The FDA is attempting to require full-scale clinical trials on substances which have been used without incident for thousands of years. If they succeed in passing this legislation, many nutritional supplements would not be available except by prescription, and most doctors do not know how to use them and so will likely prescribe drugs instead, which is what the FDA seems to want. The FDA which took the amino acid tryptophan off the market after an incident involving one contaminated batch is the same FDA which allowed mass marketing of the drug Prozac for the same use (anti-anxiety) after only six weeks of testing. There seems to be a pattern here. The question you must ask yourself is, can you really count on the FDA to represent your interests?

The price of freedom is eternal vigilance -- be aware of what's going on. Be informed and let your elected representatives know your viewpoint if you feel your rights are in jeopardy.

Can't nutritional supplements be tested in clinical trials?

Technically, nutritional supplements can be tested clinically, with vitamin placebos and double-blind trials. However, clinical trials can take years and cost millions of dollars per product. A company making supplements would not be inclined to spend that kind of money on a product which cannot be patented and thus has a low profit margin. Such a company would never recoup the testing money and would soon be bankrupt.

It is possible that the FDA's real intention is raising prescription drug sales by eliminating the competition. Regardless of intention, this is in effect what could be the likely outcome, and in the process your freedom of choice in using substances which have been proven safe over hundreds, and in some cases thousands, of years will be seriously compromised.

A plan to make supplements available by prescription only would raise supplement prices beyond affordability for the majority of American citizens. For example, when Captomer (DMSA) became a drug the wholesale price went from about $20 a bottle to about $200, a ten-fold or 1000% increase.

Are there other sources of bias in studies?

As noted, a study can cost millions of dollars. This money has to come from somewhere, and a corporation would not be inclined to pay this much money if it did not stand to gain financially from its investment, or, more accurately, from the achievement and documentation of certain results. Given this, it is unlikely that there are many studies which are **not** biased.

Bias in this sense refers to the fact that a certain outcome is desired from the studies, and the study may be designed to increase the odds of that outcome. Thus there are:

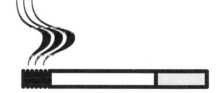

- *Studies funded by tobacco companies showing that cigarette smoke may not be as harmful as popularly believed.*

- *Studies funded by chemical companies showing that chemicals contribute little if at all to cancer development.*

- *Studies funded by the sugar and candy industries showing that sugar does not lead to obesity and dental cavities.*

- *Studies done by drug manufacturers showing that the tested drug they produced is safe and effective.*

The Council for Tobacco Research, a neutral-sounding name, is financed by tobacco manufacturers. By neither denying nor confirming that tobacco causes cancer and other diseases, they have kept the controversy alive for over forty years in spite of overwhelming evidence of the health risks. About 434,000 people die per year of smoking-related causes, yet four billion dollars per year is spent on advertising promoting smoking and tobacco products. Other chemical and dental lobbying groups use similar tactics, including the funding of questionable studies, to generate controversy and keep their products on the market. Public health is sacrificed on the altar of profit.

One such questionable study was done by the company that makes Bayer aspirin. In a deliberately poorly designed study, fish oils were shown to have little or no protective or curative effect on cardiovascular problems. Bayer paid a great deal to have these study results publicized, and results from over forty studies showing fish oils to have a beneficial effect were ignored because the groups funding these studies did not have the money that Bayer had for publicity. Bayer then conducted the well-known aspirin study described earlier in this chapter, and again spent a lot of money promoting the results. Having used a questionable study to "prove" that fish oils were useless against heart disease, they then used another questionable study "proving", apparently, that heart problems are the result of an aspirin deficiency.

Testing bias is often found in studies sponsored by trade groups, special interest groups, and chemical societies. The American Council on Science and Health (ACSH) -- which sound like an unbiased agency representing "we the people" -- is funded by many junk food, pharmaceutical, and chemical manufacturers, including Ciba Giegy, Searle, and Pfizer (pharmaceuticals); General Mills, PepsiCo, and Kraft (processed foods); DuPont, Union Carbide, and Dow (chemicals), among many others [2]. Not surprisingly, their studies find that no food, drug, or chemical is harmful if consumed in moderation, in contradiction of most other studies and common sense. Some groups have deceptive neutral sounding names such as Consumer Alert, but are funded by companies that have an interest in the publication of biased findings. Big business corporations are forming front groups to influence legislators [2]. There are 40,000 lobbyists and 23,000 special interest groups that have a lot to gain financially by misleading the public.

There are "quackbuster" organizations and individuals in the news who go after and denounce alternative treatments (i.e. those which don't involve drugs or surgery) which have proven to be helpful and safe but which don't happen to be FDA approved. These same individuals say nothing at all about the sometime ineffectiveness of, as well as the harmful side effects of, orthodox treatments such as cancer chemotherapy. It might be an interesting exercise to find out what vested interests are signing the (probably large) paychecks of these people.

Given the high stakes involved, it is not surprising that deliberate fraud in testing exists [3,4].

In one study of monosodium glutamate (MSG), a food additive connected with numerous reaction symptoms, volunteers were accepted into the study only after they answered "no" to a long list of questions regarding both general health and problems relating to restaurant meals. This virtually ensured that the 71 study participants would not react to MSG, "proving" absolutely nothing applicable to the general population. The study was funded by a group called the International Glutamate Technical Committee [5].

In another study, funded by Merck and Co., a pharmaceutical giant which manufactures the prostate drug Proscar, it was found that the herb *serenoa repens*, or saw palmetto berries, was not effective in treating prostate disorders, although studies that were not funded by a pharmaceutical competitor found that saw palmetto was indeed effective and without the drug's side effects [5].

What studies are <u>not</u> being done?

It is equally interesting to note which studies are **not** being done. There were studies in the 1930s showing that fluoride added to drinking water reduces tooth decay in children. These studies have been thoroughly disproved, but while there has been much gathering of existing data to show the link between fluoride, lack of effect on tooth decay, and fluoride-related health problems, no major controlled clinical study has been done. Why? There is nobody who would have enough to gain financially by proving that fluoride is ineffective and dangerous to fund such a study.

The American Dental Association would have much to gain in the way of silencing its critics by showing once and for all that mercury is harmless, as they claim. They easily have the financial resources to fund such a study, if they believed that a study which would hold up under scrutiny would actually prove that mercury is not dangerous. Yet this is not being done. The lack of such a study provides information in itself.

What other types of bias are there besides those in studies?

Bias is inherent in professions such as medicine. When a person invests heavily of themselves - in time, money and talent - they are strongly motivated to hold on to the beliefs that were installed as a result of this investment. For example, the owners of pharmaceutical or tobacco companies, who have spent many years and millions of dollars building up their companies, are likely to hold on to their belief that their product is beneficial or at least not harmful, even in the face of mounting evidence to the contrary or even common sense. Those who have gone to professional schools such as medical and dental schools have likewise invested much of their time, effort and money in certain belief systems such as "Drugs and surgery are the only ways to cure disease" or "Mercury amalgam fillings are harmless", and they have a lot of motivation to hold on to their ideas and biases.

There are three steps to creating bias:

1. **Sacrifice** - a person will be less likely to give up something they have sacrificed for, whether it is a possession, a company, or an idea. The more you give up to get something, the harder you will fight to keep it.

2. **Invest** - After years of time, money, energy and talent, it is again hard to have to give up something and admit you were in error.

3. **Own** - Once something is yours, and you identify with it, it is hard to give it up.

Since nearly everyone has invested heavily in something, it is very rare to find a person who is not biased.

How can professional education resemble a cult?

Any belief system with most or all of these characteristics can be said to be a cult:

- There can be a central living person - a charismatic leader, guru, or priest - that followers worship and try to emulate. This person makes the rules that you are expected to obey. Without this person's leadership the organization may well fall apart.

- Considerable amounts of your money or the value of your work could end up invested in the organization.

- You could be told what to believe, and limited in what you are allowed to read or what other points of view you are allowed to embrace.

- Information that conflicts with that which the organization wants to promote is denounced as being wrong and unacceptable. You could be strongly discouraged from making up your own mind. Those who promote conflicting information are to be shunned, and rules are often made to keep their "heretical ideas" away.

- People are kept isolated from family members as much as possible, and isolation from the outside world in general is typical of a cult.

- Cults are known for using sleep deprivation and poor nutrition to keep their adherents' minds too clouded to think or question.

An organization does not have to be religious to exert the same controlling characteristics of a cult. It's not surprising to realize that advanced education and professional schools have some characteristics strongly reminiscent of those associated with a cult mentality. With the possible exception of the strong leader, all of the other characteristics of a cult mentality fit very closely:

- Money, investment - many schools are so expensive that students are often in debt for years or even decades to pay off the loans. The only way they can make this much money is to actively promote that which they were taught.

- Students are kept too busy to read any but required texts or attend any but required lectures. Questioning and other points of view are actively squelched.

- Isolation - Students, by virtue of their demanding and rigorous regimen, find that almost the only human contact they have may be those within the academic culture.

- Sleep deprivation - Students often have to study through the night to keep up with their workload.

- Poor nutrition - Students are usually at the mercy of the school cafeteria, lacking the time or money for alternatives. Nor are nutritional studies on most curricula of medical students, except to a cursory degree, to provide some sort of balance to the allopathic orientation.

In fact, the above scenario closely parallels the way mainstream medical doctors are educated. In addition to the above points common to most professional education, laws are made which restrict alternative practitioners (keeping out conflicting information, in many cases forcefully and punitively). And 24- to 36-hour shifts are not uncommon during residency (sleep deprivation).

The isolation from the outside world and their families is so total due to the 24 hour a day immersion in the mainstream medical school and hospital that marriages often don't survive. [6]

Is this how your doctor, the one you trust your health and welfare to, was educated? Think about it.

Summary

A study is an experiment designed to test something that a research person or team would like to prove or disprove. The conclusion reached may or may not be correct. Studies may be improperly designed either inadvertently or to bias the results for profit.

Understanding the study process in general will help you to evaluate study results based on whether the study was done thoroughly and appropriately. This understanding will in turn allow you to know whether results can be believed, and to modify your decisions accordingly.

Drug trials, also called clinical trials, go through several stages. These stages are mandated by the Food and Drug Association (FDA) to theoretically show that a drug is both safe and effective. However, the FDA can determine on an individual basis how closely these guidelines must be followed.

Double-blind placebo-controlled trials have their place in drug testing, but this type of testing is often not appropriate for evaluating many supportive therapies.

There is much evidence that suggests that the FDA reflects the interests of the financially and politically powerful pharmaceutical companies rather than those of the consumer.

The millions of dollars a study costs has to come from somewhere, and a corporation would not be inclined to pay this much money if it did not stand to gain financially from it. Given this, it is unlikely that there are many studies which are **not** biased. Bias in this sense refers to the fact that a certain outcome is desired from the studies, and the study may be designed to increase the odds of that outcome.

Believe study results at your own risk. If you feel you are floundering and now don't know who you can trust, you will rarely err by doing that which is most natural and best supports the way your body was designed to work.

References and Resources

- Breggin, Peter R., *Toxic Psychiatry*, St. Martin's Press, New York, 1991.

- Megalli, Mark, and Andy Friedman, *Masks of Deception: Corporate Front Groups in America*, Essential Information, Washington DC, 1991.

- Braithwaite, J., *Corporate Crime in the Pharmaceutical Industry*, Routledge and Kegan Paul, Melbourne Australia.

The Supporters

GENERAL PRINCIPLES OF NUTRITION

More Than What You Eat

Chances are you have read and heard a great deal of conflicting information about diet and nutrition.   Let's test your nutritional knowledge:

1. Cooked or raw?
   - a. Raw food is healthier
   - b. Well-cooked food is healthier
   - c. Lightly cooked food is healthier
   - d. A variety of raw and cooked foods is best

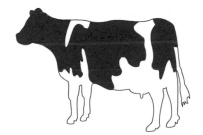

2. Cows' milk is
   - a. Good for you
   - b. Not needed after weaning
   - c. Bad for you
   - d. Not a problem if you are not allergic

3. Reducing the cholesterol in the diet
   - a. Reduces body cholesterol
   - b. Does not reduce body cholesterol
   - c. Tends to reduce body cholesterol, but not directly

4. Calories
   - a. Are the only things that matter in weight loss
   - b. Are important only for a minority of people
   - c. Are not very important for weight loss

5. Fruit
   - a. Is one of the necessary food groups
   - b. Should be eliminated because it causes yeast growth
   - c. Can be tolerated by some people
   - d. Is best eaten by itself

6. Vegetable and fruit juices
   - a. Are good for you because they contain beneficial enzymes
   - b. Are bad for you because they contain sugar

7. Vitamin and mineral supplements
    a. Are necessary
    b. Should be taken for insurance
    c. Are not necessary
    d. Can be harmful
    e. Can be useful, harmful, or necessary depending on individual needs

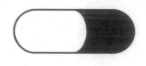

8. Oils and fats are
    a. Bad for you
    b. Necessary
    c. Good or bad depending on type
    d. Of no concern if your weight and cholesterol are normal

9. Eggs are
    a. Full of cholesterol and therefore bad
    b. Full of nutrients and therefore good

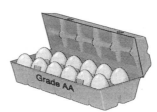

10. Stir-fried foods are
    a. Good because they are not overcooked
    b. Bad because they contain oil
    c. Bad because they contain heated oil

11. Pastas and breads are
    a. Simple carbohydrates
    b. Intermediate carbohydrates
    c. Complex carbohydrates

The answers to these questions may surprise you. In some cases the answers are indefinite, or different answers may be correct depending on circumstances. These answers are discussed in detail in the chapters that make up this book section.

1. (d.) Raw or cooked? Raw food contains enzymes which are needed by the body for digestion and other functions. Although some digestive enzymes are found in the body, a diet consisting of only cooked or microwaved foods will quickly deplete them. On the other hand, raw foods are difficult for some people to digest, and they pass through the body without being broken down completely. A mixture of raw and cooked foods is usually best. Cooked vegetables should be lightly cooked or steamed, never overcooked.

2. (c.) Cows' milk is intended for consumption by calves, not humans. While human milk is not needed after weaning, cows' milk is not usually digested well by humans of any age. Cow's milk can promote allergies in those who do not already have them.

3. (c.) Cholesterol is made in the body in the amount needed, and dietary cholesterol plays little part in this. Fats and especially sugars contribute to the making of cholesterol, and cutting down foods with cholesterol will usually incidentally reduce the amount of fat in the diet.

4. (b.) Excess calories are the main cause of weight gain for only a minority of people. Most people who are overweight are retaining water to dilute toxins in the body.

5. (b., c., and d.) Fruit contains sugar and ferments in the intestines, which contributes to yeast growth. Some people who are very healthy can tolerate fruit with no adverse effects. Fruit is best eaten by itself so that it will quickly be eliminated. Fruit eaten with other foods will slow its progress through the intestines, increasing fermentation.

6. (b.) Fruit and vegetable juices do indeed contain beneficial enzymes, but these enzymes can be obtained without the overabundance of harmful sugar by eating raw vegetables.

7. (e.) is most nearly correct because it takes into account individual differences in vitamin and mineral needs.

8. (b. and c. combined) Essential fatty acids are necessary for the body's proper functioning, and these are found in oils which are fresh, expeller or cold-pressed, not rancid, and not heated. Saturated or hydrogenated (semisolid) fats, old rancid oils, and heated oils (heated in processing or cooking) are harmful and of no benefit.

9. (b.) Eggs have gotten a bad press due to their high cholesterol content, but cholesterol in the body is only slightly related to cholesterol in the diet. Eggs are one of the most complete sources of protein, more so even than meat.

10. (c.) Foods quickly fried in oil are crisp and nutritious, but heating the oil will cause it to undergo a chemical change from a nutrient to a toxin. An approximation of stir frying can be done with water or broth, retaining the nutrition benefits without the toxic oil.

11. (b.) Sugars are simple carbohydrates which should be eliminated from the diet, and whole grains are beneficial complex carbohydrates. Pastas and breads are in the in-between category of intermediate carbohydrates.

How did you do on this quiz? There is so much nutritional misinformation around that many people may not have done well on the quiz. The chapters in this Supporters section will explain many of these references and will help clear up many of the areas of confusion and explode many of the myths about nutrition.

Is there a difference between diet and nutrition?

Many people use the terms "diet" and "nutrition" interchangeably. This is incorrect or at least incomplete; diet is only one component of nutrition. Diet is what you eat, including supplements and beverages. Nutrition is that which you are actually able to utilize from your diet. It is possible to eat all the right foods and avoid all the bad ones and still be undernourished.

> **Nutrition is more than just what you eat.**

What is nutrition?

Nutrition can be broken down into four components:

- *Diet*   *What you eat*
- *Digestion*   *What is broken down into its primary parts*
- *Absorption*   *What passes through the intestinal wall into the blood*
- *Utilization*   *What the body actually uses at a cellular level*

Nutrition, therefore, is diet, minus that which is not digested, minus that which is not absorbed, minus that which is not utilized. What remains is the actual food that is used by your cells.

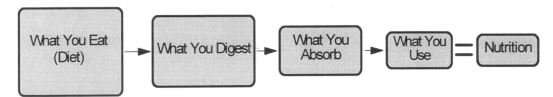

After food is eaten, it must be broken down by a combination of chemical (enzymes) and physical (mixing and moving) digestive processes. The body can use only the basic nutrients - glucose, amino acids, fatty acids, vitamins, and minerals. If these are not broken down or extracted from the food eaten, the food will complete its digestive journey without doing you a bit of good. If you have ever seen whole food in your stool or recognizable pieces such as grains, peas, or seeds, poor digestion my be contributing to nutritional deficiencies and resulting health problems.

After digestion, food must be absorbed through the wall of the small intestine (and sometimes the stomach) into the bloodstream, and from there into the cells. Even if nutrients get this far, they can still float around uselessly without the fourth step, utilization.

As with everything else in the body, the basic nutrients do not exist in isolation. For example, sunlight is necessary for the conversion and absorption of vitamin D. And vitamin C (along with bioflavonoids, its cofactors) is necessary for iron to be used by the cells. As you can see, all four steps are necessary for proper nourishment of the cells which make up your body.

How important is nutrition?

Nutrition is considered by many to be "...the single most important component of preventive health care." Diet has been associated with both the cause and the treatment of cancer, heart disease, diabetes, stroke, hypertension, arteriosclerosis, and cirrhosis of the liver [1].

Dr. Joel Wallach stated that nearly all deaths (other than accidents) are related to nutritional deficiencies [2]. However, nutrition alone won't fix most problems. Toxicology and microbiology (parasites) usually need to be addressed to achieve lasting benefit.

Former Surgeon General C. Everett Koop has estimated that, of 2.1 million annual U.S. deaths, 1.6 million, or about 75%, are related to inadequate nutrition [3].

For example, 39% of hypertensives were shown in a recent study to be able to use nutrition instead of blood pressure medication to normalize their blood pressure for over four years [4].

Everybody's a nutrition expert! So who's really right?
Information from many sources, including this book, often appear to conflict with each other. For every book or magazine article that says that fruit, juices, eggs, meat, butter, margarine, bread, or milk are bad for you, there seem to be an equal number of sources saying these are health-promoting. How can you know what to believe?

The problem with many of these sources is not necessarily incorrect information, but the assumption that all nutrition information is one-size-fits-all, or that there are silver-bullet solutions. Suppose you went to the doctor, and he gave you a prescription for medication before finding out what was wrong with you. This is obviously not an effective way to practice medicine. Yet nutritionists routinely say "eat this, don't eat that" and expect the information to apply to everybody. Just as no one medication will help all people who are sick, very few items of nutritional information will meet the needs of everyone. For example:

- Fruit and juices are a good source of nutrients and vital enzymes. However, people with a yeast problem should avoid these as they tend to feed fungus.

- Dairy products contain nutrients, but are also yeast feeders as well as being allergenic for many people.

- Salt intake should be restricted in many, but not all, cases of high blood pressure. In fact, some people, especially those on salt-restricted diets, may be *deficient* in sodium, and this deficiency could actually lead to high blood pressure in some cases.

- It is better to have low cholesterol levels (less than 200 mg/dl) if you have cardiovascular problems. However, low cholesterol levels have been associated with a higher risk of certain cancers. To further confuse matters, the amount of cholesterol in foods has very little effect on your blood cholesterol, while the intake of foods such as sugar can actually raise cholesterol levels more than eggs (poached or soft-boiled) or hamburger.

As you can see, popular health beliefs such as restricting salt, not eating eggs, eating lots of fruit, or keeping your cholesterol level down are valid for some people but not for everyone. The attempt to fit certain nutritional wisdom to the entire population accounts for many of the conflicting claims.

> **A diet that is optimal for someone else may not be optimal for you.**

One nutrient line, put out by Professional Preference, has four customized products to address some of these differences. These products combine vitamins, minerals, amino acids and herbs.

- ***Perfect Equation for Women***

- *Perfect Equation for Men*

- *Hi Balance for those with high blood pressure over 120/80 or who tend toward weight gain.*

- *Lo Balance for those with low blood pressure under 120/80 or low energy and malabsorption .*

How much of an oyster shell do you think you can digest?

Another source of conflict is a reliance on laboratory analysis. For example, oyster shells have a lot of calcium according to lab tests, and are sometimes recommended on this basis, but this calcium is nearly indigestible or useless in the body.

What really works nutritionally?

Another problem lies in the analysis of nutritional information by those who do not have enough training in how the body works as well as an understanding of biochemistry to be able to put all the pieces together accurately. The evidence for what does work can be found in the improvement in both symptoms and blood chemistries of thousands of patients who have followed the recommendations in this book.

Your particular health needs, deficiencies, age, gender, digestion, metabolism, food sensitivities, and toxic burdens will dictate to a large extent what your nutritional needs are. Information in this book will help you determine what type of diet is optimal for **you**.

What are some differences between men and women?

Men and women are not created equal, nutritionally speaking. Different hormonal composition leads to different nutritional needs in some respects. For example, women may need more magnesium, potassium and iron than men to support them through their menstrual cycle, while men often need extra zinc, which is lost in semen. Zinc supports the prostate; since prostate cancer is the number-one cancer in men, it is best to support the prostate before there is trouble. As the cliché goes, an ounce of prevention is worth a pound of cure.

	High Blood Pressure	Low Blood Pressure
Men	80%	20%
Women	20%	80%

As another example of gender differences, women tend to burn out (chronic fatigue, for example), while men tend to blow out (heart attacks, strokes). In general, women burn out their adrenals with worry, while men blow out with anger and spurts of adrenaline. To further confuse the picture, a man with hypertension (high blood pressure) and a woman with chronic fatigue may have the same underlying cause. Ideally, nutritional supplementation would take gender differences into account.

What are some other differences that should be taken into account?

- **Body type** is another consideration. For example, the amino acid aspartic acid can be beneficial to someone who is overweight, since it turns fat into energy. However, someone who is low in body fat (although not necessarily underweight) would be advised to avoid aspartic acid, as it can take fat from the myelin sheath surrounding the nerves. This can affect the nervous system and lead to multiple sclerosis-like symptoms. (Aspartic acid is in Aspartame, or NutraSweet, which is found as an artificial sweetener in many products on the market today. Let the buyer beware.)

- **Microbiology** - Having been breastfed populates the intestines with beneficial bacteria which reduce the population of fungus, worms, and parasites. Those who have not been breastfed are more likely to have these various microorganisms, which can take nutrients from your body.

- **Allergies** - Allergics increase the need for certain nutrients.

- **Size** - Larger people need more calories and other nutrients because they have more cells to feed.

- **Age** - At an early age, calories for growth, carbohydrates for energy, and nutrients for bone and brain development are most crucial. Antioxidants such as vitamins A, C, and E and other nutrients to prevent or slow down degenerative diseases are more important in later years.

- **Endocrine patterns** - Glands, such as the thyroid which requires iodine for proper function, may have higher or lower needs for certain nutrients based on high, low, or normal activity.

- **Digestion** - Certain foods such as beans or raw vegetables may be wonderfully nutritious for most people. However, an insufficiency of hydrochloric acid or certain digestive enzymes necessitate a change in diet to optimize nutrition and prevent discomfort such as gas.

- **Metabolism** - Some people burn off calories and convert food to nutrients faster than others, and intake should be adjusted accordingly.

- **Other nutrients** - Balance is necessary for optimal functioning. For example, if a person has a high sodium (salt) intake, more potassium will be needed for balance. In another example, too much iron can lower zinc and copper levels.

- **Drugs** - Many drugs destroy, reduce the effectiveness of, or increase the need for, certain nutrients. A smoker, for example, is more likely to be deficient in most nutrients than a nonsmoker with the same diet.

- **Toxic burdens** - Other toxic burdens, such as heavy metals (e.g. from dental fillings), increase nutrient needs, especially for minerals such as zinc due to fight-for-site reactions as discussed in the Metal Toxicity chapter in *Surviving The Toxic Crisis*.

- **Stress** - Stress increases nutrient needs, especially for the B vitamins and vitamin A.

- **Activity level** - The more physically active a person is, the more nutrients are needed, especially calories which are burned up as fuel, and electrolytes (minerals) which are lost through sweat and urine.

- **Illness** - Nutrient needs increase in general when illness is present. A person with a cold needs much more vitamins A and C and bioflavonoids, the minerals zinc, iodine, and copper, and the amino acid lysine. There are optimal diets for people with certain diseases, as detailed in the *Alternative Medicine* book [5] listed at the end of this chapter.

Should people who live in different areas eat differently?

The nutrients that you need to handle local weather, parasites, and overall environment are best found in foods which naturally grow in that area, especially if they are eaten at the time they naturally ripen. This is called bioregional farming.

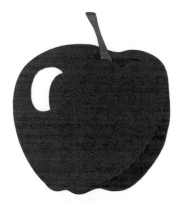

For example, apples grow in the northeastern quarter of the U.S., the part of the country with the coldest winters. The apples ripen in the fall, just before winter. Apples contain sugars which raise the triglyceride level, which in turn raises the insulating fat level and thickens the blood. Winter's cold causes shivering, which stimulates the release of triglycerides to keep warm. Apples, therefore, are best suited to people who live in the climate where the apples grow. Apples eaten in sunny California, however, can cause problems and weight gain due to the raising of the triglyceride level.

Tropical fruits such as papayas and guavas grow in tropical regions where the weather doesn't freeze in winter and parasites are a problem. Such fruits have a high level of enzymes which help to kill the parasites in the body.

Are there any nutritional rules of thumb which fit everyone?

There are some basic rules regarding nutrition agreed upon by nearly everyone, including the authors and many research sources used in this book:

- Food should be as whole, natural, and unprocessed as possible.

- Refined sugar, white flour, processed foods, and most food additives such as nitrates and MSG should be reduced or eliminated.

- Most food should be eaten raw or lightly cooked, but not overcooked.

- Nearly everyone (barring rare conditions or allergies) should eat complex carbohydrates, vegetables, and complete proteins.

What kind of diet are we supposed to have?

A look at human teeth is an excellent indication of the type of diet that we are intended to have, the claims of vegetarians notwithstanding. We have three types of teeth: the canines of meat-eating animals, the incisors (front teeth) of plant-eating animals, and the molars of grain- and nut-eating animals. We are apparently intended to eat all three types of foods.

What about vegetarian diets?

A word about vegetarian diets - proponents of these diets have many valid reasons for following their regimens such as:

- *One can feed about sixteen people on the amount of grain needed to produce enough meat for one person*

- *Slaughtering methods can be brutal to the animals*

- *Meat is more harmful than healthful due to additives such as steroids and antibiotics*

There are a number of different types of vegetarian diets - live or raw food, macrobiotic, vegan, and those which are semi-vegetarian due to the addition of dairy products (lactovegetarian), eggs (ovovegetarian), and/or seafood. A vegetarian diet is probably more healthful overall than the standard American diet. A vegetarian diet along with exercise and stress-reduction measures can prevent and even reverse heart disease [6].

However, there are two drawbacks to a strict (no animal products at all) vegetarian diet:

- It is difficult to get all nutrients, especially vitamin B12, manganese and iron unless one is very knowledgeable and careful.

- Some people, due to digestive or other problems, are not able to get all the nutrients they need without animal products no matter how careful they are.

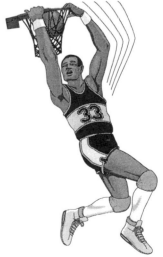

Bill Walton, a pro basketball player with the San Diego Clippers for ten years, had recurrent broken foot injuries. He was a strict vegetarian, and after a while he became manganese deficient. Manganese is a necessary mineral, and a person who is manganese deficient can't assimilate calcium to make bones strong. He added meat back into his diet, and got his career back with a Boston team.

One patient, a karate instructor in his 30s, followed a vegetarian diet for years. He was so tired he could hardly stand, got frequent colds, was very thin, and his hormones were off. Adding meat protein to his diet remedied this within a few weeks. He regained full energy and started putting on muscle weight.

The body is like a bank account. You can't keep making withdrawals without making deposits.

Some people who have health problems such as cancer would be better off on a vegetarian or macrobiotic diet. Others can do well on either type of diet. Many people, however, need animal products for optimum nutrition, and these people may need to choose between their ideology and their health. Only they can make this decision.

What are the basic diet rules?

The basic diet rule is: eat more of the good stuff, and reduce or eliminate the bad stuff. The good stuff includes complex carbohydrates, raw or lightly steamed vegetables, complete proteins such as eggs and white meat, and healthful oils that are not rancid, heated or hydrogenated. These are necessary for life, and are discussed in detail in the following chapters in this section.

A corollary of the basic diet rule is: the closer to its original nature a food is, the better. The more a food is refined, processed, stripped, devitalized, technologically manipulated, or mixed with additives, the worse it is. There are a few exceptions to this - we are not equipped to digest whole raw grains straight from the field, raw meat may contain parasites, and some preservatives such as antioxidants can make food safer. The general rule, however, holds in most cases.

Why are bad foods sold?

If refined foods are so bad for us, and government agencies exist to protect us, then why are these foods, or nonfoods, sold? Consumer demand dictates what is sold, as should be the case, and most people buy food for taste and trust that it will keep them alive and healthy if they think about nutrition at all. There is also much consumer miseducation, propagated by advertisers' claims. Many if not most people erroneously believe, for example:

- *"enriched" white bread is just as good as whole wheat bread*
- *sugar is harmless unless one is diabetic*
- *milk is necessary for all children and even adults*
- *taking one multivitamin supplement a day allows people to eat what they want without fear of deficiency.*

Another reason for the sale of refined and processed foods is their longer shelf life, which often translates into lower costs for the consumer. What does longer shelf life mean? Bugs and microbes, if they get into food and eat it and multiply, will spoil food and end its shelf life. Bacteria and bugs know what is and isn't food, and there is little in white flour, sugar, most commercial cereals, or irradiated milk that would interest them. There is little in these foods that would interest our cells, either. For thousands of years we were able to make bread rise with certain bacteria as leaven, but today's flour is so depleted that yeast is now needed to make bread rise. If food can go bad, that's good.

> **If food can go bad, it's good.**

How can good food be made bad after purchase?

Foods can also be devitalized, or deprived of nutritional value, by the consumer after purchase. Although cooking makes most foods more digestible, there is a tradeoff in terms of nutrients lost. It is nearly always undesirable to overcook foods. Vegetables and grains boiled to a mush, or meat cooked until tough, has lost many of the enzymes and other living nutritional components that these foods originally contained. Microwave cooking, although faster than conventional heat, can do other cell damage. Cell mutation of microwaved food is possible. Light and air can also inactivate some enzymes or cause harmful oxidative changes. Food should not be cut, ground, or cooked until ready to use, and should be refrigerated or frozen where appropriate.

Food additives can deplete nutrients. For example, EDTA is often added to frozen vegetables to retain their color, but EDTA, a chelating agent, often strips zinc and other minerals from these foods [7].

Can nutrition help specific ailments?
Many chronic problems and symptoms are caused at least in part by nutrient deficiencies. It follows that remedying the deficiencies will help these ailments to the extent that they are deficiency-related. In addition, many foods and nutrient supplements have been shown to help prevent or treat a large number of ailments. These applications are discussed further throughout this book and the *Alternative Medicine* book [5].

In particular, dietary suggestions are discussed in the chapter on Cancer. Comparison studies of cancer patients who did and did not follow nutritional protocols showed a dramatic difference in favor of nutritional support [8], as detailed in the Cancer chapter.

According to a member of the Academy of Rheumatoid Diseases, over 250,000 people have used nutritional supplements in arthritis treatment, with 80-90% of patients reporting improvement [9].

How is nutrition related to behavior and learning?
Three research studies involving 60,000 delinquent children and teens have linked malnutrition to juvenile delinquency. Anger, depression, tension, fatigue and confusion were all linked to vitamin and mineral deficiencies. Diet modification produced 47-54% lower rates of antisocial behavior, and the simple administration of multiple vitamin/mineral tablets at RDA levels changed most delinquents into normal kids. In a study of 803 public schools, making school lunches more nutritious reduced the number of learning disabled children from 120,000 to 49,000 [10].

Intelligence levels of school children actually rose measurably with vitamin and mineral supplementation, according to *The Lancet*, a well-known and prestigious medical journal [11].

What are the basic nutritional components?
The basic nutrient groups are:

- Macronutrients (macro means large in Greek, and these are taken in large portions) include proteins and amino acids, carbohydrates, and oils.

- Micronutrients (micro means small, and these are taken in small amounts, much less than an ounce) include vitamins and minerals.

- Enzymes and other components are needed for digestion.

- Other things needed for life, but which are not strictly food nutrients, include pure water, air, exercise, light, and sleep.

All of these are discussed in greater detail in the chapters in this book section.

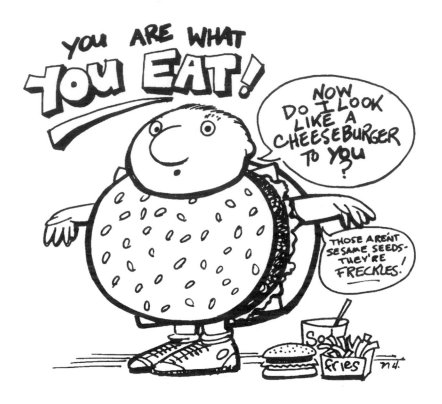

References and Resources

- Airola, Paavo, *How To Get Well*, Health Plus Publishers, Phoenix AZ, 1974.

- Appleton, Nancy, *Secrets of Natural Healing With Food*, Rudra Press, Portland OR, 1995. *Provides a knowledgeable exploration of body chemistry as it relates to diet.*

- Atkins, Robert C., *Dr. Atkins' Nutritional Breakthrough: How To Treat Your Medical Condition Without Drugs*, William Morrow and Co., NY, 1981.

- Balch, James F. and Phyllis A., *Prescription for Nutritional Healing*, Avery Publishing Group Inc., Garden City Park NY, 1990.

- Barnard, Neal, *Eat Right, Live Longer*, Harmony Books, NY, 1995.

- Bland, Jeffrey, *Medical Application of Clinical Nutrition*, Keats Publishing, New Canaan CT, 1983.

- Bland, Jeffrey, *Your Health Under Siege: Using Nutrition to Fight Back*, Greene, 1982.

- Bogert, L. Jean, *Nutrition and Physical Fitness*, W.B. Saunders Co., 7th ed., 1960.

- Braverman, Eric R. and Carl C. Pfeiffer, *The Healing Nutrients Within*, Keats Publishing Inc., New Canaan CT, 1987.

- Broder, Roy, *Discovering Natural Foods*, Woodbridge Press Publishing Co., Santa Barbara CA, 1982.

- The Burton Goldberg Group, *Alternative Medicine: The Definitive Guide*, "Nutritional Supplements", pp. 385-397, Future Medicine Publishing, Puyallup WA, 1994.

- Carlson, Wade, *Hypertension and Your Diet*, Keats Publishing, New Canaan CT, 1990.

- Carper, Jean, *Nutrition Pharmacy*, Bantam Books, NY, 1988.

- Chaitow, Leon, *The Body/Mind Purification Program*, Simon And Schuster, NY, 1990. *Fasting.*

- Colgan, Michael, *The New Nutrition: Medicine For The New Millennium*, Apple Publishing Co. Ltd., Vancouver BC Canada, 1995.

- Davis, Adelle, *Let's Eat Right To Keep Fit*, Harcourt Brace Jovanovich, NY, 1970.

- Diamond, Harvey and Marilyn, *Fit For Life*, Warner Books, NY, 1985.

- Dunne, Lavon J., *Nutrition Almanac*, McGraw-Hill Publishing Co., NY, 3rd edition, 1990.

- *East West Journal*, editors of, *Shopper's Guide to Natural Foods*, Avery Publishing Group, Garden City Park, NY, 1988.

- Garrison, Robert H. and Elizabeth Somer, *The Nutritional Desk Reference*, Keats Publishing Inc., New Canaan CT, 1985.

- Gittleman, Ann Louise, *Super Nutrition for Men and the Women Who Love Them*, M. Evans and Co., Inc., NY, 1996.

- Gruberg, E.R. and S.A. Raymond, *Beyond Cholesterol: Vitamin B6, Arteriosclerosis and Your Heart*, St. Martin's Press, NY, 1981.

- Haas, Elson M., *Staying Healthy With Nutrition*, Celestial Arts Pub., Berkeley CA, 1992.

- Haas, Robert, *Eat Smart, Think Smart*, Harper Collins, NY, 1994.

- Heidenry, Carolyn, *Making the Transition to a Macrobiotic Diet*, Avery Publishing Group, Garden City Park, NY, 1988.

- Heumer, R.P. (ed.), *The Roots of Molecular Medicine: A Tribute to Linus Pauling*, WH Freeman and Co., NY, 1986.

- Hoffer, Abram and Morton Walker, *Nutrients to Age Without Senility*, Keats Pub. Inc., New Canaan CT, 1980.

- Hoffer, Abram and Morton Walker, *Smart Nutrients: A Guide to Nutrients That Can Prevent and Reverse Senility*, Avery Publishing Group, Garden City Park, NY, 1994.

- Hoffer, Abram, *Orthomolecular Medicine For Physicians*, Keats Publishing, New Canaan CT, 1989.

- Hoffman, Jay M., *The Missing Link in the Medical Curriculum*, Professional Press Publishing Co., Valley Center CA, 1981.

- Kilham, Christopher, *The Bread and Circus Whole Food Bible*, Addison-Wesley Publishing Co., Reading MA, 1991. *Discusses how to find relatively safe, additive-free foods.*

- Krause, MV, L. Kathleen Mahan, *Food, Nutrition and Diet Therapy*, W.B.Saunders, Philadelphia PA, 1984.

- Kuchi, Mishio, *The Book of Macrobiotics*, Harper and Row, NY, 1986.

- Lesser, Michael, *Nutrition and Vitamin Therapy*, Parker House, Berkeley CA, 1982.

- Lieberman, Shari, and Nancy P. Bruning, *The Real Vitamin and Mineral Book*, Avery Publishing Group, Garden City Park NY, 1990.

- Mindell, Earl, *Earl Mindell's Safe Eating*, Warner Books, NY, 1987.

- Null, Gary, *The Complete Guide to Health and Nutrition*, Delacorte Press, NY, 1986.

- Ornish, Dean, *Stress, Diet and Your Heart*, Holt, Rinehart and Winston, NY, 1983.

- Ornish, Dean, *Dr. Dean Ornish's Program for Reversing Heard Disease*, Ballantine NY, 1990.

- Passwater, Richard, *Supernutrition*, Dial Press, NY, 1985.

- Pauling, Linus, *How To Live Longer and Feel Better*, Avon Books, NY, 1987.

- Pfeiffer, Carl, *Mental and Elemental Nutrients: A Physician's Guide to Nutrition and Health Care*, Keats Publishing, New Canaan CT, 1975.

- Pfeiffer, Carl, *Nutrition and Mental Illness: An Orthomolecular Approach to Balancing Body Chemistry*, Healing Arts Press, Rochester VT, 1987.

- Price, Weston A., *Nutrition and Physical Degeneration*, Keats Publishing Inc., New Canaan CT, 1945.

- Rector-Page, Linda, *Cooking for Healthy Healing*, Griffin Printing, 2nd ed. 1991. *Cookbook.*

- Rogers, Sherry R., *Tired or Toxic?*, Prestige Publishing, Syracuse NY, 1990.

- Rogers, Sherry R., *You Are What You Ate*, Syracuse NY

- Rose, Mary Swartz, *A Laboratory Handbook for Dietetics*, MacMillan Co., NY, 1921.

- Salaman, Maureen and James F. Scheer, *Foods That Heal*, Statford Publishing, Menlo Park CA, 1989.

- Schauss, Alexander, *Diet, Crime and Delinquency*, Parker House, Berkeley CA, 1980.

- Schmid, R. *Traditional Foods Are Your Best Medicines*, Ocean View Publications, Stratford CT, 1987.

- Smith, Lendon, *Feed Your Kids Right: Dr. Smith's Program For Your Child's Total Health*, McGraw-Hill, NY, 1979.

- Steinman, David, *Diet For A Poisoned Planet*, Ballantine Books, NY, 1990.

- Swank, Roy L. and Barbara Brewer Duncan, *The Multiple Sclerosis Diet Book*, Doubleday, NY, 1987.

- Watson, George, *Nutrition and Your Mind*, Harper and Row, NY, 1972.

- Weissman, JD, *Choose To Live*, Grove Press, NY, 1988.

- Werbach, Melvyn R., *Nutritional Influences on Illness*, Keats Publishing, New Canaan CT, 1988.

- Wigmore, Ann, *Recipes For Longer Life*, Avery Publishing, Garden City Park, NY, 1982.

- Williams, Roger J., *Nutrition Against Disease, Environmental Protection*, Bantam Books, NY, 1971.

- Williams, Roger J., *Nutrition Against Disease: Environmental Prevention*, Bantam Books, NY, 1972.

- Williams, Roger J. and Dwight K. Kalita, *A Physician's Handbook on Orthomolecular Medicine*, Keats Publishing, New Canaan CT, 1979.

- Worthington-Roberts, BS, J. Vermeersch and SR Williams, *Nutrition in Pregnancy and Lactation*, Times/Mirror Mosby College Publishing, St. Louis MO, 1985.

- Wright, Jonathan V., *Dr. Wright's Book of Nutritional Therapy*, Rodale Press, Emmaus PA, 1979.

- Wright, Jonathan V., *Dr. Wright's Guide to Healing With Nutrition*, Keats Publishing Inc., New Canaan CT, 1990.

- **American College of Advancement in Medicine**, P.O. Box 3427, Laguna Hills CA 92654. Phone 714-583-7666. *Provides worldwide listing of practitioners trained in nutritional and preventive medicine, as well as an extensive list of books and articles on nutritional supplementation.*

WEIGHT CONTROL AND CALORIES - EXPLODING THE MYTHS

Why Most Weight Programs Just Don't Work

Things in this chapter that can change your weight - and your health:

- *There are many myths surrounding weight loss. This chapter can explode some of them.*

- *Weight gain or retention is a symptom, not a primary problem. Identify and treat the underlying problem(s) to have lasting success with the symptom.*

- *How you can tell what your primary weight-gain problem is.*

- *Overweight is due to fat in only about 20% of cases.*

- *Some oils can actually help you lose weight.*

- *Weight problems are not about lack of willpower.*

- *Why most weight-loss programs don't work, at least not permanently.*

- *What exactly is a calorie, and what do calories have to do with weight gain or loss.*

- *Taking in more calories can actually increase weight loss.*

- *How you can gain weight if needed.*

- *Why men lose weight more easily than women.*

- *What is compulsive overeating, and how can you get control.*

- *Anorexia and bulimia - what can help.*

- *How dieting can be harmful.*

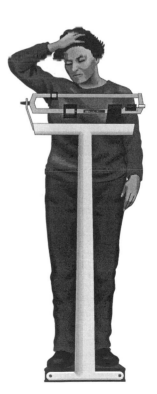

Why is weight control of such concern?

This is a very weight-conscious society we live in, and this is especially true for women. If a poll were taken, it is likely that most of the women and many of the men would consider themselves overweight. Up to 45 million Americans, or 20% of the population, are considered to be medically overweight or obese. Obesity is defined as a weight 20% or more over the medical (not fashion) ideal.

People actually seem to be getting bigger than they used to be. New stadiums are built with seats two inches wider than the previous standard. As a result of this actual and perceived weight gain, the diet and weight loss industry is booming.

There are many books, programs, magazine articles, diets, diet drugs, spas, and prepackaged diet foods that promise the pounds will melt away. They all have one thing in common -- they don't work, especially over the long term. The experience of about 95% of those who lose weight with these programs is that they gain it all back, and then some, within a year or two, a pattern called the yo-yo syndrome. Clearly the wrong approach is being taken.

Why don't most weight loss programs work?

Overweight is a symptom, not a primary problem. Any program that treats all overweight as the problem to be overcome only through physical (lowering calories) or mental (willpower, behavior modification) methods is doomed to failure. If the real problem is not identified and treated, the symptom - the overweight - will continue to reoccur.

> **Overweight is a symptom, not a primary problem**

Weight, like smog, is the byproduct of an out-of-tune system.

Weight loss approaches may work short term, but the underlying problems will not be treated long term and may even worsen. Diets can cause new problems of their own, which are discussed in this chapter.

What most diets have in common is that you end up fighting your body's self-protective mechanisms (against fungus and chemicals) instead of working with your body.

Causes of Overweight

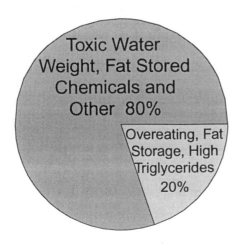

What is the real problem that causes the symptom of overweight?

There is no one problem, just as there is no single underlying cause of headaches or fatigue. Much overweight (about 70%), but not all, is due to retention of excess fluid, rather than fat caused by the overeating of fat, although both can be combined in one person. Toxins in the body can lead to fluid retention as the body attempts to dilute the toxin. Allergies can cause the same effect, as the body perceives the allergen as a toxin and tries to dilute it. A mineral deficiency causes the body to hold on to whatever minerals it can. Unfortunately, water and toxins are also held in the body.

Although physical causes are responsible for most overweight, the overweight person usually feels guilty about cravings and overeating and obsesses about food and dieting. Psychological problems such as low self-esteem and self-punishment can then follow, and added to the physical problems can further complicate recovery.

Do you ever wonder why you crave sugar?
Microorganisms such as fungi (yeast) use sugar as their food. If the fungi grab the sugar and nutrients before they can be assimilated by the body, you can crave more sugar since your body never got to use the last glucose from food that you ate. This can lead to a vicious cycle:

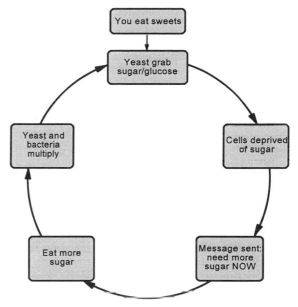

    1. You eat sweets

    2. Yeast grab the sugar before your cells can get it

    3. Your starving cells send the message: more sugar, now!

    4. You eat more sugar

    5. The fermentative yeast and bacteria multiply and need even more sugar

    6. The problem is self-perpetuating

The microorganism connection to overweight, a significant factor for many people, is discussed in greater detail later in the chapter.

Why do some overweight people eat as if they were starving?
Have you ever seen an overweight person shoveling in the food at a restaurant as if s/he were starving? It is possible that, even with the overweight and the amount of food consumed, the person is deficient in certain nutrients and is, in effect, actually starving. The nutrient deficiency can be due to poor diet (discussed in chapters in this book section), to a digestive problem (see Digestion chapter), to allergies, or to microorganisms (see Microorganisms section in ***Surviving The Toxic Crisis***) that grab the nutrients before they reach the bloodstream, leaving you with, in effect, the table scraps. The body responds as if there were not enough food available, and the person feels compelled to eat.

Remedying the nutrient deficiency by correcting the underlying cause for it will often lessen the feelings of starvation and the consequent overeating.

What are some of the dangers of being overweight?
Some health problems such as heart disease and diabetes are weight related. A person with a lot of extra fat has to have more blood vessels to supply the person's greater bulk. The heart must

then work harder to serve all of the extra blood vessels, which can weaken the heart over time. It is commonly believed that overweight can lead to cardiovascular problems, since the two are often seen together. However, both cardiovascular problems and overweight can be due to free radical and other damage, rather than a simple cause-and-effect relationship.

Obesity is a factor linked to cancer, especially in women. Overweight women are more likely to develop cancer of the uterine lining and do more poorly with breast cancer. Higher levels of fat usually correlate with higher levels of estrogen, which can worsen many female cancers. Obesity in women can also contribute to cervical, uterine and gallbladder cancer. Obesity in men may contribute to colon and rectal cancer [1].

Real or perceived overweight can lead to harmful dieting practices, such as self starvation (anorexia nervosa), nutritional deprivation, and the binge and purge cycle known as bulimia. These types of eating disorders can create problems such as nutritional deficiencies or fungus where none existed previously. These disorders are discussed later in this chapter.

How can you tell if weight is toxic water weight?
Water weight is more likely to make up the excess poundage if:

- Excess weight is disproportionately concentrated in certain parts of the body, most notably the hips and thighs (the usual female pattern), on the abdomen (sometimes female but usually male), or around the waist (men's "love handles").

- The skin over the areas of overweight is lumpy, puckered, and dimpled rather than smooth. This is often referred to by the nonmedical term "cellulite" or as "cottage cheese thighs". These dimples and lumps are actually lymph nodes and toxic fat between dermis and epidermis. You can starve yourself and exercise faithfully but the cellulite will remain until the toxins are cleared.

- There is allergic / toxic puffiness under the eyes or on the ankles and feet.

- A detoxification diet, or limited commercial diet (all the rice you can eat, for example, but not much else), can cause a water weight loss of a pound or more per day for a week or so accompanied by increased urination. But the weight is often regained, and then some, because an allergy can develop to the single food eaten daily.

- There are known food allergies or toxic burdens.

- The amount of weight gain seems excessive in relation to the amount of food regularly eaten. In theory at least, 3500 calories equal one pound.

- Calorie reduction diets result in little or no weight loss.

- Thyroid test results (T3, T4) are normal or elevated, which would be inconsistent with fat-based overweight.

- Triglyceride levels in a blood test are less than 100 mcg/dl.

- Triglyceride:thyroid ratio is less than 10:1. For example, if triglycerides are 70 and thyroid (T4) is 10, the ratio is 7:1 and fat is unlikely to be the primary cause of overweight. In such a case the thyroid is strong enough to handle the triglycerides.

- If you rarely sweat, even when hot or working hard, this is a sign that your body is holding onto water.

What causes water weight gain or retention?

If there is a toxin present, such as pesticides, mercury, or the waste byproducts of microorganisms, the body's natural response is to try to dilute the poison with water or fat. An excess of salt or the related deficiency of potassium can also cause water to be retained. The liquid in the body is primarily salt water of a certain concentration, and if the salt level in the body goes up, so will the amount of water increase to maintain the optimal concentration. If too little water is taken

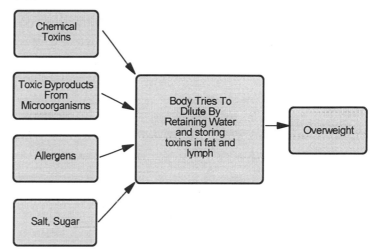

in, it has the same effect as too much salt and again water will be retained. One of the body's self-preservation mechanisms is to hoard water if it senses that there is a water shortage.

An allergen, interpreted by the body as being a toxin, will have the same effect. Interestingly, aminophyllin cream is promoted as a weight loss aid. The specific claim is that it "dissolves" cellulite. Aminophyllin is an allergy medication, so part of its mechanism of action may be symptomatic treatment of allergies which in turn can reduce puffiness.

In some cases water retention can be caused by too little salt. One patient, a doctor, was overweight (260 pounds) and had high blood pressure (240/130). His own doctor had him on a low salt diet, which didn't help. Another doctor, who was more knowledgeable about the way the body really works, took note of the low sodium level on his blood test. He *increased* the patient's salt intake, going against conventional wisdom in doing so. The water weight was quickly dropped and his blood pressure returned to near normal. The kidneys may not let water out of the body until the electrolytes such as sodium and potassium are rebalanced, a process complicated by the fact that sodium is lost in sweat and vomit. It is desirable to let water out of the body so new water can come in, much like an oil change allows your car to run better and protects the engine.

> **Water retention can actually be caused by too *little* salt.**

Paradoxically, one way to encourage the elimination of too much water is to drink even more of it. This makes sense in light of the above discussion on excess salt. The body will sense that there is plenty of water available, so it is not necessary to hoard it. Additional water also flushes out excess salt and some water soluble toxins, which is beneficial both weight-wise and health-wise.

Attempts to defeat the body's self-protective mechanism of diluting toxins by losing water and fat through dieting, exercise, diuretics or liposuction can lead to the toxins' becoming more concentrated in the body and in the brain and central nervous system, or being released into the blood and lymph. This in turn can lead to fatigue and other symptoms of toxicity and to stronger attempts by the body to retain water and fat.

Two patients, women in their 30s and early 40s living in the Los Angeles area, released fat-stored chemicals when they lost weight, with resulting central nervous system symptoms such as shakiness, fatigue and headaches. Removal of dental metals, sauna to remove chemicals, treatment for microorganisms, and emotional/spiritual counseling was part of their treatment so they could both lose the weight and decrease their toxicity.

What kinds of testing can help to determine the root cause of overweight?
Blood tests can be done for the following:

- Thyroid function - whether food is metabolized at the proper rate

- Triglyceride level - whether weight is due to fat (if elevated over 100 or the triglyceride to thyroid ratio is over 10:1) or water (triglycerides are low - below 80 - or normal)

- Glucose - if high, this could indicate diabetes, which is sometimes associated with obesity.

- Liver function - low or high LDH, SGOT, SGPT, or GGTP - how well toxins are eliminated

- High LDL (bad cholesterol), total cholesterol, or triglycerides can indicate fatty liver or fat-based overweight.

- Nutrient deficiencies - these can be determined by low albumen (protein), glucose (sugar), triglycerides (fat) and minerals.

- Chemical and metal toxins - high SGOT is one indication.

- Allergies - a five day rotation diet and other allergy tests. A low A/G ratio, high chloride, or high eosinophils on a blood panel are other indications.

- Parasites - liver enzyme tests and blood and stool tests can point to parasites. High SGOT may be indicative of parasites in the gallbladder, and high SGPT can mean fungus. These measurements are made relative to each other. Urine pH over 7 can also indicate fungus.

- White blood cell (WBC) differential - for example:
  - high eosinophils can indicate chemical / metal toxicity, parasites or allergy
  - high lymphocytes can indicate a viral infection

- high neutrophils can indicate a bacterial infection

- Urine pH, taken towards the end of the first urination of the morning after dawn, can indicate chemical or metal toxicity if less than 5.0. A urine pH of 7.0 or greater can indicate fungus, bacteria, fermentation or allergy. Both types of toxicity can be interpreted by the body as being something that needs to be diluted with water or fat. A pH that goes up and down can indicate both problems. Ideally pH should stay at 6.0 to 6.2 for at least two weeks straight. If you are on a restricted dietary regimen for yeast problems, once you are able to maintain this pH level, you can then begin to add some foods back into your diet, beginning with those foods with the lowest sugar content first. But you would need to confirm this with your Nutritionist who is monitoring your program and progress. (The *Toxic Immune Syndrome Cookbook* discusses this in more detail)

Once the cause is found, treatment of the problem can begin.

How can oil be a weight loss aid?

It may seem strange to tell a person who is overweight and who has probably thought of oil as being the enemy to eat oil - the right oils - to lose weight. But it's true. Beneficial oils - see the chapter on Oils and Fats - will help to dissolve and carry oil-soluble toxins out of the body, again decreasing the body's need to retain water in addition to benefiting your general health. The way this works is similar to the way changing your car's oil and filter can help the new oil clean dirt from your engine.

Eliminating allergens will help for the same reason. If a person who lost water weight on a detoxification diet stays away from food allergens and toxins, much of the weight should stay off.

Are there other reasons why oils are important?

Adults need good non-rancid oils for health and survival. Fatty acids from oils are needed for cell membranes and for the outer layer of nerve cells, among others. The importance of oils and sources of good oils are discussed in the chapter on Oils and Fats. An adult needs at least 5% of total calories from fat, preferably about 15-20%, and a child needs up to 30% because so many new cell membranes are forming.

Often when a person is attempting to lose weight, oils and fats are the first to be eliminated from the diet. Eliminating unhealthy fats (semisolid, hydrogenated or saturated fats, heated oils, rancid oils) is a good idea, but care must be taken not to eliminate all sources of necessary fatty acids such as seed, nut and fish oils.

What if some or all of the excess weight is due to fat, not water?

This should be dealt with on two levels - physical and mental. Physically, what is happening is that more calories are taken in than are expended, but the picture is much more complex than that. Actual numbers of calories are not necessarily the important part.

What is a calorie?

A calorie (correctly called a kilocalorie) as the term is used here is a unit of energy for the body. If all of the potential energy is not used, the excess is stored as fat. By way of analogy, suppose you brought in five fireplace logs but only burned three. There would be two left to store for future use. If you brought in four or five logs every time you wanted to burn three, you would soon have quite a pile of logs that may never get used up.

How do they know how many calories are in food?

In the laboratory, a calorie is the unit of energy needed to raise one gram of water one degree Celsius. A device called a bomb calorimeter is used to measure the number of calories in a certain amount of food or other substance. In a bomb calorimeter, a flash current ignites the material tested, which vaporizes the substance and produces a certain amount of energy, expressed as calories.

Why doesn't calorie counting work most of the time?

Our bodies are not bomb calorimeters. Traditionally, calorie arithmetic goes like this: 3500 calories equal one pound of fat. If you eat 1700 calories per day and expend 1200 through your daily life cycles and exercise, you will gain a pound a week (500 extra calories times 7 days = 3500 calories). If the numbers are reversed, you lose a pound a week. This makes sense, but there's one problem - it doesn't work this way. We all know people who eat more than others without exercising much, yet they gain less weight or none at all. Other factors are clearly at work here. Calorie counting is the ultimate symptom suppressor. It is also, for some people, the ultimate myth.

> **Calorie counting is the ultimate symptom suppressor**

Symptom-suppressing reducing diets are like symptom-suppressing medications - they work only as long as you're on them. In both cases this is a sign that the root cause is not being addressed.

What are some things that can complicate the calorie-counting picture?

The use of artificial sweetener offers one of many examples of how the weight gain and loss picture is much more complex than calories. In an attempt to reduce calories, many people substitute artificial sweetener, which has essentially zero calories, for sugar, which has about 19 calories per teaspoon. As far as they are concerned the only change has been a reduction in the number of calories, and they sit back and await their anticipated weight loss. Again, NutraSweet is the artificial sweetener used predominantly in most commercial products on the market today. And, as already mentioned, there is a real concern for the damage you could eventually incur to the myelin sheath of the nerves.

Then you need to be aware that taking in all that artificial sweetener can actually cause weight <u>gain</u> for the following reasons:

- Artificial sweeteners obviously taste sweet, and the sweet taste signals the pancreas to produce insulin. Blood sugar drops without any or enough actual sugar to buffer the insulin, and the hunger level rises. More food is then eaten.

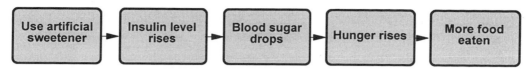

- Psychological factors can also cause one to eat more, as the person using artificial sweeteners may give her/himself permission to eat more of other things to compensate, such as apple pie with their artificially sweetened coffee.

- Artificial sweeteners are not simply an inert substance with an absence of calories. They are toxic substances that the body is not designed to use. As this chapter discusses, the body will often retain water and fat to attempt to dilute toxins, resulting in weight gain.

Are all calories created equal?

Consider the difference between brown rice, a complex carbohydrate, and rice syrup, a refined concentrated rice product (discussed, with an accompanying chart, in the Carbohydrates chapter). Portions of each are chosen that have the same number of calories. In theory, both products would cause the same weight gain. In actuality, the rice syrup would lead to greater weight gain.

Why is this? The pancreas and digestive enzymes can't work fast enough to keep up with the rice syrup or with any refined sugar. Too much insulin is produced and the undigested sugar

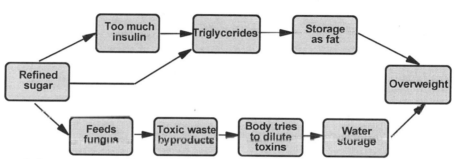

is turned into triglycerides and then stored as fat. In addition, the syrup ferments and feeds fungus, which gives off toxic waste products which the body tries to dilute by retaining water.

In addition, concentrated sugar releases insulin, which in turn releases inflammation-promoting prostaglandin E2. On the other hand, complex carbohydrates promote the release of glucagon, which is involved in the production of "good" prostaglandin E1, which promotes the release of stored fat to burn for energy, which in turn promotes weight loss.

A bomb calorimeter measures the amount of energy given off instantaneously, with no regard to time. Since the body is set up to metabolize food slowly, time is important in digestion of food and weight gain.

How important is metabolic rate?

Metabolic rate is one of the missing links, although less important than many would suppose. Only about 20% of overweight is due to excess fat, and only a portion of these people have a metabolic problem.

Some people burn up calories faster than others. A car running at a high idle speed uses up more gas than one at low idle. If a low metabolic rate is your problem, chances are that you have one or more of the following:

- *Fatigue*
- *Dry skin*
- *Sluggishness*
- *Hair loss*
- *Mental dullness*
- *Cold hands and feet*
- *Low thyroid function test results (T3, T4)*

Any of the following can help to speed up a sluggish metabolism:

- *Essential fatty acids (see chapter on Oils and Fats)*

- *Iodine along with copper and zinc if a thyroid imbalance is present, indicated by the ratio of T4 to triglycerides (less than 1:10)*

- *Improved nutrition*

- *A complex carbohydrate:protein ratio of 40% to 30%, or 1/3 more carbohydrate than protein by weight. Figure on a fist-size serving of protein with a fist plus a couple of knuckles worth of carbohydrate.*

- *More food, especially whole grains, if on a very low calorie or limited diet. Cook fresh until chewy, not soggy.*

- *Exercise*

Is there a fungus among us?

As mentioned previously, the body can retain water to dilute toxins. It can also retain fat to try to dilute and store oil-soluble toxins.

In addition to toxins, time and metabolism, microbiology is an important player in the weight gain and loss game. Fungus often grows out of control due to diets that are too high in sugars and intermediate carbohydrates, combined with a shortage of protective bacteria. As the fungus ferments, it gives off toxic waste products that the body tries to dilute by holding water. A vicious cycle is created, as the body craves more sugar to feed the hungry fungus. Women are more likely to have a fungus problem than men due to their higher estrogen levels. Estrogen promotes the storage of sugar, leading to lower blood sugar levels, sweets cravings (especially premenstrually), and more fungal growth.

Low intake or absorption of good oils, common in women who are trying to lose weight, can also lead to a hormonal imbalance and high estrogen / low progesterone ratio.

Why are starvation-and-feast diets a problem?

Dieting can make a fungus situation worse. If you starve the body through dieting, the fungus can put down deeper roots and become more firmly entrenched like a tree that is not being watered enough. The fungus then thrives when more food, especially sugar, is eaten.

How can taking in more calories help one to lose weight?

The body, in its wisdom, senses a famine situation when insufficient calories and nutrients are consumed and reacts by conserving energy usage. You then feel tired because so little fuel is being burned, and fat is hoarded to use as fuel during the anticipated period of shortage. A lesser decrease in calories from the usual rate is more likely to result in long term weight loss than a drastic decrease.

Can thyroid hormone help in weight loss?

Natural (not synthetic) thyroid hormone, prescribed by a doctor, can be useful in the short term if thyroid output is inadequate and if all else fails. It is important to realize, however, that a lowered metabolism is generally a symptom of a deeper problem, which should be addressed. Thyroid hormone in this case is merely a symptom suppressing measure which can ultimately make matters worse by suppressing your own thyroid's hormone production. It does this by telling your pituitary that you have plenty of thyroid hormone, so it doesn't send any thyroid stimulating hormone (TSH). Your own thyroid no longer has to work, so it can atrophy.

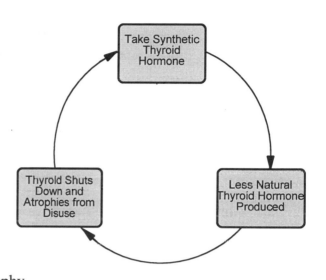

How can poor nutrition cause weight gain?

Insufficient calories can cause the body to sense a famine situation and hoard whatever it can. Insufficient nutrients can cause the body to react in the same way. If you fill up on junk food, your body senses an insufficiency and grabs onto what it can. A deficiency of good oils can cause the body to hang onto bad oils and body fat in an effort to remedy the situation. A high intake of fruit juice, in addition to feeding fungus, can chelate and deplete minerals, causing the body to try to hoard what it has.

Do all foods burn calories at the same rate?

All calories are not created equal! Some foods burn more calories for digestion than others. A cup of brown rice has about the same number of calories as a cup of white rice, but the brown rice requires more work (energy) to digest it, which is desirable, and so consumes more calories (units of energy) in digestion than white rice. As a bonus, brown rice provides far more nutrition than white rice - 24 nutrients in brown rice compared to only one nutrient in white rice.

What happens when you lose and then regain weight?

When weight is lost, especially through starvation diets, lean muscle mass is lost along with fat and water. The amount of lean muscle lost varies from 5% of the total with heavy exercise to 25% of the total with no exercise [2]. If the lost weight is regained, nearly all of it is fat. If a person loses and regains repeatedly, her/his body will have a progressively larger fat to lean ratio. After the age of about 25-30, it is more difficult to replace lean muscle mass.

The amino acids arginine and ornithine stimulate the growth of lean body mass. However, they also promote viral growth and so the amino acid lysine is needed for balance. Arginine and ornithine are like fertilizer that promotes the growth of both flowers and weeds. Arginine, ornithine and lysine are three of the basic amino acids that, like some minerals, fight for the same biological pathways.

How can one gain weight?

Ironically, a good way to **gain** weight is to do what weight-**loss** dieters do. In experiments with mice, researchers let a control group of normal weight mice eat when and as much as they chose. The experimental group of mice were limited in what they could eat by the researchers, and then allowed to eat as much as they wanted, in cycles. This replicates the long term diet and binge cycles followed by many dieters. The control mice maintained normal weight. The experimental mice gained weight when eating at will and then lost it progressively more slowly when their intake was controlled. People who alternately diet and eat at will usually experience the same dismaying results.

Many people who want to gain weight have tried to do so by stuffing themselves with high calorie foods, without getting the results they want. Some doctors working with such people take their ideas from those on the lose-and-gain roller coaster, and reduce the food intake of their thin patients. They then allow the patients to eat what they want, in cycles. The patients are amazed and skeptical of this advice, but it works. The thin patients start gaining weight.

This mechanism suggests one possible reason there are so many overweight people, especially women, in this country. Most of them started out at a normal weight, but started dieting because they wanted to be a few pounds thinner. Even Junior High school girls proudly admit to being on diets. Soon a real weight problem has replaced the imagined one.

Why would you have trouble gaining weight?

Some causes of insufficient weight gain are

- *Hyperthyroidism (too high a metabolic rate due to too much thyroid hormone). This is sometimes called Graves' disease.*

- *Digestive problems (food not being absorbed properly).*

- *Leaky gut and its associated allergies and malnutrition.*

- *Worms and parasites take in nutrients that your body should be getting.*

- *Allergy keeps the body in sympathetic fight-or-flight mode rather than parasympathetic digestion mode. Poorly digested food may not be used by the body to maintain weight.*

- *Toxins may cause the same problem as allergy, and for the same reason.*

- *Cancer patients often lose weight and have trouble gaining it because they are in sympathetic fight mode, and because the tumor itself often steals fat.*

What are some dietary suggestions to gain weight?

A 30/40/30 diet - 30% protein, 40% carbohydrates, and 30% vegetable oils (by calories, not weight) - is recommended to both those who would like to lose weight and those who would like to gain. Such a diet helps the body to work optimally and such a body would seek its own best weight [3]. The carbohydrates, protein, and oils should be of good quality - see the chapters in this section on those food groups.

Enzymes and hydrochloric acid (HCl) can help digestion. Take enzymes at the beginning of the meal and HCl towards the end of the meal.

If digestion of complex carbohydrates is a problem, try grinding the grains in a grain or coffee mill. The appearance of recognizable grains in the stool is a clue that this may be going on. One patient, an art teacher in her 30s, was losing weight and had low energy. When she started grinding her grains before cooking, she got her weight and energy back.

Predigested rice-based protein powder is recommended if protein digestion is a problem.

A 20 year old male patient who wanted to gain weight used an oil mix, protein and carbohydrate mixes, calcium, and the amino acids arginine, ornithine, leucine, isoleucine and valine. He was able to absorb the nutrients and gain the muscle weight.

What is the importance of exercise in losing and keeping off weight?

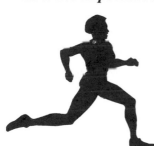

Nearly all researchers in this field agree that exercise and diet work better than diet alone. The cells of our bodies contain mitochondria, which are the power plants of the cell. They convert food to energy rather than storing it as fat. The more mitochondria a person has, the more efficiently the body will burn off food. Exercise will increase the number and efficiency of mitochondria a person has, since more energy is now needed.

Aerobic (oxygen using) exercise starves the cells of oxygen, and larger and more efficient mitochondria are grown to meet the increased demand for cellular oxygen. In addition, exercise raises the body's metabolic rate to meet the increased demand for energy. More food is then burned, just as turning up the thermostat increases furnace fuel consumption.

Exercise also works the lymph glands, which helps the body eliminate toxins. This toxin elimination is good for you overall and decreases the chances of retaining water to dilute the poisons.

Diet here refers to a healthy diet, not merely a low calorie one. A healthy diet is like using higher octane fuel in your car, which burns more completely and is more efficient. Restricting calories (fuel) and exercising is like deliberately reducing the amount of gas you put into your car and then expecting it to get you where you want to go anyway.

Is it possible to exercise too much?

It is possible to exercise too much, and the body will actually lower its metabolism to protect itself. This point is usually reached when body fat drops to a level which is unhealthy. Women often stop menstruating at this point.

If your albumen protein level is less than 4.0 (4.5-4.8 is optimal), strenuous or prolonged exercise can steal protein from your heart muscle, actually causing heart attacks in susceptible people.

Why do men lose weight more easily than women?

Many women who have embarked on a weight loss program along with a man have found that he will lose weight faster than she will. This infuriating (for women) fact is due to the fact that men have 40% more muscle cells than women, and muscle cells have a larger number of food-burning mitochondria than most other cells. In addition, women are built to store fat more easily to ensure the survival of her offspring, since body fat stores can make the survival difference if she is pregnant or breastfeeding during a famine. Although times have changed, bodies have not, and most women still retain fat more than most men [2].

> **Times have changed, but bodies have not.**

This is not all bad. It is believed that woman's 40% more fat is partially responsible for woman's longer life expectancy. 11 out of 12 married women outlive their husbands. However, there is both protective and toxic fat for women, although men's fat is usually toxic or allergic.

What is the mental/emotional aspect of overweight?

The mental/emotional aspect of overweight is involved when a person eats to fill an emptiness that is not caused by lack of food, such as loneliness, unworthiness or boredom. Food can be used as a drug to relieve anxiety or depression. Ironically, the refined carbohydrates that are usually chosen for this purpose can make the anxiety or depression - and hunger - worse in the long run.

Compulsive eating can result from constant obsessing about food, weight, and diets. This is in part because the mind cannot comprehend a negatively phrased thought. If you say to a toddler, "Don't touch the light switch", the child will immediately go to the light switch as if the word "don't" did not exist. Try this mental exercise: I won't think about a yellow canary. I'm not allowed to think about a yellow canary. I'm trying to think about anything but a yellow canary.... You weren't thinking about a yellow canary before, but you are now, right? Trying to program your mind to *not* think about food is likewise doomed to failure.

It's better to replace the thoughts of food with other thoughts, such as work or helping others.

How do natural body signals work?

Another way in which the usual mental approaches to diet and overweight fail lies in the lack of respect for natural body signals. Consider the way you think about water as compared with your approach to food:

- *You at first don't think about water*
- *You get thirsty*
- *You want a glass of water*
- *You drink some water*
- *You are no longer thirsty*

This doesn't become an emotional issue, nor do you judge yourself to be a bad person for wanting or drinking too much water, nor do you slosh around uncomfortably from overindulgence. You are simply aware of, and responding appropriately to, your body's natural thirst signals. These signals tell you when to drink and when to stop.

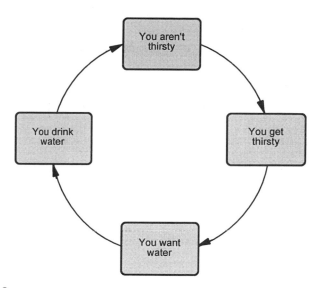

What happens when you don't listen to your body?
Natural hunger signals work the same way as natural thirst signals. Unfortunately, most people with weight problems reacted to the first actual or anticipated unwanted pound by attempting to suppress hunger signals. When the natural urge to start eating is suppressed, so is the natural urge to stop. Eating or the desire for food then starts when food is seen or smelled, when the clock says dinnertime, when one is bored, when the TV is turned on or the book is opened. Eating stops when the food is gone, the plate is empty, or the stomach is uncomfortably distended. It is ironic that a technique which is supposed to result in less food consumption actually results in more.

Another contributor to a lack of awareness of hunger signals is the childhood experience of having your food intake - time, type, and amount - determined by someone else, usually a parent. You may have gone through childhood rarely having ever felt and responded appropriately to a hunger start or stop signal because this was not your decision to make. As an adult, you have lost touch with what true hunger feels like. Many people with a weight problem actually do not know the feeling of true hunger, as distinguished from a craving.

Your body is more likely to tune into natural hunger signals if you eat breakfast and lunch with complex carbohydrates and vegetables. Natural eating, in general, leads to more natural body responses.

The ability to tune in to what type of food your body wants can also suffer. Your cells may be saying "send broccoli", but the message you receive might be "gee, a donut sounds good".

It is a good idea to chew your food thoroughly. If there isn't enough chewing, insufficient HCl may be produced in the stomach, leading to increased sugar which feeds fungus and helicobacter pylori, a bacteria which is involved in the formation of stomach ulcers. The sugar/microorganism cycle can contribute to overweight as well.

Many refined foods, including juices, will not allow the stop-eating signal to kick in until too much of the food has been eaten. Eating too fast can have the same result. There are books and programs designed to teach, or reteach, a person to recognize true body hunger [4].

What is compulsive overeating?

Compulsive eating is regularly eating for any reason other than physical hunger, although cellular hunger for certain nutrients due to poor diet or hungry fungus or bacteria can express themselves as cravings. Everyone occasionally eats for reasons other than hunger, such as social occasions, boredom, comfort, and others. The problem arises when such eating becomes a regular habit. Compulsive eaters often do not know what real physical hunger feels like, and confuse it with cravings. When the weight starts piling on and you want to eat less, but can't seem to be able to, this is compulsive eating. Eating certain foods or in a certain way then becomes an addiction like alcoholism or drug addiction.

Are you a compulsive overeater?

If you can answer "yes, I regularly do that" to several of the following statements, you are probably a compulsive overeater.

- *I step on the scale in the morning to determine how I am going to feel about myself that day.*

- *I eat when I'm tired, bored, angry, or I feel guilty.*

- *I eat when the clock says it's mealtime.*

- *Comfort foods are very important to me.*

- *I'm going on a diet on Monday / the first of the month / my birthday / New Year's Day, and I don't want "bad" foods around in the kitchen to tempt me, so I'll eat them now.*

- *I'm going on a diet on Monday (or whenever) and I won't be allowed to eat certain foods, so I'll eat them now whether I want them or not to make up for the anticipated deprivation.*

- *If "bad" foods are around, I'll eat them whether I want them or not.*

- *There are certain foods that I simply can't give up.*

- *I eat to postpone doing something that I don't want to do.*

- *I feel that I was never allowed to eat enough _____ when I was a child, so I'm making up for lost time.*

- *I will eat everything on my plate even if I am uncomfortably full rather than throw anything away.*

- *I treat myself with food to make myself feel good. I use food as self-medication and consolation after a bad day.*

- *I eat until I'm stuffed to the point of discomfort, especially at all-you-can-eat buffets.*

Why are some people compulsive overeaters?

There are several possible root causes of compulsive overeating. One or more of these may apply to you.

- **Allergic addiction** - Allergy and addiction are closely linked. In fact, if an allergist suspects a food addiction, s/he will often ask what your favorite food or food group is, the one you feel you can't do without. That food is usually the culprit. A strong daily craving for a particular food or food group is an indication that allergy to the food may be the problem. Eating the craved food almost daily will often worsen the allergy by putting you in a daily allergic fight-or-flight reaction so you can't digest very well, then you react to the incompletely digested food in a vicious cycle. If you feel you have to have the food at least once in a 72 hour period (3 days), you may have an allergic addiction. It takes at least three days to clear an allergen from the body.

- **Nutrient deficiencies** - If you crave certain foods, this may be due to a nutrient deficiency. For example, many people are deficient in the mineral magnesium, especially women in the week before their periods. Chocolate, a source of magnesium, is a common craving. A deficiency of beneficial oils can lead to a craving for fried or fatty foods. Eat almonds if you are having a chocolate craving - they contain both magnesium and good oils.

- **Emotional hunger** - Food can be a substitute for love, self esteem, meaningful activity, or sleep. It is not uncommon for people, especially women, to stuff their anger by stuffing themselves with food. Some people overeat to get even with a parent or spouse who wants them thin. Rebellion against "shoulds", such as "I should diet" or "I should be thin" can also be a factor. A feeling of scarcity in general - that there isn't enough love, money, time, or food to go around regardless of the actual situation - can motivate one to eat food she doesn't want rather than waste it, or overeat to make up for the deprivation of past and future diets.

- **Fungus infection** - A systemic fungus infection can set up a craving for sweets, fruit, or refined flour, which feeds the fungus, which sets the stage for more cravings.

- **Sugar imbalance** - Hypoglycemia, meaning low blood sugar, results when too much insulin or too little adrenaline is released, causing shakiness, mood swings, lack of energy, and craving for sugar. Eating sugar in any form will cause more insulin to be released in a continuous cycle.

What can be done about compulsive overeating?

First identify the cause, then treat the problem. To identify and treat the above causes, explore the following:

- **Allergic addiction** - Go on a detoxification diet (described later in this chapter), and then add back foods one food group at a time, monitoring your symptoms. Those foods which cause symptoms (e.g. fatigue, cravings, bloat, headaches, mood swings) are probably the allergens. Alternatively, get tested by an allergist, preferably a clinical ecologist who will give you only dilute amounts of the allergen (some allergists give huge amounts which can cause a severe reaction). NAET allergy testing and treatment, developed by Dr. Devi Nambudripad [5,6] can also help to identify and eliminate allergic addiction.

- **Nutritional deficiency** - Get tested for nutrient status (blood, hair, or saliva testing). Some of these tests include albumen, glucose, triglycerides, and mineral tests. These are not necessarily on a standard blood panel. When looking at these and any blood test results, look for deviations from the midpoint, not just out-of-range values. See the Testing chapter (called A Visit To The Doctor) for more information on reading blood test results.

- **Emotional hunger** - When you want food, first ask yourself "What am I feeling" - bored, angry, etc. Deal more appropriately with these feelings. Ask yourself: what does the food buy you versus the cost to your well-being? Better yet - write down cost vs. benefit in two columns to make the issue more visual and clearer. Take the focus off yourself by serving people (but not necessarily serving them *food*). Counseling may be helpful.

- **Hypoglycemia** - The sugar craving is similar to the craving for alcohol experienced by an alcoholic when the blood alcohol level drops. The alcoholic needs to quit using alcohol, and the hypoglycemic needs to quit using sugar. The first few days are the hardest, and then the craving usually subsides.

- **Fungus infection** - Treat the fungus, and the sweets cravings should diminish. A good detoxification diet (next paragraph) can reduce the numbers of fungi because all forms of sugar, its food, are eliminated, and enzymes used eat up the roots of the fungus.

Can anything else be done?

A detoxification diet helps to eliminate and detoxify from the body allergens and fungus feeders. The diet is a strict one for this reason. A knowledgeable health practitioner or clinical ecologist should monitor any diet like this. The basic eight day detox diet involves:

- For the first four days, eat only non-sweet vegetables, good oils, hypoallergenic protein powder, and supplements. Enzyme tablets assist digestion and help digest and kill microorganisms. Colon cleansing powder absorbs toxins and cleans out the colon.

- For days 5-8, add non-gluten or low-gluten grains, which are less likely to be allergenic, one per day: brown rice, quinoa, millet, amaranth, or buckwheat. Start with the grains eaten the least frequently.

- Oral use of aloe vera with potassium sorbate helps to change pH and kill yeast and pathogenic bacteria in the mouth and digestive tract and helps prevent upper respiratory infections. It may taste unpleasant at first due to microorganism die-off, but if you persevere the taste will usually improve and you will lose your sweets cravings.

After the eight days, certain foods are carefully added back to the diet on a five day rotation basis to monitor for and lessen the chance of allergic reactions. Due to the possibility of die-off reactions this diet program should be done under the care of a qualified professional. The program is good only for problems in the small intestine and large intestine, where 65% of problems exist. The diet is a strict one and is not meant to be followed for more than eight days.

One patient, a woman who was overweight and had heavy cellulite on her thighs, tried many diets and up to two hours a day of exercise with no success. The detoxification diet helped her get rid of both the excess weight and the cellulite. Treatment for allergies and microorganisms allowed her to keep the weight off.

A man in his early 20s had colon cancer. His doctor recommended chemotherapy but he went on the detox diet instead. His cancer cleared in six months. This was verified by an oncologist. Meanwhile, the doctor who recommended lifestyle changes rather than chemotherapy was charged with malpractice.

The **Toxic Immune Syndrome Cookbook** [7], written and edited by the authors of this book, gives nutritional information and recipes useful to those who want to eliminate allergenic and yeast-feeding foods.

What are some other eating disorders?
In addition to compulsive overeating, there are two other serious and even life-threatening eating disorders of concern. Anorexia nervosa and bulimia can cause death if untreated.

What is anorexia nervosa?
Anorexia nervosa is a disorder in which the victim diets to the point of starvation and sometimes death. The disease is most likely to affect teenage girls and women in their twenties. Anorexia nervosa usually starts with a diet to lose a moderate amount of weight, and becomes a compulsion to become progressively thinner. The dieter will take

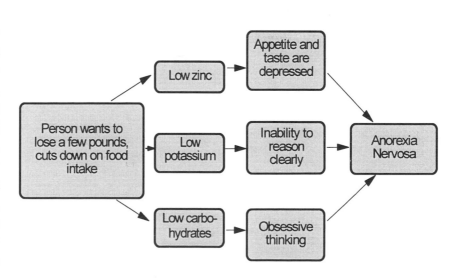

in far fewer calories than what is needed to sustain life for very long, and she may also induce vomiting or use laxatives (bulimia) to rid herself of some of what little she does eat. The person can be very emaciated and yet still see herself as fat.

Traditional treatment for anorexia nervosa has been to feed the patient, by force if necessary, to prevent her decline and death. Next, a counseling approach is used to determine the psychological reasons for the disease. This approach is incomplete. Remedying the nutrient deficiencies is the first step in helping a patient with anorexia nervosa.

The changeover from relatively normal dieting to anorexia nervosa can be partially due to biochemical causes. Nutrient deficiencies can cause brain, and therefore mental, changes. Most notably, the mineral zinc, which helps to maintain a healthy appetite and sense of taste, can become deficient. The result is a loss of appetite. One patient, a 17 year old female with anorexia, was helped by zinc supplementation combined with treatment for roundworm. She regained her sense of taste and smell and her appetite returned to normal, plus the food she ate stopped causing pain and bloating.

The word anorexia refers to loss of appetite from any cause. Low blood sugar (hypoglycemia) from insufficient carbohydrates or low potassium can cause obsessive thinking and an inability to reason clearly, as well as possible anxiety and sleeplessness. Lack of magnesium can lead to heart arrhythmias which can lead to death from heart failure.

What is bulimia?

A patient with bulimia may appear to be of normal weight. However, her way of staying at that weight is hazardous to her health and life. The bulimic binges and then purges. She can eat an incredible amount of food, and then make herself vomit and/or take laxatives to eliminate it. She may be motivated by fear of weight gain or by fear of how she feels when full - bloated, sick etc.

This method seems wonderful at first, as the person can eat all she wants and not gain weight. After a while, however, the bingeing and vomiting becomes an addiction that she feels she can't stop even when she wants to.

The dangers of bulimia include:

- Damage to the stomach from repeated vomiting.

- Damage to the enamel of the teeth from stomach acid coming into contact with the teeth while vomiting.

- Severe depletion of necessary electrolytes from vomiting and laxative use. Heart arrhythmias can result from loss of magnesium, for example. Salt depletion can cause heavy fatigue.

- As with anorexia nervosa, low blood sugar can perpetuate the compulsive behavior.

What are some of the harmful diets?

In general, diets which are rigid and limited, and eliminate whole food groups or types, are likely to be harmful. Many of these start with a good idea (for example, that raw foods are healthful) and take it too far (eat nothing but raw vegetables, fruits, nuts, and seeds). Nutritional deficiencies are almost certain to result sooner or later. The Western mind-set of "if a little is good then more is better" can lead to extreme all-or-nothing diet approaches.

Many rigid diets promote a feeling of health and well-being as well as weight loss. This is because the diet is balancing out the previous dietary excesses. After a while on the diet, the person moves from diseases of excess, through better health, to diseases of deficiency. What often happens, unfortunately, is that the mind is affected by the nutrient deficiencies, and the person is too impaired to even notice the impairment. You may have encountered someone who has been on one of these diets long enough to be quite thin. This person may be spacey, speak slowly, have difficulty making coherent conversation, and seem tired and run-down, and yet insist that s/he is just fine.

Some very low carbohydrate diets can put the patient into ketosis, an abnormal metabolic state. At least one death has been reported from such a diet.

Near-starvation diets of 1000 calories or less can lead to life-threatening deficiencies. One patient who weighed about 500 pounds had been put on a very low calorie diet. His albumin was 3.2, which meant he was starving. Continuing the diet could have killed him. A root cause oriented approach was implemented, and he went down to 300 pounds in a little over a year, with an albumin level of over 4.4, which is more near normal. The albumin/globulin ratio should be 1.8-2.0, and is a reliable indicator of whether one is getting enough food.

What are some other harmful approaches? - What you don't know can hurt you

Drastic measures are sometimes taken in the quest for thinness. Liposuction, the surgical removal of fat, is one of them. Toxins are held in body fat, and removing the fat but leaving the toxins will only make the person sicker and more likely to retain water to try to dilute the poison. Liposuction is like removing the barrels for holding toxic waste while doing nothing to stop the flow of new toxic waste. In addition, liposuction can cut nerves, leading to numbness and pain; can cause scars which can block the body's skin surface energy pathways as well as being unattractive; and can cause infection which can lead to antibiotic use and the resulting overgrowth of fungus.

Nearly all drugs have a rebound effect as the body tries to counteract the effect of the drug. Diet drugs are no exception, and those who take them, whether prescription or nonprescription, will usually experience reduction in hunger, then no effect, then rebound hunger as the cellular starvation causes a ravenous hunger that is stronger than the drug.

One patient in her mid 30s who combined sauna (which releases toxins) with a body wrap (which prevents toxin release through the skin) developed liver problems so severe that she needed a liver transplant. The liver, which processes toxins, was overloaded beyond repair.

What do allopathic medicine and weight loss programs have in common?
One characteristic of allopathic medicine is its focus on symptom suppression. Another characteristic is its parent/child role playing. The doctor is the active partner, the one who has the knowledge and gives the orders. The patient is forced into a childlike, passive role; she/he has no responsibility for her/his own health other than obedience.

Most diet programs follow the allopathic model in terms of symptom suppression, pseudo-parent/child roles, and lack of personal responsibility. The dieter follows rules set up by someone else - follow the diet sheet, eat the diet program's overpriced frozen dinners, see the diet counselor once a week. Fear of displeasing the white-coated diet counselor is intended to be a motivator but often has the opposite effect. Weight loss is rewarded by a verbal pat on the head, a "good girl!". These programs have another thing in common - they usually don't work - at least not for very long with permanent weight maintenance. And you're back to the "yo-yo" syndrome again.

What You Can Do

What mental approaches are best? - Is success dependent on who's in charge?
A study was done on the subject of successful and unsuccessful diet regimes [8]. In this study, a large number of people who had lost at least twenty pounds and had kept the weight off for at least five years were interviewed to see what they attributed their success to. The authors hoped to find some common patterns. It turned out that nearly all of the successful dieters followed a program devised or modified by themselves to fit their own preferences and lifestyles. They didn't report to an outside authority figure, nor did they allow a book or program to become their authority figure. They maintained an adult rather than a childlike role, taking responsibility for the success or failure of their regimen rather than crediting or blaming a doctor or program. In addition, most of the dieters learned to trust their body's signals rather than following even a self-made list of rules. Self education and understanding is also an important component of success.

Other successful mental approaches include:

- Find out what the root cause(s) of your overweight is/are (chemicals, allergy, fungus or other microorganisms), and correct these rather than trying to suppress the symptom through calorie reduction.

- Change your mindset from dieting to health. Aim for health and eat accordingly, and weight loss should follow if you were meant to lose the weight (i.e. if your goal is realistic).

- If you are healthy your body will do what is best for you. You and your body will both be on the same side instead of working at cross purposes as with traditional diets.

- Give up the negative focus on dieting, deprivation, and how much you don't like your body. Get back in touch with real hunger. Have positive reasons for lifestyle changes (caring about yourself, looking and feeling young) rather than negative ones (hating your appearance).

- Reduce stress and deal with emotional problems such as anger, guilt, worthiness, obligation, or inability to say no.

What physical approaches are helpful?

There are a number of physical approaches to weight loss. Which ones will work for you depends on your root causes, although nearly all of these will be of benefit to anyone.

- Detoxify the body via detox diet, chelation to remove toxic metals from the body after they are removed from the teeth (see Metal Detoxification chapter in *Surviving The Toxic Crisis*), sauna to eliminate chemicals, and colonics to clean sludge out of the digestive tract.

- Remove mercury fillings and root canals properly (see chapter on Mercury in *Surviving The Toxic Crisis*). Mercury can contribute to fungus growth by killing your protective bacteria, which can stimulate cravings.

- Get nutritional testing and professional advice and take supplements as needed.

- Eliminate or cut down on sugar, caffeine, artificial sweeteners, harmful fats, processed foods, and refined starches.

- Get treatment for allergies.

Those people who lose weight do not simply want to lose weight. They refuse to be fat - or unhealthy - and do whatever it takes to reach their goal.

Summary

Overweight is a symptom, not a primary problem. The symptom can be alleviated for good only if the root causes are identified and addressed.

Overweight is due to fat in only about 20% of all cases.

Overweight can be due to one or more of the following root causes:

- *Toxic water weight to dilute poisons in the body*
- *Eating too much relative to the amount of energy expended*
- *Underactive thyroid or adrenals*
- *Nutritional deficiencies from eating bad foods or not eating good foods.*
- *Hypoglycemia due to sugar consumption fungus, or parasites*

- *Emotional hunger*
- *Allergic addiction*

The solution to overweight (or underweight) lies in finding the root causes through testing, and then correcting the source of the problem.

References and Resources

- Bruch, Hilde, *The Golden Cage*, Vintage, 1979. *Anorexia nervosa.*

- The Burton Goldberg Group, *Alternative Medicine: The Definitive Guide*, Future Medicine Publishing, Puyallup WA, 1994. *The following chapters deal with weight control issues:*
  "Obesity and Weight Management", pp. 762-772
  "Bulimia", p. 893
  "Anorexia Nervosa", p. 885
  "Hypothyroidism", pp. 936-7

- Cannon, Geoffrey, and Hetty Einzig, *Dieting Makes You Fat*, Pocket Books, NY, 1983.

- Chernin, Kim, *The Obsession: Reflections on the Tyranny of Slenderness*, Harper and Row, NY, 1983.

- Chernin, Kim, *The Hungry Self: Women, Eating and Identity*, Perennial, NY, 1985.

- Colvin, Robert, and Susan C. Olson, *Keeping It Off*, Simon and Schuster, NY, 1985.

- Jensen, Bernard, *Slender Me Naturally*, Published by Bernard Jensen, Escondido CA, 1986.

- Hunt, Douglas, *No More Cravings*, Warner Books, NY, 1987. *Physical reasons behind food cravings.*

- Kano, Susan, *Making Peace With Food*, Harper and Row, NY, 1989. *Discusses myths related to overweight.*

- Kellas, W.R., *Toxic Immune Syndrome Cookbook*, Comprehensive Health Center, Encinitas CA, 2nd ed., 1995.

- Levenkron, Steven, *Treating and Overcoming Anorexia Nervosa*, Warner, NY, 1982.

- Marsden, Kathryn, *The Food Combining Diet: Lose Weight The Hay Way*, Thorsons, Hammersmith, London England, 1993. *Based on the work of Dr. William Howard Hay, who developed this system in the 1930s. The author's quote: "Aim for good health and weight control will follow".*

- Nambudripad, Devi, *Say Goodbye To Illness*, Delta Publishing Company, Buena Park CA, 1993.

- Nambudripad, Devi, *The NAET Guidebook*, Delta Publishing Company, Buena Park CA, 1994.

- Orbach, Susie, *Fat is a Feminist Issue*, Berkley Books, NY, 1982 (Vol. I) and 1987 (Vol. II). *Acceptance of one's body and how to lose weight without dieting.*

- Orbach, Susie, *Hunger Strike - The Anorectic's Struggle as a Metaphor for Our Age*, Norton, 1986.

- Pipher, Mary, ***Hunger Pains***, Adams Publishing, Holbrook MA, 1995. *Discusses obesity, anorexia, bulimia and cultural influences.*

- Pope, Harrison and James Hudson, ***New Hope For Binge Eaters***, Harper and Row, NY, 1985.

- Roth, Geneen, ***Feeding The Hungry Heart***, New American Library, NY, 1982. *Compulsive overeating and how to overcome it.*

- Roth, Geneen, ***Breaking Free from Compulsive Eating***, Signet Books, New York, 1984.

- Schoenfielder, Lisa, ***When Food is Love: Exploring the Relationship Between Eating and Intimacy***, Signet, NY, 1992.

- Sears, Barry, ***The Zone***, HarperCollins, NY, 1995.

- Waterhouse, Debra, ***Outsmarting the Female Fat Cell***, Hyperion, NY, 1993.

- Welbourne, Jill and Joan Purgold, ***The Eating Sickness***, Harvester, 1984.

- Zerbe, Kathryn, ***The Body Betrayed: Women, Eating Disorders and Treatment***, American Psychiatric Press, 1993.

- **American Anorexia/Bulimia Association**, 293 Central Park West, Suite 1R, New York, NY 10024, phone 212-501-8351.

- **ANRED** (Anorexia Nervosa and Related Eating Disorders), P.O. Box 5102, Eugene OR 97405, phone 503-344-1144.

- **Institute for the Study of Anorexia and Bulimia**, 1 West 91st Street, New York, NY 10024, phone 212-595-3449.

- **National Eating Disorders Organization**, 445 East Granville Road, Worthington OH 43085-3195, phone 614-436-1112.

CARBOHYDRATES

Fuel For The Body

In this chapter you can learn:

- *Why carbohydrates are so important.*

- *What are the best carbohydrate sources, and which ones are harmful or not so good.*

- *What's the big deal about refined food anyway?*

- *Why is sugar harmful?*

- *Did you know how many people get drunk on sugar?*

- *Sugar - you'll find it where you least expect it.*

What are carbohydrates?

Carbohydrates are one of the three macronutrient groups (nutrients needed in large amounts). They are composed of the elements carbon, hydrogen, and oxygen, accounting for the name carbohydrate. Carbohydrates are sometimes abbreviated CHOs, from the first letters of the chemical elements that form them. Carbohydrates are the fuel for your body as gasoline is fuel for your car.

What do carbohydrates contain that is useful to the body?

Unrefined or minimally refined carbohydrates contain the following, although not all carbohydrates have all of these:

- *Fiber, which provides bulk, stabilizes blood sugar (and therefore energy), and aids in digestion*

- *Vitamins and minerals, provitamins such as beta-carotene, bioflavonoids, vitamin E*

- *Water for detoxification and cooling of the body*

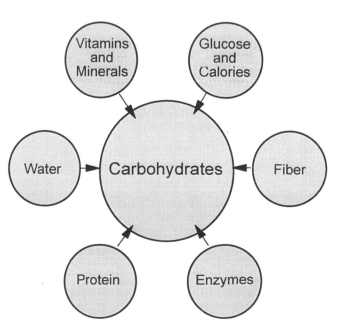

229

- *Glucose (sugar)* and **calories**, *needed for short-term energy (fuel) and brain function*

- *Protein (building blocks), which is found in some carbohydrate foods and which supplies raw material for cell walls. Protein is found especially in nuts and seeds*

- *Enzymes necessary for digestion*

Where do carbohydrates come from?
All carbohydrates come from plants, with the exception of lactose (milk sugar). They are the material from which plant cell walls are made. When ingested, complex carbohydrates help to build our own cell walls and tissues.

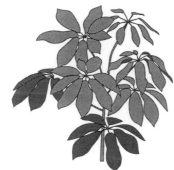

Photosynthesis is the process by which plants take the energy of the sunlight and make green chlorophyll, a substance which is remarkably like the hemoglobin of our blood. The major difference between the two is the iron atom in the center of hemoglobin which makes it red, and the magnesium atom in the center of chlorophyll which is responsible for its green color. It is thus not surprising that what green vegetables provide matches so closely what we need.

The sunlight also causes plants to make sugar, needed by our bodies for life and function. The eating of carbohydrates is like taking in the stored energy of the sun. Carbohydrates give us energy, and the fiber component of the plant cleans house (our colons and bodies) afterward. Carbohydrates slow the uptake of sugar, saving us from sugar spikes that lead to fungus growth and then hypoglycemia.

What is glucose and why is it so important?
Glucose is a simple six-carbon sugar. It is the basic carbohydrate unit extracted from more complex carbohydrates and used by the body. Once the larger carbohydrate molecules are broken down into glucose through the digestive process, the glucose is absorbed through the wall of the small intestine. Glucose then provides fuel, or energy, for necessary cellular processes as gasoline does in a car.

Up to 1200 calories (energy units) of excess glucose enters short term storage (less than 24 hours) as glycogen, which is stored in the muscles and the liver. The nervous system's sympathetic fight-or-flight response to threatening stimuli causes the rapid conversion of glycogen back to glucose, which is released by the liver to provide energy to deal with the impending crisis.

An excess of glucose beyond that which is needed for storage as glycogen is converted to and stored as triglycerides and fat. Body fat can be used for energy when other sources are not available or are used up, although the conversion process is much slower than for glycogen. It takes at least a twenty minute workout before you actually start burning fat.

What kinds of carbohydrates are there?

Carbohydrates can be grouped as complex, intermediate, and refined (or fast). Complex carbohydrates are not processed other than through simple cooking, or they may be raw as in the case of some vegetables and fruits. They contain many nutrients and enzymes needed by our bodies. Refined carbohydrates are highly processed, and include sugar and white flour. The less of these that are eaten, the better. Intermediate carbohydrates, as the name suggests, includes those foods that are somewhat refined such as pasta, bread, and white rice.

The more complex (un-tampered-with) the carbohydrate is, the better it is for you.

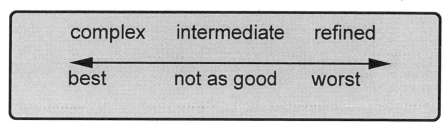

Where do carbohydrates come from?

- The primary food sources of carbohydrates listed with some examples, are:

- *Grains*   *rice, wheat, quinoa, oats*
- *Roots and tubers*   *beets, carrots, yams, potatoes*
- *Beans and legumes*   *lentils, peas, garbanzos*
- *Vegetables*   *leafy greens, squash, broccoli, onions*
- *Fruits*   *apples, citrus fruits, bananas*

Seeds, nuts, and dairy products contain significant amounts of both carbohydrate and protein, and are usually listed in the protein food group.

Grains

What are the grains?

Grains are the seeds of a variety of grasslike plants, and range in size from up to 1/3 inch long (rice) to not much larger than the period at the end of this sentence (amaranth). Grains include:

wheat	***rice***	*oats*	*barley*
spelt	*quinoa*	*amaranth*	*teff*
kamut	*rye*	***millet***	*triticale*

Wheat, quinoa, amaranth, spelt (related to wheat), rye, oats, and barley contain gluten, a sticky protein which holds bread together and that some people have an intolerance to. Millet contains less gluten than these. Rice, millet and buckwheat groats (a grass) are non-gluten or very low gluten grains.

Celiac sprue is one form of gluten intolerance, characterized by bloat and gas when eating wheat or other gluten grains. About one sixth of the population of North European extraction have a predisposition to gluten intolerance, and alcoholics and sugar addicts are the best candidates. One patient, a man in his early 40s, had these characteristic symptoms, along with fatigue, weight gain and a constant feeling of hunger - no matter how much he ate he just never felt satisfied. The symptoms were relieved when wheat was eliminated from his diet.

Contrary to popular belief, understandable due to the similarity in names, buckwheat and wheat are not the same, nor are rice and wild rice. A person with a wheat allergy may not have a problem with buckwheat, or a person who is sensitive to wild rice may not be allergic to brown or white rice.

How are grains prepared?

Grains can be cooked as is, or can be ground into flour to make a variety of intermediate carbohydrate products such as breads and pasta. Although wheat is the grain that is primarily used in this country for these products, nearly all of the grains can be used as cereals or in breads, pastas, crackers, and other products. A health food store is a good source for these alternative grains and grain products. Many whole grains are sold in bulk food bins or packages that include cooking directions and recipe suggestions. Whole grains are significant sources of incomplete proteins, as discussed in the Proteins chapter, and are also sources of the B vitamins.

Some people have difficulty digesting grains, and symptoms of this are gastrointestinal distress (gas, bloat) or recognizable grains such as rice in the feces. Grains can be ground in a grain or coffee mill just before use for easier digestion.

Roots

What are the root vegetables?

Roots and tubers, another source of carbohydrates, have the edible portion of the plant underground. They are a quicker source of carbohydrates than grains. Some roots are:

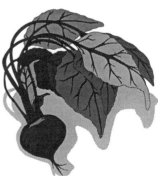

- Potatoes
- Carrots
- Beets
- Turnips
- Parsnips
- Sweet potatoes or yams

White potatoes are primarily starch, although they contain enough vitamins, potassium and protein to be useful in the diet. Most of the nutrition is in and close to the skin, although sprouting potato "eyes" are poisonous, as are green areas in the potato skin to a lesser extent. Carrots and other yellow or orange vegetables contain vitamin A or beta-carotene, its precursor.

Which are better, roots or grains?

Both roots and grains contain valuable nutrients and fiber in their unrefined forms. Roots tend to be sweet, and may worsen a fungus problem. Grains are usually more allergenic than roots. Grains are therefore better than roots for those with fungus, and roots may be better than grains for those with allergic tendencies. Ideally the diet should contain both if you can handle both.

Beans and Legumes

What are beans and legumes?

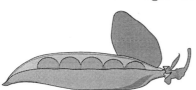

Beans and legumes are larger than grains and grow several to a pod. Beans are generally sold either dried or canned. Dried beans must be soaked and cooked before use to be edible, either by the end user or by a processing company that sells them in canned form. Beans include black, navy, pinto, kidney, garbanzo, and nearly anything else that is called "bean" as part of the product name. Legumes can be sold and eaten raw, such as peas, or cooked. Peanuts are considered to be legumes rather than true nuts. The consumption of peanuts is not recommended because peanuts can contain mold and mold's carcinogenic byproducts aflatoxins, as well as sometimes being rancid. Beans and legumes are also sources of incomplete protein and vitamins.

Beans have a reputation for producing gas, diarrhea, bloating, and other gastrointestinal symptoms. Many people do not digest beans well, resulting in fermentation and allergies. If beans cause discomfort, it is best not to eat them, or to eat them along with proteolytic or pancreatic enzymes or an enzyme product such as Beano, which can help digestion. Cooking beans with a seaweed such as Kombu has also been reported to help with the gas problem, as has rinsing and draining the beans frequently along with soaking overnight, before cooking.

Vegetables

What kinds of vegetables are there?

Vegetables are of several basic types:

- Leafy greens, such as kale, parsley, collards, cabbage, lettuce

- Roots and tubers, such as potatoes, yams, taro, carrots, radishes, beets. These are sometimes considered to be a separate category as are grains.

- Squash family, such as squash, cucumbers, pumpkins, zucchini

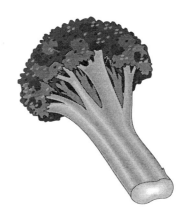

- Vegetables in the Cruciferous family, such as broccoli, Brussels sprouts, cauliflower, and bean sprouts

- Others, such as onions and garlic

What are leafy greens good for?

Leafy greens are important vitamin and mineral (especially calcium) sources. In general, the darker green the leafy vegetable is, the more nutritious it is. Cooked greens are more digestible, while their raw form contains enzymes and a higher level of vitamins. Your diet should contain both.

Which is better, romaine or iceberg lettuce?

Even foods that seem similar can vary greatly in nutritional value, for example romaine vs. iceberg lettuce. One cup contains [1]:

Vitamin	Romaine lettuce	Iceberg lettuce	
Vitamin A	1000 IU	180 IU	
Vitamin B2	0.04 mg	0.02 mg	
Vitamin C	10 mg		2 mg

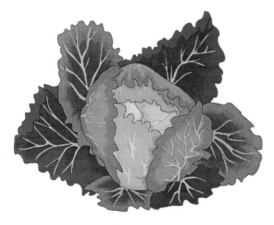

Romaine is also much richer in minerals such as calcium. Iceberg lettuce provides plenty of water but negligible amounts of anything nutritional. The clear choice here seems to be romaine lettuce over iceberg lettuce.

However, things are not that simple. Iceberg lettuce is an excellent metal chelator, and is a good way to clear heavy metals from the body. A person whose body needs cleansing may develop a healthy craving for iceberg lettuce, and this craving should be indulged. Iceberg lettuce, then, takes out the bad and romaine puts in the good. Both are equally important and would work well together in a salad.

What are the squash vegetables?

The vegetables in the squash family grow on vines and contain multiple seeds, usually inedible, in the center. Cucumbers are the least nutritious of the group, resembling iceberg lettuce in that respect. There are many types of squash, including zucchini, Italian, spaghetti squash, butternut, banana squash, and others. These are yellow, orange, or green, and vary in sweetness and calorie content. Yellow and orange vegetables, including carrots, contain beta-carotene, the vitamin A precursor.

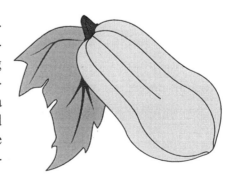

Summer squash, which generally have edible skins, include zucchini and yellow squash. Summer squash are usually less sweet and more easily tolerated by those with a yeast problem than the sweeter winter squash such as butternut or acorn. Winter squash usually have thick inedible skins.

Which vegetables can help prevent cancer?

Cruciferous vegetables have been in the news as being possible cancer fighters. It is speculated that the compound glucarate, present in these vegetables, regulates hormone production which in turn regulates cell growth. Breast cancer is most likely to be influenced [2], as the breasts are mostly lymph tissue. These vegetables contain other nutrients, especially vitamin C.

Fruits

Are fruits good for you?

Citrus fruits are best known as good sources of vitamin C and associated bioflavonoids. Other fruits, such as apples, contain soluble fiber in addition to other nutrients. Fruits, which include berries and melons, contain more natural sugar than most vegetables. For this reason, they are fungus feeders which should be avoided if you have a fungus or yeast problem.

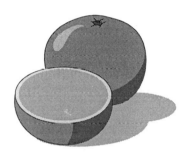

Some people feel that fruits, if eaten at all, should be eaten alone and in the morning when the stomach is empty so they speed through the digestive tract. If proteins or fats are eaten with fruit, the transit time of the fruit is slowed down, giving it time to ferment. An alternative argument, however, is that fruits eaten alone can cause the blood sugar to go too high too fast, resulting in the release of too much insulin. Which advice should you follow? As with other conflicting claims, choose the advice that most closely fits your health situation - eat fruit with protein if blood sugar surges are a problem; eat low-sugar fruit alone first thing in the morning if fermentation is a problem (urine pH above 6.0 is a reliable indicator), or avoid fruit altogether if fermentation or fungus is a problem.

Refining

What are complex, intermediate, and simple carbohydrates?

| **Health food store food is not necessarily healthy.** | All rice is not created equal, nor are all wheat products. Most food sold in America today, other than in health food stores, is highly refined. Actually, so are some "health" foods, so careful label reading is necessary. |

Complex carbohydrates are those which are as close as possible to the way they are found in nature. These include whole grains which still contain the outer husk, such as brown rice, whole beans, fresh vegetables and fruits. Any grain, bean, legume, nut, or seed that can be sprouted is a whole food, still full of enzymes and vital life energy. Refined foods are lacking this vital energy. White rice, for example, will not sprout, or attract bugs, or do anything except sit there. It won't provide much nourishment, either.

Refining of foods refers to any type of processing done to increase shelf life, speed cooking time, or attract consumer attention. It isn't simply a matter of refined vs. unrefined; there are different degrees of refinement. The more refined a product is, the farther away it is from its original form, and the poorer it is nutritionally.

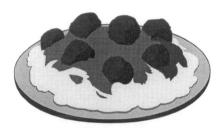

Complex carbohydrates are, as mentioned, as close as possible to the natural state. Simple carbohydrates are sugars which need little or no breaking down. Intermediate carbohydrates are, as the name suggests, a category between simple and complex. Intermediate carbohydrates include pasta, bread, white rice, pretzels, and others. Some intermediate carbohydrates are closer to the complex end of the spectrum (e.g. whole wheat pasta), while others are closer to the simple end (e.g. white flour).

What happens when wheat is refined?

Wheat, like all grains, consists of three parts:

- The outer hull, which provides fiber to clean you out

- The germ, which contains nutrients and enzymes and without which the grain cannot sprout. The germ is the highest protein source.

- The starchy endosperm, which makes up the bulk of the grain and has almost no nutritive value other than calories and a source of glucose

When refined, the husk and germ are removed leaving a pure starch. At this point even further refining is possible. Wheat, for example, can go through a series of steps, each of which is more refined than the previous one:

- The husk and germ are removed

- The devitalized wheat grain is ground into flour

- The flour is mixed with water and other ingredients and pressed into flakes

- The flakes are cooked and dried

- Vitamins and artificial flavors and colors are added to bring it up to the minimum level necessary to be called a food, along with the addition of miscellaneous chemicals and large quantities of sugar.

Voila! Breakfast cereal. It may taste like food - after all, what do most Americans have to compare it with? - but it has about the same nutritive value as a bowl of wallpaper paste combined with a handful of sugar cubes and a multivitamin tablet.

Wouldn't refining food be helpful to the body?

If you recall that the body's goal is to break complex carbohydrates into the smallest unit, i.e. glucose, that can be used by the body, the question may arise: wouldn't refining help the body by performing some of the breaking-down steps? The answer is no. For one thing, refining removes most or all of the valuable nutrients and fiber. Brown rice has 24 nutrients, while white rice, with the husk and germ removed, has only one. In fact, the hull of the rice, removed to make white rice, is such a concentrated source of vitamins that the hulls are used to make vitamin pills. Even "enriched" processed foods have only a small amount of these added back, usually in synthetic (not natural) form. Enriching food is like having a burglar steal $100 from you and then give you back bus fare.

So much for "All calories are created equal" (calorie-wise, a cup of brown rice has about as many calories as a cup of white rice). This is a myth perpetrated by the food processing industry, embraced by dieters and the end result is hospital food.

How much nutrition is lost in refining?

When wheat flour is refined to white flour, the following percentages of nutrients arc lost [3]:

Vitamin E	*96%*	*Iron*	*76%*
Vitamin B1	*88%*	*Zinc*	*73%*
Vitamin B6	*84%*	*Copper*	*65%*
Niacin	*80%*	*Calcium*	*64%*
Magnesium	*80%*	*Folic acid*	*63%*
Phosphorus	*78%*	*Vitamin B5*	*62%*
Potassium	*77%*	*Vitamin B2*	*54%*

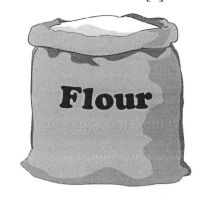

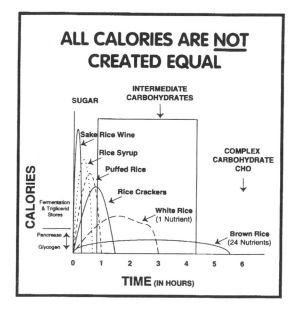

ALL CALORIES ARE NOT CREATED EQUAL

Why else is refining bad?

The other reason that refining is bad has to do with the smooth, constant delivery of glucose to the body. Refined products such as sugar and white flour provide a large amount of glucose in a short time, while unrefined carbohydrates allow a slower, more consistent release. If the speed of sugar entering the bloodstream is increased, this in turn raises the insulin level, which can raise the unwanted conversion of sugars to triglycerides and fat. The difference in sugar release from a single product can be shown in graph form with progressively more refined forms of rice, as shown in the chart to the left.

How well would your car run if your fuel injection system alternately delivered too much and too little gasoline to the engine? Your body doesn't do much better with refined carbohydrates, even with the help of the glycogen storage and release system. The release of insulin also helps to moderate blood glucose, but can itself cause fluctuations between too much and too little glucose. Hypoglycemia or adult-onset diabetes (which may begin as hypoglycemia) can result over time.

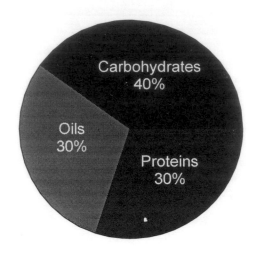

The best balance of carbohydrates to other dietary components is: 40% carbohydrates, 30% protein, 30% healthful vegetable oils (by percentage of calories, not weight).

Why else are refined carbohydrates bad for you?
In summary, refined carbohydrates are useless, nearly useless, or even harmful because:

- Refining has removed most or all of the nutrients and enzymes.

- Sugar (glucose) concentration is too high, and its consumption all at once leads to inefficient energy spurts and lows, as well as hypoglycemia and diabetes.

- Fiber, which helps to clean the colon, has been removed.

- Filling up on nutrient deficient (non)food can take away the appetite for healthful foods, at the same time leaving you unsatisfied and craving more.

- Refined sugar (sucrose) is so far removed from the original natural source that it acts as a drug if consumed in excess, complete with addiction and withdrawal symptoms in some people.

- Refined flour and sugar provides food for yeast, other fungus, and bacteria in our bodies.

- Refined carbohydrates can be made into alcohol in the body, a phenomenon called the auto-brewery syndrome.

Sugar

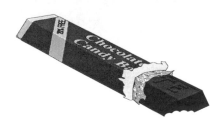

Is there a difference between refined and unrefined sugars?
Sugars are converted rapidly into glucose. They are present in all carbohydrates to some extent, especially fruits and sweet vegetables such as carrots, corn and peas. In unrefined form they cause less trouble than refined forms, although problems can arise when fruits are consumed by people who have problems with yeast overgrowth and fermentation. Refined sugar of

any type, on the other hand, provides only glucose and calories. For a number of reasons, the less refined sugar in the diet the better, and one can easily do without it altogether. Although your body needs glucose, you can get all the glucose you need from vegetables and complex carbohydrates like grains and roots.

How can sugar become fat even more than fat does?
Sugars can be rearranged by the body's good bacteria to form necessary short-chain fatty acids if the sugars come from unrefined sources which make the conversion slowly. Refined sugars are more likely to become sticky harmful triglycerides, which can cause weight gain from the deposit of fat, insulin swings, and eventually blockage of arteries.

Is sugar really bad for you?
Since refined sugar both is unnatural to the body and has a profound effect on body systems, it can properly be classified as a drug or toxin. In fact, sugar addiction is possible, and is quite common. Sounds extreme? The characteristics of addiction from the chapter on Drugs in *Surviving The Toxic Crisis* include:

- *Feeling of being "high", at least for a short time after ingestion*
- *Tolerance - ever-increasing amounts are taken for the same effect*
- *Withdrawal symptoms - tiredness, depression, irritability*
- *Strong craving for the substance on a repeated, daily basis*

While many people can consume sugar occasionally and nonaddictively, these signs of addiction may be very familiar to those who feel incomplete without their morning donut, the chocolates in the desk drawer at work, or the constantly replenished ice cream in the freezer. Like the three legal drugs coffee, cigarettes and alcohol, sugar is extremely addictive.

Stress tends to increase sugar consumption, much as stress increases the chances that a person will turn to other drugs for relief. Actually, sugar *increases* stress from the inside so that even figurative speed bumps look like the Matterhorn to hypoglycemics. It is probably a coincidence, but it is interesting to note that "stressed" spelled backwards is "desserts".

> "Stressed" spelled backwards is "desserts".
> Coincidence?

Yeast overgrowth, or candida, is a problem for many people. If you have ever baked bread, you know that sugar must be added to the mixture or the yeast won't grow and multiply as fast. Sugar in the body is likewise food for yeast. Refined flour, white rice, and other processed foods break down into sugar so fast that they cause effects similar to those of pure sugar - the high, the addiction, the yeast overgrowth.

Lucille, a 30 year old woman, found that her candida (yeast) and PMS symptoms cleared when she stopped eating sugar and started taking acidophilus. Mark, a preteen child with Attention Deficit Disorder (ADD), was taken off sugar, wheat and dairy and became calmer and was better able to study. He stopped disrupting the class, and the teacher was so amazed that she assumed that he was on the drug Ritalin.

Researchers at Yale University School of Medicine found that sugar causes a noticeable physical and psychological reaction in normal healthy children. Children's adrenaline levels rose twice as high as adults' to counteract the effect of insulin which is released to counteract the effect of sugar. The ability to pay attention is also affected [4,5].

Monkeys fed sweets and pastries develop bones that are porous, weak and brittle - this is osteoporosis [6].

Refined sugar may contribute to irritable bowel syndrome by shortening bowel transit time and increasing the fecal bile acid concentration [7].

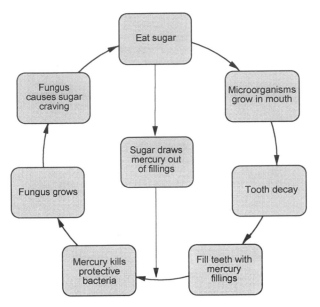

Why do some people become hypoglycemic?

When people eat too much sugar, it feeds the microorganisms in the mouth which cause tooth decay and plaque on the teeth. They then need more mercury amalgam fillings to fill the cavities. When they eat more sweets, the acidic sugar pulls mercury out of the fillings into the body. Mercury is an antibiotic which kills the protective bacteria, allowing the fungus and pathogenic bacteria to proliferate. The fungus steals your sugar causing hypoglycemia and sweets cravings in a vicious cycle.

Sugar, including fruit, upsets the body's mineral balance because the acidic sugar chelates out the minerals so that mineral dependent enzymes are unable to function properly. Food then does not digest properly, leading to leaky gut, allergy, and immune depletion and disease. When you eat as little as two teaspoons of sugar per day, equivalent to two ounces of soda or a tablespoon of jam, mineral balance can change. Typically calcium increases in the blood to buffer inflammation, stealing copper from the long bones, and phosphorus decreases [8]. This can lead to arteriosclerosis, arthritis and other degenerative conditions.

Can you get drunk on sugar? or: What's the difference between you and a wine bottle?

Do you know how alcoholic beverages are made? A carbohydrate such as grapes, barley, or malt is incubated with yeast in a warm dark wet place until fermentation occurs. In fermentation, the yeast and bacteria break down the starch into sugar, and the sugar into alcohol. Our digestive tract is a warm dark wet place, and we all have yeast and bacteria in our bodies. Since a diet high in refined foods is also usually low in fiber, and a low fiber diet can cause foods to sit in the digestive tract for days before being eliminated, all the ingredients are present to turn a body into a brewery!

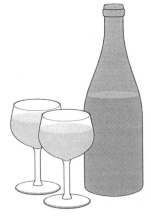

An intake of alcohol usually causes a high - a feeling of increased energy and alertness - followed by a feeling of fatigue and depression. Thinking is foggy, reaction time is sluggish, sleep is disturbed. Addictive symptoms both follow and result in increased intake. If you have ever gone on a sugar binge, you will probably recognize all of these symptoms, differing only in intensity from those of alcohol. The recovering alcoholic, ending an Alcoholics Anonymous meeting with a cup of heavily sugared coffee and a donut or two, may not be as sober as he thinks he is - he may be making his own alcohol! This is sometimes called the auto-brewery syndrome or a dry drunk. High SGOT (over 30) or GGTP (over 40) in a non-drinker can be a sign of auto-brewery syndrome.

The bloat and gas that often results is similar to the gas that can pop the cork off a bottle of homemade wine.

As in the alcohol fermentation industry, the consumption of the following grains or fruits can produce the following alcoholic beverages in your body, differing from commercial products only in concentration:

- *Apples   hard cider*
- *Barley   malt whiskey (Scotch)*
- *Rye   rye whiskey*
- *Grapes   wine*
- *Corn   bourbon*
- *Potatoes   Irish whiskey*

Apart from the harmful effects of sugar, its presence in large quantity in the diet means that proportionately less nutritious food is being eaten. Also, once a person is used to the concentrated sweetness of sugar, fruits and vegetables can taste so dull by comparison that they may be omitted from the diet.

Where is refined sugar found?

If you have decided to reduce or eliminate refined sugar from your diet - and this is highly recommended - you may find it more difficult to do than you thought. There is more to abstinence than foregoing candy, cookies, cake, and sugar in your coffee. Sugars are found in nearly all processed, packaged, canned, and frozen foods, even the most unlikely ones. Sugar is defined here as excluding natural sugars already present in the product, and including refined sweeteners other than sucrose (table sugar). Some ketchup, for example, contains more sugar than it does tomatoes. Commercial cereals that look unsweetened, such as plain flakes or granola, also contain quite a bit of sugar, as do canned and frozen vegetables and fruits, and chewable vitamins. Some salad dressings contain more corn syrup than oil. Some common foods and their sugar content include [9,10]:

Some ketchup contains more sugar than it does tomatoes.

Food	Serving size	Teaspoons of sugar
Cola and sodas	12 ounce can	10-12
Pudding mix	1/2 cup	10
Fruit pie	1 slice	10-14
Layer cake	1 slice, iced	9-15

Chocolate bar	1 average	7
Hard candy	1 ounce	7
Fruit yogurt	1 cup	7
Sherbet	1/2 cup	6-8
Ice cream	1 scoop	5
Donut, plain	1	4
Vanilla yogurt	1 cup	3.5
Jam or jelly	1 Tbsp	3
Marshmallow	1 large	1.5

One teaspoon of sugar is equivalent to three feet of sugar cane, and one can of soda therefore contains the equivalent of 30 feet of sugar cane!

Put another way, sugar makes up the following percentage of the total weight of the food [11]:

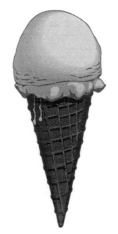

Hard candies	88% of total weight
Choc. chip cookies	75%
Apple Jacks cereal	52%
Raisin Bran	30%
Ketchup	23-35%
Ice cream	23%
100% Bran cereal	22%
Fruit flavor yogurt	18%
Mayonnaise	15%
Donuts	15%
Coca-Cola	10%

By contrast, most vegetables have 0-5% sugar (natural sugar) by weight. Even the relatively sweet vegetables have very little [12]:

Carrots	4%
Tomato juice	3%
Corn	2%
Peas	1%

> **The average American eats 48 teaspoons of sugar per day.**

The average American eats 48 teaspoons of sugar per day in various products - the equivalent of one teaspoon every half hour around the clock [3]. This adds up to 120-130 pounds of sugar per person per year, which is 20-25% of all calories consumed, or 500-600 calories per day [11]. This 48 teaspoons of sugar multiplied by three feet of sugar cane per teaspoon equals the equivalent of 144 feet of sugar cane per day without its beneficial nutrients and roughage to support and regulate processing. Is it any wonder that we have so many candida-caused cases of hypoglycemia which can lead to adult-onset diabetes?

What kinds of refined sugar are there?
Refined sugar comes in many types and forms. Although minor differences exist, especially in taste, your body's microorganisms considers them all to be about the same. These include:

- *Sucrose, fructose, and any other ingredient ending in -ose*

- *Raw or turbinado sugar, date sugar*

- *Any type of syrup, such as corn, maple, or rice. Corn syrup may also be called high fructose corn syrup or corn sweetener.*

- *Molasses, sorghum, honey, malt, barley malt*

- *Sorbitol, mannitol, xylitol*

What are the differences between these kinds of sugar?

Sucrose is plain white table sugar. Confectioner's sugar is powdered sucrose with cornstarch added. Sucrose is a disaccharide, meaning that it is made up of two types of sugar, glucose and fructose.

Raw or turbinado sugar, which is a light brownish tan color, is sucrose which is slightly less refined than white sugar, or white sugar that has been sprayed with a small amount of molasses. It contains a small amount of minerals, but the nutritional affect is comparable to using white sugar and biting off a tiny corner of a mineral supplement tablet.

Fructose is fruit sugar, but is not much more natural or desirable in refined form than sucrose. Fructose bears the same relationship to an apple as table sugar does to a sugar beet. Most commercial fructose is made from sucrose with the glucose component chemically removed or from corn rather than being extracted from fruit. Lactose is milk sugar, which has a high allergic potential, especially if you don't have the enzyme lactase which requires the presence of healthy bacteria. Dextrose is another name for glucose.

Molasses, sorghum, and honey are closer to nature than most other sugars, but the difference in the body is slight - the sugar is released somewhat more slowly. Honey is not recommended for infants under one year, as a form of infant botulism is possible. Honey's primary sugar is fructose, which is even simpler than sucrose, but the honey base causes it to be released more slowly. All things considered, honey is usually the best choice if refined sugar is used at all.

Mannitol, xylitol, and the other -itols are sugar alcohols that are similar to fructose. They are less sweet than sucrose and are metabolized more slowly. They penetrate cells to a greater degree than sucrose and are therefore more toxic.

How is sugar disguised in food labeling?

Food labeling requirements stipulate that product ingredients be listed in descending order. Sometimes more than one sugar is used in a product so that none of them would have to be listed first or second. If all of the sugar were listed together, sugar may be the first and most plentiful ingredient. Another labeling trick to disguise the amount of sugar present is to use sugars with names which are unfamiliar to many consumers, such as malto-dextrin or levulose.

How can sugar cravings be reduced?

The following have proven to be useful in reducing sugar cravings:

- *Protein*
- *Complex carbohydrates for slower sustained release of blood sugar*
- *Chromium for blood sugar regulation*
- *Vanadyl sulfate for blood sugar regulation*
- *Orifresh (aloe vera with potassium sorbate) for controlling yeast*
- *Other treatments for yeast*
- *Zinc*
- *Grapefruit seed extract - Nutricidal or Citricidal brands*
- *Myrrh*
- *Black walnut*
- *Caprylic acid*

Fiber

What part of the grain does cleanup work?

Fiber is the relatively insoluble part of complex carbohydrates. Fiber is found in all unrefined carbohydrates, although the type and amount differ. Bran, fiber that is removed from grains as part of the refining process, can be added to other foods to increase the fiber content. Fiber is a necessary component of a healthful diet for a number of reasons, including

- *colon health*   • *detoxification*   • *weight loss*
- *blood glucose regulation (slows down sugar highs and lows)*

What are the types of fiber?

There are two basic types of fiber: water soluble and water insoluble, with several fiber subtypes in each category.

- *Insoluble - Cellulose, hemicellulose, lignin, waxes*
- *Soluble - Pectins, gums, mucilages, sterols*

Grains and bran and some fruits supply insoluble fiber, while fruits, vegetables, beans, and psyllium seed supply soluble (gel forming) fiber.

How does fiber aid in weight normalization, appetite suppression, bowel regularity, and lowering of cholesterol?

The effects of fiber are both mechanical and metabolic. Mechanical (non-chemical) effects include regulating (increasing or decreasing) transit time of food through the intestines and absorption of water. The absorption of water by both soluble and insoluble fiber leads to increased fecal bulk and increased bowel movement frequency, both important in cleaning out the digestive system and in preventing fermentation and putrefaction in the gut. Increasing water absorption tends to correct both diarrhea and constipation, as the fiber will absorb liquid from either the fecal matter or the colon walls as needed.

Fiber acts as a sponge to absorb harmful fatty acids. Some fiber attracts fats through electrical charges, and some are fermented by bacteria and yeasts into acids that change pH (acidity) of the intestinal tract and block the making of cholesterol in the liver [13]. One patient with high cholesterol and blood sugar swings had both of these problems which were helped by the addition of fiber to his diet.

Metabolic effects are a property of water soluble fiber only. These effects include:

- *Reducing serum cholesterol and fats*
- *Stabilizing blood sugar*
- *Lowering blood pressure*
- *Blocking the absorption of fat*
- *Promoting growth of friendly intestinal flora*
- *Fiber causes the "I've eaten enough" signal to kick in sooner and stronger and to last longer, which helps in weight control.*

Degenerative and other diseases known or thought to be helped or prevented by fiber include [14,15,16]:

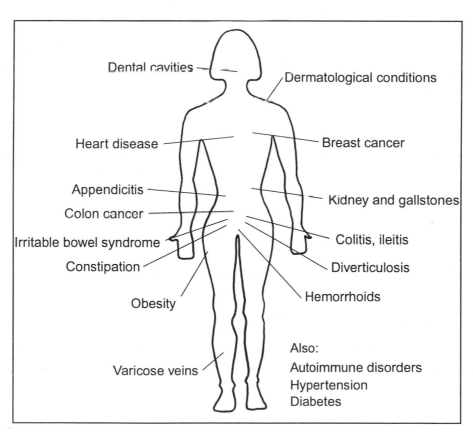

Fiber tends to lower and/or prevent age-related increase in blood pressure, even without weight loss [17-19].

What has been shown to reduce diabetes deaths by over 50%?

The British ate only brown bread by government stipulation from 1941 to 1955 due to reduction of wheat imports as a result of World War II. Diabetes deaths fell by 54% between 1942 and 1954 [8]. The bulk, or fiber, of whole food gives the intestines the work they were designed to do and the whole body functions better as a result. The increased nutrient content of brown bread very likely also played an important part.

Lack of what can cause up to four times the increase in colon cancer?

Low fiber diets (as well as gallbladder removal) increase colon cancer risk because carcinogens are more concentrated when there is a smaller mass of food to dilute them. The slower transit time of food through the colon gives the carcinogens and toxins more time to contact each portion of the colon wall and also increases the possibility of allergic reactions.

Should fiber be added to the diet rapidly?

When introducing fiber into the diet, do it gradually. If you abruptly go from a sedentary lifestyle to marathon training, your body will hurt and complain. Similarly, adding a lot more fiber to the diet without a transition period is asking your body, especially your digestive system, to work harder than it is used to, and it may complain. Gas and abdominal cramps can be reduced by adding more fiber to the diet gradually.

If too much fiber or the wrong kind of fiber is added to the diet of those who are ill, elderly, or severely constipated, or if the fiber is taken without enough water or oil, the fiber can cause blockages and worsen the situation.

Summary

Carbohydrates are fuel for the body as well as providing other necessary functions.

To get the most out of carbohydrates:

- Reduce or eliminate refined foods such as sugar, white flour products, and white rice.

- Eat more vegetables and complex carbohydrates

- Eat carbohydrates in balance with other types of foods - 40% carbohydrates, 30% each protein and healthy oils.

References and Resources

- Appleton, Nancy, *Lick The Sugar Habit*, Avery Publishing Group, Garden City Park, NY, 1989.

- Cheraskin and Ringsdorf, *Psychodietetics*, Stein and Day, 1974.

- Damen, Betty, *New Facts About Fiber*, Nutrition Encounter Inc., Novato CA, 1991.

- Harrington, Geri, *Real Food, Fake Food*, MacMillan Publishing Co., New York, 1987.

- Lowell, Jax Peters, *Against the Grain: The Slightly Eccentric Guide to Living Well Without Gluten or Wheat*, Henry Holt, NY. *Practical guide to dealing with the psychological challenges of living with a restricted diet, restaurants, airline food, label reading etc.*

- Murray, Michael and Joseph Pizzorno, *A Textbook of Natural Medicine*, John Bastyr College Publications, 1989.

- Trowell, H., Denis Burkitt and K. Heaton, *Dietary Fibre, Fibre-Depleted Foods and Disease*, Academic Press, NY, 1985.

- Yiamouyiannis, John, *High Performance Health*, Health Action Press, Delaware OH, 1987.

PROTEINS AND AMINO ACIDS

Our Body's Building Blocks

In this chapter you can learn:

- *Why protein is so necessary, even though it's expensive, allergy-causing and hard to keep fresh.*
- *What to be sure of when taking amino acid supplements.*
- *How you can make a complete protein, and why this is important.*
- *How the body's recycling system works.*
- *Does everyone, or even children, really need cow's milk?*

What is protein?

Protein is the body's major building material. The word protein comes from the Greek word "proteios", meaning "of prime importance", a well chosen name considering its importance in the body. Up to 75% of our body solids are protein.

What is protein used for?

Protein is used in the body for:

- *Growth of hair and nails*
- *Wound healing*
- *Connective tissue*
- *Enzymes and hormones*
- *Fetal development and human milk production*
- *Tissue growth and maintenance*
- *Immune system antibodies*
- *Transportation of nutrients*

What are proteins made of?

Proteins are made up of amino acids that are joined together chemically by linkages called peptide bonds. Amino acids are nitrogen-containing compounds that can work either alone as amino acids or combined as proteins, which are large groups of amino acids. If protein can be compared to a house, amino acids are the bricks it's built with.

Just as any type, number, and combination of boxcars can be linked together to form a train, so can amino acids be linked together to form proteins. The twenty basic amino acids can be combined to form many thousands of proteins, each of which has a specific function in the body.

When protein is eaten, it is broken down by the body into amino acids. These can be used as is or recombined into new proteins necessary for body function, like recycling building materials.

If the body is not efficient at breaking down protein into amino acids, they may be broken only into polypeptides - small amino acid groups - that can cause allergies.

Amino Acids

Are all amino acids essential?

The term essential as used here is not the same as necessary. All amino acids are necessary, but essential amino acids are the amino acids that must be supplied by the diet, while the others can be synthesized by the body. Amino acids are thus divided into two groups, essential and nonessential. There are about 22 major or commonly found amino acids discussed here [1,6]; however, over 150 lesser-known amino acids also exist.

Not all sources agree on the number of major amino acids or which ones are essential or nonessential. For example, some sources include cystine and cysteine as either two separate amino acids [2] or as one [3]. Other sources include carnitine [4], taurine and GABA (gamma-amino butyric acid) [5], or ornithine [2]. All of these are made in the body from the other amino acids, and all are necessary. The discrepancy lies only in whether they are listed as separate major amino acids vs. minor amino acids or combinations.

There are four basic groups of amino acids [7]:

- *Glycogenics (glucose producers): alanine, glycine, proline, glutamine, lysine*

- *Sulfur based for detoxification: cystine, cysteine, methionine, taurine*

- *Branched chain used for protein synthesis, build muscle mass: Leucine, isoleucine, valine. These are also important constituents of the liver, an organ which is critical in detoxification [8]*

- *Neurotransmitter (nervous system): phenylalanine, tyrosine, tryptophan, glycine, taurine, GABA*

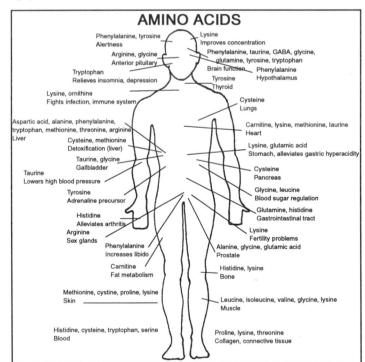

What are each of the amino acids used for?

The major amino acids (in alphabetical order), some of their uses, and other information include the following. Essential amino acids are marked (E). The nutrients they work best with are also called synergists.

Alanine (E)

Used for: Maintains blood glucose levels

Arginine (E)

Used for:
- Immune stimulation, helps immune response
- Growth
- Blocks tumor formation
- Increases male sperm count
- Aids in wound healing
- Metabolizes stored body fat
- Ammonia detoxification
- Liver regeneration

Works best with: Vitamin B6, manganese, magnesium, zinc

Found in: Nuts, seeds, brown rice, oatmeal, whole wheat, gelatin

Supplement information:
- Available as tablets or powder.
- Best taken before bed on an empty stomach with water in a two gram dose.

Asparagine

Used for: Metabolic control of brain and nervous system cells

Aspartic acid

Used for: Increases resistance to fatigue, converts fat to energy, protects central nervous system, expels harmful ammonia from body, protects liver from drug damage.

Caution: Can strip fat from nerve cells, especially in those who are quite thin, causing symptoms of multiple sclerosis (MS). Aspartic acid is found in harmful excess in the artificial sweetener Aspartame (NutraSweet) and in mineral chelates such as **calcium aspartate.**

Supplement information:
- Available as 250 and 500 mg tablets.
- Take 1-3 times daily with water and no protein.

Carnitine

Used for:
- Improves fat metabolism

- Increases use of fat as energy source
- Helps to manage ischemic heart disease
- Prevents accumulation of ketones (waste products) during weight loss
- Reduces blood triglycerides

Cystine and cysteine

One is converted to the other as needed.

Used for:

- Good for body detoxification
- Resistance to free radical damage, chemicals, and heavy metals
- Antioxidant
- Protection against cancer
- Protection from radiation
- Promotes healing from injury
- Disease resistance
- Aids in iron absorption
- Skin formation.

Works best with:

- Vitamins B6, B12, and C; folic acid, magnesium

Caution:

- Diabetics should avoid cysteine, which can inactivate insulin.
- In excess, cystine can chelate heavy metals and allow them to pass through the blood-brain barrier.
- It should be used with glutathione, methionine and vitamin C.

Glutamic acid, Glutamine (E)

Used for:

- Brain fuel, improves intelligence
- Relieves fatigue
- Shortens healing time for ulcers
- Potassium transport
- Ammonia detoxification by turning glutamic acid into glutamine
- Glutamine reduces craving for alcohol and sugar
- Protection against alcohol's toxic effects

Works best with: Vitamin B6, folic acid, magnesium

Supplement information:

- Available in 500 mg capsules.

- 1-4 grams recommended daily in divided doses.

Glycine (E)

Used for:

- Aids in pituitary and prostate gland function
- Blood sugar regulation
- Relaxes muscles
- Alleviates gastric hyperacidity

Works best with: Vitamin B6, folic acid, zinc, sodium

Histidine (E)

Used for:

- Reduces high blood pressure
- Blood cell production
- Used to treat allergies, ulcers, anemia, and rheumatoid arthritis
- Stabilizes allergic reactivity
- Used to chelate trace minerals

Leucine

Used for:

- Found in high concentration in muscle tissue
- Lowers blood sugar
- Promotes wound and bone healing

Lysine

Used for:

- Fights viral and herpes infections (especially with copper as copper lysinate)
- Promotes better concentration
- Affords cardiovascular protection
- Utilizes fatty acids for energy production
- Alleviates some fertility problems
- Promotes bone growth
- Forms collagen
- Aids in calcium absorption

Works best with: Vitamins B6 and C, copper, iron.

Found in: Fish, milk, cheese, eggs, yeast, and soy.

Supplement information:
- Usually in 500 mg capsules.
- Take 1-2 capsules daily between meals.
- Taken with copper to form anti-viral copper lysinate.

Of interest:
- Lysine and arginine are shown to enhance immune function by increasing the number of lymphocytes and IgG levels [9]. This combination of amino acids can help reverse age-related decline in thymus function, and is effective in children with recurrent upper respiratory infections [10].

Note: Arginine aids viral growth while lysine controls virus; arginine should not be taken without lysine by viral patients.

Methionine (E)

Used for:
- Detoxification of metals and chemicals
- Reduces cholesterol deposits
- Antioxidant
- Fights fatigue
- Lowers blood levels of histamine which can produce allergic symptoms
- Helps protect against certain tumors
- Helps prevent skin and nail disorders and hair loss
- Helps prevent fat accumulation in the liver

Works best with: Vitamin B6, B12, C, folic acid, magnesium, molybdenum

Ornithine

Used for:
- Immune system builder
- Protects against free radical damage
- Releases growth hormone
- Promotes wound healing
- Liver regeneration.

Works best with: Vitamin B6, manganese, magnesium, zinc

Phenylalanine (E)

Used for:
- Reduces hunger
- Increases libido

- Mental alertness
- Alleviates depression
- Used in manufacture of the neurotransmitters norepinephrine (noradrenaline) and catecholamine
- Has painkilling properties.

Found in: Milk products, soy, nuts, and seeds. Also found in the artificial sweetener Aspartame, whose use is not recommended.

Supplement information:
- Available in 250 and 500 mg tablets. Should be taken with water an hour before meals.

Proline (E)

Used for:
- Maintains and repairs joints and tendons
- Collagen formation.

Works best with: Vitamins B6 and C, copper, iron.

Taurine

Used for:
- Controls electrical discharge in brain (epilepsy) and heart (arrhythmia)
- Increases bile flow
- Anticonvulsant
- Breaks down fats
- Lowers high blood pressure

Works best with: Vitamins B6 and B12, magnesium, zinc.

Threonine

Used for:
- Helps prevent fatty buildup in liver
- Constituent of collagen and tooth enamel protein

Tryptophan (E)

Used for:
- Helps induce sleep and relaxation by producing the neurotransmitter serotonin
- Antidepressant, relieves anxiety
- Treats migraine headaches

- Muscle growth
- Reduces blood pressure by dilating blood vessels
- Reduces blood fats and cholesterol
- Improves ability to go to sleep by converting to melatonin, which requires sunlight to produce.
- Produces nicotinic acid (niacin) which helps counteract nicotine in cigarettes.

Found in:

- Meats and poultry, especially turkey.
- Dairy products - this is why a glass of warm milk has long been used as a sleep aid.
- Bananas, peanuts.

Works best with: Niacin, vitamin B6

Of interest:

- When tryptophan was banned, many patients who couldn't sleep turned to Prozac instead, and many became addicted to it. Melatonin is a natural sleep aid that can be used instead.

Supplement information:

- No longer available as supplement in the U.S for political/legal reasons. Should be taken at night.

Tyrosine

Used for:

- Precursor of adrenaline and thyroid hormones
- Promotes ability to stay asleep
- Helps control depression and anxiety
- Helps in dealing with physical and emotional stress
- Appetite suppressant
- Stimulates growth hormone
- Antioxidant
- Production of melanin (skin colorant and protectant)

Works best with: Vitamins B6 and C, copper, magnesium, manganese

Supplement information:

- Should be taken in the morning to provide adrenal support and energy, or in small amounts before bed.
- Tryptophan and tyrosine are antagonists and should not be taken together.

More detailed information on each amino acid can be found in many standard nutritional reference books, including those listed at the end of the chapters in this section.

Any complete protein source as discussed in the following pages will provide all of the essential amino acids and many of the nonessential ones.

Let's resolve some labeling confusion - What are L and D forms of amino acids?

Amino acids are found in both D and L forms. L means levo, or left-handed, while D means

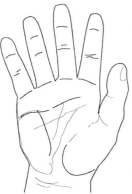

dextro, or right-handed. D and L refer to the rotation of the molecule, and one is the mirror image of the other, like a screw or bolt and its mirror image. L forms are found naturally and are most useful to the body, while D forms, with few exceptions, are not utilized and may even be harmful. DL forms refer to a combination. You may have encountered terms like L-lysine or DL-phenylalanine; this should resolve the confusion. L-forms of amino acids are preferable as they are more normal to the body. There are exceptions; DL-phenylalanine is sometimes taken for pain relief.

Buyer beware

Amino acids must be balanced to work correctly. A common mistake is to take one or two single amino acid supplements based on perceived need and end up worse off because an imbalance has been created. All cells

Buyer Beware!

need all nutrients, and a higher dose of one or two may influence health effects. For example, if you take a lot of arginine to build muscle mass, less lysine, which uses the same metabolic pathways, gets to the cells. This created deficiency in lysine, an amino acid which is a virus fighter, can lead to more colds and even herpes outbreaks. The best course for supplementation is to take amino acids on the advice of a knowledgeable health practitioner, preferably after taking a blood test called an amino acid panel.

How can amino acid supplementation help?

In a clinical study, chronic fatigue patients were given amino acid supplements for three months. The particular amino acid mixture was individualized by each patient's fasting blood plasma values. The most commonly deficient amino acids were phenylalanine and tryptophan; 75% of the patients reported a 50-100% improvement in their symptoms, and some experienced a substantial increase in energy within several days to two weeks [11].

What conditions can benefit from which amino acids?

Some diseases and probable amino acid therapies include [5]:

Disease or problem	Probable therapy
Aging	methionine, tryptophan
Appetite control	tryptophan, phenylalanine
Arthritis	histidine, cysteine
Cancer	cysteine, taurine
Cholesterol, high	methionine, taurine, glycine, carnitine, arginine

Chronic pain	tryptophan, phenylalanine
Cigarette addiction	tyrosine
Depression	tryptophan, phenylalanine, threonine, tyrosine
Diabetes	alanine, tryptophan
Epilepsy	glycine, taurine
Hair loss	cysteine, arginine
Heart failure	taurine, tyrosine, carnitine
Herpes	lysine (with copper)
Hypertension	tryptophan, GABA, taurine
Hypoglycemia	alanine, GABA
Insomnia	tryptophan
Liver disease	isoleucine, leucine, valine
Manic depression	tryptophan, glycine
Osteoporosis	lysine
Radiation toxicity	cysteine, taurine, methionine, glycine
Stress	tyrosine, histidine
Viral infections	lysine (taken with copper)

Correcting amino acid deficiencies normally starts with correcting albumin protein deficiencies, being sure there is sufficient hydrochloric acid (HCl) and avoiding allergens.

Protein

How does protein become amino acids, and then become new proteins?

Protein is made up of amino acids, and must be broken back down to amino acids through the digestive process to be utilized by the body. Stomach acid and enzymes in the stomach and small intestine break the chemical bonds holding the amino acids together. Cooking and marinating animal products start this process and make the protein easier to digest, but themselves cause the loss of natural enzymes from the meat.

Should you just look for amino acid content on the side of a can of protein powder?

There is more to the picture than just the amount of total protein. Some proteins are easier to digest than others, and digestibility is very important or the protein will be useless or even allergy producing in the body. For example, there is enough protein in the average wooden desk (as assayed in the laboratory) to supply your protein needs for a year, but only a termite is equipped to make use of it.

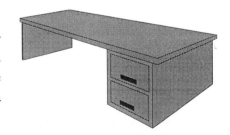

Some protein powders with soy or milk protein, especially without enzymes, are hard to digest and are therefore lower in *usable* amino acids, regardless of the amino acid content listed on the package. Rice-based protein powder with enzymes is usually easiest to digest. Those who have trouble gaining weight from degenerative disease such as cancer or AIDS, or those with allergies, should especially consider digestibility when choosing protein powder.

One patient, a 49 year old bicycle enthusiast, failed to get any noticeable energy with cheap protein powder. In fact, allergy to the ingredients made him even more tired. Predigested rice-based protein powder with electrolytes solved the problem. His stamina has increased to the point that he is now beating the 20 and 30 year olds who regularly outrode him in the past.

Once in the body, amino acids can be used as is or recombined into proteins necessary for body function. These proteins can then be broken back down to the component amino acids and reformed into yet other proteins. The body's amazing recycling process does not operate at 100% efficiency, however, so protein must be ingested on a daily basis to keep the system going.

What are complete proteins?

There are both complete and incomplete proteins. Complete proteins contain all of the essential amino acids. If even one is missing the protein cannot be fully utilized by the body. Foods containing complete protein include eggs (one of the best sources), meat, poultry, fish, milk products, and to a lesser extent soy products, which are less digestible and are allergenic for many people.

How can incomplete proteins be made complete?

Incomplete protein foods do not contain all of the amino acids by themselves. However, there are many food combinations which, when eaten together, complement each other and form a complete protein. Nearly any whole grain combined with nearly any bean or legume forms a complete protein, although grains or beans by themselves are incomplete. This allows vegetarians to get adequate protein with little difficulty, assuming that they have a healthy digestive system. An incomplete protein combined with a small amount of animal protein is also complete. It is interesting that nearly every culture has developed a grain and bean combination characteristic of that culture long before formal nutrition studies were possible. Some examples are:

- *Mexican*   *beans and tortillas, enchiladas*
- *Middle Eastern*   *chick peas and bulghur wheat*
- *Asian*   *tofu (from soybeans) and rice*
- *East Indian*   *dahl (split peas or mung beans) and rice*
- *Italian*   *minestrone (soup with beans and macaroni)*
- *American*   *baked beans and corn bread, peanut butter sandwiches*

Is milk a desirable food?

Cow's milk is not desirable as a food for people of any age, in spite of the fact that it is a complete protein. Milk is a substance which is designed to make a calf grow to 1000 pounds in a relatively short time. The cow or bull then dies at about age 20. To compound the effect, beef and milk cattle are routinely given hormones to bring them to market even sooner, and those who drink milk are ingesting these as well.

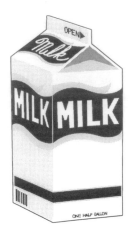

People who drink a lot of milk as children can suffer from a number of problems as a result. If certain hormones are supplied or oversupplied by food, the glands which normally make these hormones become dysfunctional and even atrophied with disuse. Testosterone and progesterone are lowered, resulting in women and men with low motivation and sex drive. Milk may well exacerbate the hormonal and emotional storms weathered by teenagers today, as hormonal peaks and dips contribute to teenage depression, violence, and suicide. Immune system problems often start to develop at around age 20, the age at which a cow or bull normally dies. Since growth hormones cause the growth of cells, it is possible that these hormones are related to cancer, which is an uncontrolled growth of cells.

Parents and doctors have noticed that the physical changes of puberty are occurring about two years earlier than in previous generations. Also, many people are now taller than either of their parents, and up to 5 or 6 inches taller than relatives in the "old country". There may be a correlation between these phenomena and the double dose of growth hormones (natural and industry-supplied) provided in milk.

Dairy products are thought of as a good source of calcium. Although they contain calcium, they raise phosphorus levels and actually deplete calcium in the body.

World-famous child care expert Dr. Benjamin Spock warned parents about the dangers of milk at a 1992 press conference. Milk is implicated in diabetes, ovarian cancer, cataracts, iron deficiency and allergies [12]. Milk consumption has been associated with greater frequency of lymph system cancer [13].

In lactase-deficient patients, lactose can cause not only the more common gastrointestinal symptoms, but also migraines and asthma [14].

Sinusitis is commonly caused by allergy to milk products. In a study of 135 multiple sclerosis (MS) patients, 66% had histories of sinusitis [15].

Allergy to milk is common but is not generally detectable by many allergy tests such as skin tests because milk sensitivity is not IgE (or airborne) mediated [16].

Homogenizing milk, which is routinely done so cream doesn't separate and go to the top, breaks milk into smaller particles which can sometimes pass through the intestinal wall, causing allergies; a major cause of most of the tonsillectomies in the 50's, but some of us now know better.

Why is albumin so important?
Albumin (sometimes spelled albumen) is a protein in the body which has several important functions. It is one of the highest antioxidants in the body, protecting against free radical damage. Cultured cells in albumin live far longer than those in regular culture medium. It is a chelating agent, helping to remove toxic metals. Albumin also helps to carry minerals and nutrients to their cellular destinations.

In general, the higher the albumin level, the better. The amount of albumin is usually expressed as a ratio with globulin, another protein. The optimal albumin/globulin (A/G) ratio is 1.8. A ratio higher than 2.2 can be a sign of viral infection. These values are usually part of a standard blood panel test.

Infections and allergies can lower the albumin level - the A/G ratio may go to 1.4 or below. If the albumin level (not ratio) is less than 4 the body is in effect starting to digest itself.

Good sources to increase albumin in the diet are eggs (one of the best sources), chicken, and fish. These can increase the A/G ratio. However, if there is insufficient hydrochloric acid (HCl) in the stomach, albumin levels may be low due to poor digestion of protein. Allergies and infection, by keeping the body in fight-or-flight mode rather than digestion mode, can also lower levels of food albumin, which plays a part in immune response.

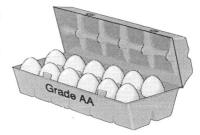

How much protein do we need?
The Recommended Daily Allowance of protein is 0.8 grams per kilogram (2.2 pounds) of ideal body weight. This figure is for healthy adults. A 150 pound person (68 kg) would then need about 54 grams (only about two ounces) of protein per day. Pregnant and lactating women need ten and fifteen grams (about 1/2 ounce) additional per day respectively. For reference, four ounces of protein is about one fistful. Infants, children, and teenagers need more protein per unit of body weight to support growth. A higher protein level has been associated with a higher IQ. However, a South American study showed that too much protein can cause kidney problems. The 30/40/30 diet (30% protein, 40% carbohydrate, and 30% vegetable oil by calories) is a good one for those with kidney problems. Even less protein than this might be desirable for treating kidney problems.

Is all meat created equal?
One of the major sources of protein is meat. However, protein from larger animals is harder to digest. Stronger and more complex proteins are needed in larger animals to bear the additional weight, and this more-complex protein is harder for us to digest. Rule of thumb - avoid (but not necessarily eliminate) meat that comes from an animal larger than you are, such as beef. This is especially the case if the meat animal doesn't exercise and is on antibiotics and hormones.

What are some sources of protein?
Sources of protein and the amount provided include the following [1]. The amount of protein in a particular source was determined in a laboratory, and may not reflect how well the protein is digested and utilized in the human body. The protein digestibility index is a way to express the relative digestibility of foods, with the higher numbers more digestible and therefore more desirable. The best sources of protein as used by the body are those with both a high protein content (ounces per serving) and a high digestibility index.

Cooked food	Serving size	Protein, oz.	Dig. index
Egg	1 large	0.21	8
Broccoli	1/2 cup	0.07	8
Tuna	3 oz.	0.82	7
Brown rice	1 cup	0.18	7
Green peas	1/2 cup	0.14	7
Bread	1 slice	0.07	7
Potato	1/2 cup	0.04	7
Chicken			7
Turkey			7
Steak	3 oz.	0.93	6
Hamburger	1	0.89	6
Shrimp	3 oz.	0.64	6
Lentils	1/2 cup	0.32	6
Hot dog	1 @ 3 oz.	0.21	6
Oatmeal	1 cup	0.21	6
Enchilada	1	0.71	5
Milk	8 oz.	0.29	5
Peanut butter	2 Tbsp.	0.29	5
Tofu	1/2 cup	0.36	5
Sunflower seeds	1 Tbsp.	0.21	5
Soybeans	1/2 cup	0.50	4
Peanuts	1 oz.	0.25	4
Cheddar cheese	1 oz.	0.25	4
Beans			4
Cottage cheese	1/2 cup	0.46	3

References and Resources

- "Amino Acid Connection" (chart), Pax Publishing, San Francisco CA, 1985.

- Braverman, Eric R. and Carl Pfeiffer, *The Healing Nutrients Within: Facts, Findings and New Research on Amino Acids*, Keats Publishing, New Canaan CT, 1991.

- Herbert, Victor, and Genell J. Subak-Sharpe (editors), *The Mount Sinai School of Medicine Complete Book of Nutrition*, St. Martin's Press, New York, 1990.

- Mindell, Earl, *Vitamin Bible*, Warner Books, New York, 1985.

- Rogers, Sherry A., *Tired or Toxic?*, Prestige Publishing, Syracuse NY, 1990.

OILS AND FATS

The Most Misunderstood Part of Nutrition

Things in this chapter that can change your health:

- *Much of what you "know" about oils may be incorrect.*
- *Healthy oils are necessary for life and health.*
- *Cholesterol is not necessarily bad.*
- *Heating oil can cause a necessary nutrient to become toxic waste.*
- *Unhealthy fats and oils can contribute to degenerative diseases such as cancer.*
- *Learn the difference between healthy and unhealthy oils.*
- *Oils can actually help you lose weight.*
- *What do saturated, polyunsaturated, and hydrogenated mean?*
- *You can be overweight or eat fried foods and still be oil deficient.*
- *The right kinds of oil can help eliminate PMS and menstrual cramps*

How much do you know about oils and fats?

There is a great deal of misinformation around concerning fats and oils. For example, would you say that these statements are true or false?

- *The less fat and oil in the diet, the better.*
- *Americans get too much fat and oil in their diets.*
- *Less oil leads to weight loss, more oil leads to weight gain.*
- *Unsaturated oils are good, especially polyunsaturates; saturated fats are bad.*
- *It is healthier to use oil for frying than to use solid shortening.*
- *Cholesterol is bad.*
- *A low-cholesterol diet is the way to control cholesterol in the body.*
- *Fat in the body is mostly from consumption of fat.*

Most people would believe that all of these statements are true. In fact, they are all either false, or only partially true, or conditionally true.

Are oils and fats bad for you?

In a society that is so weight-conscious and cholesterol-conscious, oils and fats are usually lumped together and considered to be unhealthy food items to be avoided. In actuality, healthy oils are necessary to life and health. However, good healthy oils can be made into toxic oils and fats through processing, hydrogenation, heating, and improper storage (exposure to light and air).

It should come as no surprise that many Americans are unhealthy, a fact due in part to their consumption of saturated/hydrogenated fats in processed and fast foods. Surprisingly, however, many intelligent, well-read people who make deliberate food choices based on health considerations are also less than optimally healthy due to their consumption of the wrong types and amounts of fats and oils. In fact, many people who sharply restrict their oil intake to maximize their health or weight loss may be doing themselves more harm than good.

Why are essential oils needed?
Oils are needed for many body functions, including:

- We are made up of cells, and all cells and the organelles (small structures) within them have membranous outer walls made up of lipids (fats). These walls keep that which belongs inside (nutrients) inside the cell, and that which belongs outside the cell (toxins) outside.

- The production of energy in the body from food substances.

- The formation of hormones which regulate our body processes.

- The production of prostaglandins, which regulate many body processes and act as anti-inflammatory (or in some cases pro-inflammatory) agents.

- They shorten the time required for recovery of fatigued muscles after exercising by facilitating conversion of fatigue-causing lactic acid.

- They are involved in oxidation, one of the most important biological processes They participate in the transfer of oxygen from air in the lungs to hemoglobin in the blood cells, and from there to cellular locations where needed.

- Good oils also help carry out (and keep out) oil-soluble and petrochemical toxins from our bodies.

- Essential fatty acids help prevent sunburn from UV radiation. If you sunburn easily, this may be a sign of insufficient essential fatty acids (EFAs).

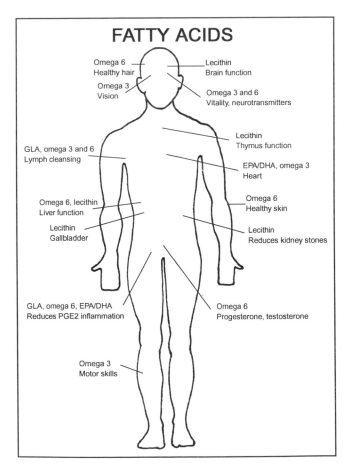

FATTY ACIDS

Omega 6
Healthy hair

Lecithin
Brain function

Omega 3
Vision

Omega 3 and 6
Vitality, neurotransmitters

Lecithin
Thymus function

GLA, omega 3 and 6
Lymph cleansing

EPA/DHA, omega 3
Heart

Omega 6, lecithin
Liver function

Omega 6
Healthy skin

Lecithin
Gallbladder

Lecithin
Reduces kidney stones

GLA, omega 6, EPA/DHA
Reduces PGE2 inflammation

Omega 6
Progesterone, testosterone

Omega 3
Motor skills

- Tissue growth and repair

- Vitality and mental state due to their involvement with neurotransmitters

- Mineral and nutrient transport

What are fatty acids?

Fatty acids are the basic building blocks of fats and oils. If amino acids and proteins are the building blocks of the body, fatty acids are the mortar which holds it together.

When good oils are eaten, they are broken up into fatty acids before being absorbed and utilized by the body. This is discussed in more detail in this chapter.

Fatty acid molecules are composed of two parts, fatty (carbon chain) and acid (carbonyl group, -COOH). The carbon chain can be as short as four carbons (butyric acid, found in butter) and as long as 24 carbons (found in fish oils and brain tissue).

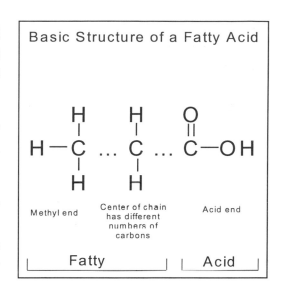

What are saturated and unsaturated fats?

You have probably heard terms pertaining to fats and oils such as saturated, polyunsaturated, and hydrogenated. What do these terms mean?

Each carbon forms four bonds total, in a combination of single bonds with hydrogen or single or double bonds with other carbons. It may be easier to think of carbon as being like a monkey with two hands and two feet, and each carbon can hold a total of four other hands or feet. Each carbon in the chain, other than at the ends, can either be double-bonded with another carbon and one hydrogen, or be single bonded and carry two hydrogen atoms.

If all of the carbon atoms are single bonded and carry two hydrogens each (or three on the end carbons), the maximum, the oil is said to be saturated, i.e. filled to capacity with hydrogen atoms. For this reason such an oil is also said to be hydrogenated. The terms saturated and hydrogenated mean the same thing as an end result, although "hydrogenated" usually refers to an oil that has been processed, while "saturated" can refer to a fat or oil that is naturally single-bonded.

The saturated molecule is then stable and does not want to change. If there is at least one double bond, there are fewer hydrogens, and the molecule is unsaturated. The terms monounsaturated and polyunsaturated refer to one or more double bonds respectively. The length of the chain and the number and placement of double bonds determines the identity of the fatty acid and its chemical properties.

What are the different shapes of unsaturated oils?

Double-bonded carbons can have either a cis or a trans configuration. In a cis configuration, the hydrogen atoms are on the same side of the molecule, while in a trans configuration, the hydrogen atoms are on the opposite sides of the molecule.

$$\ldots C = C \ldots$$
$$H \quad H$$
Cis

$$\ldots C = C \ldots$$
$$H$$
Trans

In cis-fatty acids, the adjacent hydrogen atoms repel each other, causing a kink in the molecule that is not present in trans-fatty acids. This kink changes the shape of the molecule, and therefore its chemical and biological properties. The cis form of essential fatty acids is necessary to life, while the trans form is toxic (more on this later). Unfortunately, the trans form is more stable, meaning that the beneficial cis form is easily converted to the harmful trans form, but the reverse is not the case. Unstable in this case is a good thing, as the unstable cis form is good partly because it can react with and grab oil-soluble toxins.

Saturated/hydrogenated oils have no double bonds and thus no cis or trans configurations.

What is free radical damage?

Another important chemical concept is that of free radicals, which are unpaired electrons in a molecule. Electrons want to be paired, and the unpaired electron will find another one to pair 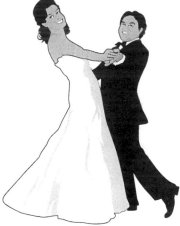 with even if it has to rip it from another molecule in your cells. The second molecule, newly missing an electron, grabs one from a third molecule, and the disruptive cycle continues. In the process, the extreme reactivity of free radicals causes a chain reaction in which one free radical can ultimately affect thousands of molecules.

Imagine a dance floor with many couples dancing. A lone man enters, cuts in on a couple, causing a new man to be partnerless. This new man cuts in on yet another couple, releasing a third man and so on. The resulting chaos adversely affects the smoothness of the dance and the harmony of the original couples. Similarly, free radicals can adversely affect the functioning of the body and can lead to cancer and degenerative diseases.

What does all this chemistry stuff have to do with fats and oils and nutrition?

Some fats and oils can contribute to free radical and other damage in the body. Other oils are both are essential to life and help to eliminate free radicals and their damage. It is important to know which ones are which, and to understand the basic principles so you don't have to carry a list with you every time you shop for oils.

Cis oils are essential, while trans forms of the same oil are toxic. But both forms are sold in the same supermarket with nothing on the label to tell you which is which - unless you know what to look for. Cis oils can become trans oils or saturated fats with improper handling (exposure to heat light, or air) during manufacture, grocery shelf storage, or use.

 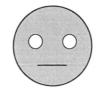

Cis oils
Healthy absorption

Saturated fats

Trans Oils
Block absorption, toxic

So now you understand how saturated fats are like monkeys with their hands and feet full of bananas - they can't grab toxins to eliminate them.

What types of oil are essential?
There are two types of essential oils:

- *Linolenic acid (LNA), or omega-3 oils*
- *Linoleic acid (LA), or omega-6 oils*

The terms omega-3 and omega-6 refer to the position of the first double bond in the molecule - on the third and sixth carbon respectively. Some other types of oils, generally longer chain, are also necessary for proper bodily functioning. While these oils can be obtained from other foods such as fish and seeds, they can also be manufactured by the body from the two essential oils, so they are not in themselves considered to be essential. However, to make the longer chain oils, the body must be in fairly good shape to do this work. If not, it is a good idea to take the fish and other oils directly. The fish, in essence, has done the work for you.

Sugars are converted in the body by beneficial bacteria, if enough are present, to certain short-chain fatty acids such as butyrates, which help to control fungus in the colon. If this is not done properly, your triglyceride and LDL cholesterol levels may rise.

What do the essential oils do in the body?
LA and LNA have a number of vital functions in the body, at least in the beneficial cis form. In addition to those listed on the second page of this chapter, Dr. Johanna Budwig, noted cancer researcher, has found that cell respiration and division require the presence of essential fatty acids. She also found that healthy people's red blood cells have a fat layer but those of cancer patients do not unless they are given essential fatty acids. She recommends flax oil, up to half a cup per day, for cancer patients [1].

How can the right oils help relieve cramps and arthritis?
Essential fatty acids are also the precursors to prostaglandins, which regulate many functions of all body tissues. Prostaglandins are short-lived hormone-like substances, of which there are three basic types, called E1, E2, and E3. Some people think of E1 and E3 as the "good guys", while E2 is in a sense the inflammatory "bad guy", although things aren't quite that simple. More accurately, E2 has useful rebuilding and protective functions and just needs to be kept in balance.

One of E2's useful functions is to keep the intestinal lining intact, and NSAID (non-steroidal anti-inflammatory) drugs, by suppressing E2, can lead to ulcers since the intestinal lining is no longer maintained by E2.

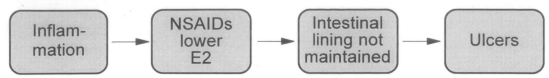

E1 and E3 help keep blood platelets from sticking together and in this way help to prevent clot-caused heart attacks and strokes. E1 also:

- *helps the kidneys to remove unneeded fluid from the body*
- *opens up blood vessels, thus improving circulation*
- *slows down cholesterol production*
- *prevents inflammation*
- *controls arthritis*
- *makes insulin work more efficiently*
- *improves nerve function*
- *gives a sense of well-being*
- *is involved in the function of the immune system's T cells*
- *may help to prevent cancer cell growth by regulating cell division rate*

E1 also prevents the release of arachidonic acid from the cell membranes. Arachidonic acid is a precursor to prostaglandin E2, which works against E1. E2, the inflammatory kind:

- *promotes platelet aggregation, which is the first step in clot formation, which in turn can lead to heart attack and stroke.*

- *causes the kidneys to retain salt, leading to high blood pressure and water retention.*

- *causes inflammation.*

- *is implicated in the formation of some cancers.*

Arachidonic acid is found primarily in butter and other animal byproducts. Vegetarians may be less likely to develop degenerative diseases for this reason, as long as they are taking sufficient oils.

Nonsteroidal anti-inflammatory drugs (NSAIDs) are medications which work by blocking prostaglandin E2. It is much better to utilize the body's control method by using essential oils to build up prostaglandin E1 and E3, which will then keep E2 under control. Linoleic acid (LA) is converted in the body to gamma-linolenic acid (GLA) which actually increases the amount of E2 but more importantly also increases progesterone (in women) or testosterone (in men) which counteracts E2.

Low-fat diets, the kind many women follow to lose weight, deplete prostaglandin E1 and E3, causing a hormone imbalance which can lead to PMS and cramps. Evening primrose oil is especially recommended to alleviate PMS. Men who follow a low-fat diet may suffer from lowered testosterone, the male sex hormone, with lowered motivation and sex drive.

> **The right kinds of oil can help eliminate PMS and cramps.**

One patient, a man in his 30s who was too tired to even talk, suffered from muscle pain and had no sex drive. He was given essential fatty acids as well as transfer factor, c-AMP, did whiplash adjustment and bite balancing, and added sea salt and minerals along with amino acids such as copper lysinate. His energy levels rebounded and he got his life back.

What happens if you are deficient in essential fatty acids?
Symptoms of linoleic acid (omega-6) deficiency include:

- *eczema-like skin eruptions*
- *behavior disturbances*
- *drying up of glands*
- *arthritis*
- *heart and circulatory problems*
- *slowness in wound healing, especially stomach / gastrointestinal*
- *hair loss*
- *thirst*
- *susceptibility to infections*
- *retarded growth*
- *lowered testosterone (male hormone) and progesterone (female hormone), which can lead to female infertility and male sterility*
- *liver and kidney degeneration as oil soluble vitamins A and D are not carried to their destinations*

Deficiency of linolenic acid (omega-3) can cause:
- *retarded growth*
- *impairment of vision*
- *impairment of learning ability*
- *numbness and tingling in arms and legs*
- *mood swings such as anger or depression, resulting in behavior changes*
- *weakness*
- *motor incoordination*
- *dandruff*

All of these deficiency symptoms can be reversed by the addition of these two essential fatty acids in sufficient quantities to the diet.

Where are essential oils found?
Sources of linoleic acid (omega-6) are primarily warm-weather seeds and nuts, grown in the southern part of the country. These include oils of:

- *safflower*
- *flax seed*
- *sesame seed*
- *sunflower*
- *soybean*
- *pumpkin seed*
- *hemp seed*
- *walnut*
- *most nuts*

Sources of linolenic acid (omega-3) include oils of :

- *flax seed*
- *canola*
- *hemp seed*
- *walnut*
- *soybeans*
- *rapeseed*

Most of these grow in cold weather and in the northern part of the country. Omega-3 oils are more sensitive to heat, which fits in with their growth locations. Their sensitivity to heat is part of why they are so reactive and effective to the body's anti-inflammatory response. These oils need to be kept refrigerated. Dark green leafy vegetables, whose oil is protected by cholesterol, and whole unroasted seeds such as sunflower, sesame, and pumpkin are also valuable sources.

What about other oils?

Other oils are needed by the body, but a body that is functioning as it should can make these oils from the two essential fatty acids. However, it is a good idea to take in these other oils directly. These oils include:

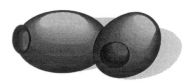

Oleic acid (omega-9 or omega-1) is found most prominently in olive oil but also in oils of peanut, almond, pecan, cashew, filbert, and macadamia nut. Both the unroasted nut and the extracted oils are valuable. Oleic acid is less likely than other oils to be damaged by heat. Olive and peanut oils are used in cooking and frying for this reason.

Olive oil helps to flush out the liver and hepatic bile duct, and breaks down gallstones and liver stones.

Dietary oleic acid such as that found in olive oil increases the resistance of LDL to oxidation. Oxidation of LDL is one of the initiating events in atherosclerosis, and so it follows that olive oil may offer some protection against atherosclerosis. Not surprisingly in light of this study, cardiovascular disease is relatively low in societies such as those in Mediterranean areas where a lot of olive oil is used [2,3]. A study published in the ***Journal of the American Medical Association*** which surveyed 4900 Italians ages 25-59 found that those who had a high intake of olive oil and a low intake of butter or margarine had lower cholesterol and blood pressure than those who ate more butter and margarine [4].

The drier (less oily) nuts such as almond oil are less likely to go rancid. Cashews and macadamias are oily and more likely to be rancid, and pistachios and peanut oil are even worse.

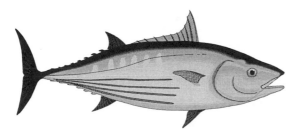

Fish oils - Eicosapentaenoic acid (EPA) and docosahexaenoic acid (DHA or DHEA) are found in fish and marine mammal oils, especially cold-water fish such as salmon, trout, mackerel, and sardines. These are omega-3, and are like the cold-weather oils. These oils are also found in animal tissues such as brain, eyeballs, adrenal glands, and testes. EPA and DHA can be made slowly by the body from LA and LNA, although the body's ability to do so may be impaired by certain degenerative diseases. Fish oils are therefore useful additions to the diet, although not all fish oils are created equal. The fatty acid cetoleic acid, which is found in herring and capelin oils and to a lesser extent in cod liver oil, is toxic. Many low fat and warm water fish contain oil which is neither toxic nor particularly useful.

Fish oil and eicosapentaenoic acid (EPA) has been shown to significantly reduce coronary heart disease death. It works by affecting prostaglandin ratios which in turn reduce blood stickiness, favorably alters blood lipid ratios, and helps lower blood pressure [5-7].

Evening primrose oil, borage oil, and black currant seed oil contain both LA (omega-6) and gamma-linolenic acid (GLA), which is a precursor to the formation of "good" prostaglandin E1. Certain metabolic and nutritional deficiencies block the conversion of LA to GLA, and so GLA in the form of evening primrose oil supplements is necessary to make prostaglandin E1 in these cases. PMS and menstrual cramps, caused in part by excess prostaglandin E2 and insufficiency of progesterone, can be eased by taking essential oils, especially evening primrose oil. Too much of this oil, however, can actually increase E2 through a regulator called delta-5-desaturase.

Conversion of LA to GLA can be hindered by [8]:

- *Vitamin B6 deficiency*
- *Common viral infections*
- *Diets high in refined foods*
- *High sugar consumption*
- *Zinc and magnesium deficiency (often secondary to mercury toxicity from amalgam fillings)*

- *Radiation*
- *Alcohol*
- *Trans fatty acids*

- *Cancer*
- *Diabetes*
- *Aging*

What oil deficiency can contribute to infertility and miscarriages?
All of these can hinder conversion of LA to GLA, with resultant prostaglandin E1 deficiency symptoms. Flax oil and borage are other sources of GLA. GLA is also the precursor of progesterone and testosterone, a lack of which can cause lowered sex drive and motivation. Lack of GLA can also cause or contribute to [8]:

- *arthritis*
- *eczema*
- *cancer*

- *hyperactivity*
- *multiple sclerosis*
- *alcoholism*

- *infertility and miscarriages*
- *autoimmune disorders*

Lecithin is valuable in nutrition for several reasons:

- It supplies choline, which is necessary for brain and liver function, and helps the body to break down fats and cholesterol properly. Phosphatidyl choline, necessary for neurotransmitter function and sometimes sold as a supplement, contains three times as much choline as lecithin. Some people report that phosphatidyl choline increases mental clarity.

- About half of lecithin's fatty acids are essential fatty acids.

- Its emulsifying action prevents and dissolves kidney stones and gallstones, and the emulsification of food fats (breaking them into small droplets) makes digestion of fats by enzymes easier.

- It helps the liver in its detoxification functions. Poor liver function is often a forerunner of cancer.

- It increases resistance to disease by boosting thymus gland function.

- It is an important part of membrane fluidity and electrical (nerve) transmission.

- It thins fats and helps in weight loss. One patient, an overweight woman in her mid 40s, was helped in this way by taking lecithin.

What else do you need to get good oils besides good oils?

Adequate levels of nutrients are needed for metabolism and utilization of beneficial oils. Magnesium, zinc, selenium and vitamins B, C and E are especially important for this purpose [9].

Is this all there is to know about good oils?

Okay, now that you know about the importance of essential fatty acids in your diet, and where these fatty acids can be found, you are ready to hit the supermarket and stock up. A person may buy oils gleaming pale and shiny from their clear glass bottles on the store shelves. This person might fry with sesame oil, spread safflower oil margarine on toast, buy roasted nuts and sunflower seeds to munch on, and live healthily ever after, right? Wrong. Read on -- there's a lot more to consider here.

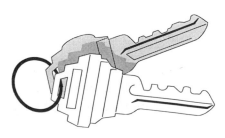

What is wrong with trans fatty acids?

All of the benefits listed for the fatty acids apply only to cis-fatty acids, not trans fatty acids. As previously mentioned, however, the cis form is easily changed to the trans form, which is toxic. The trans form, shaped differently than the cis form, tries to perform cis functions in body systems but is unable to do so. In addition, the trans fatty acids block the cis fatty acids from being able to do their job. Cis fatty acids fit into the cell membrane like a key into a lock. Trans fatty acids are like a broken key in that the key will fit the lock (cell membrane) but will not open the door. Trans fatty acids block entry of the correct key, i.e. the molecules the cell needs.

Cis fatty acids are liquid at room and body temperatures, while trans fatty acids are solid at body temperature. Just as liquid oil can be flushed down your household plumbing without incident while bacon grease will solidify in your sink trap and cause a clog, sticky trans fatty acids will clog up your arteries, liver, and other organs with fatty deposits.

An example of the conversion of cis to trans oils occurs on the outside of an oil bottle. Have you ever noticed what happens when salad oil drips down the side of the oil bottle and is not wiped up? After exposure to air, it becomes sticky rather than oily, i.e. trans rather than cis, and is very difficult to wash off. Trans fatty acids are sticky and less easily dissolved in the body as well.

Trans fatty acids are useful to the body only as energy-creating fuel. Cis fatty acids provide energy as well as the many benefits previously listed. Trans fatty acids also change cell permeability, so that things that should be kept out of the cell, such as carcinogens, can get in, and things that belong in the cell, such as nutrients, can get out. The presence of trans fatty acids can keep the cis fatty acids from making prostaglandins and other important molecules, causing deficiency symptoms. Trans fatty acids have been implicated in degenerative diseases such as athcrosclerosis and cancer.

Even when trans fatty acids are a small proportion of the total ingested, they can cause trouble, much as a small amount of water in your gas tank can cause major damage and stall your car.

> **Three things that can change good oils to bad are heat, light, and oxygen.**

How can good oils change to bad?
Both trans fatty acids and free radicals cause adverse effects on health. Both of these deleterious chemical changes are caused by three things: **heat, light, and oxygen**.

Heat Commercial oils are typically heated to high temperatures during extraction and processing, and manufacturers generally don't know or care about cis or trans forms. So-called cold-pressed or expeller pressed oils are actually pressed with heat, but with less than commercial oils. "Cold-pressed" oils may also be exposed to heat in other parts of the manufacturing or refining process such as deodorization of the oil. Oils labeled cold-pressed or expeller-pressed are still preferable to commercial brands.

Heating up or frying with oils in home cooking will also change good oils to bad ones. Ironically, as saturated (solid) fats have gained a bad reputation, some restaurants have announced that they now fry with vegetable oils, implying that this is healthier for you. Saturated fats have no double bonds and therefore no cis or trans forms. They 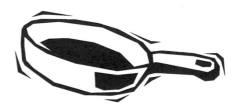 therefore have no benefit other than as energy sources, but neither are they as toxic as trans forms caused by heating oil. You are actually better off cooking or frying with solid shortening than with oil for this reason. Olive oil is least likely to be destroyed by heat, as the cis to trans conversion occurs at a higher temperature than with most other oils.

At the other end of the heat-sensitivity spectrum, flax oil starts to convert from cis to trans at about room temperature and should be kept refrigerated. Flax oil is so sensitive to conversion that it is usually sold with a three to six month expiration date.

It is recommended that oil, not just flax oil, be stored in the refrigerator. Some oils may thicken, cloud or partially solidify when refrigerated. This solidifying is harmless and reversible when the oil is brought to room temperature and is not related to the irreversible solidifying that occurs when cis oils convert to trans oils.

Heating oil to high temperatures can also cause chemical changes called polymerization. You may have noticed this in the form of a rubber-like substance on the side of the pan after frying that must be scrubbed off.

Nuts and seeds that are good sources of essential oils can undergo the same trans chemical changes during roasting, so the unroasted nuts and seeds are far more nutritious and less harmful. Cold water fish and fresh nuts and seeds are the best way to get healthy oils.

Light - Most oils, except some in health-food stores, are displayed in clear glass bottles on open shelves under fluorescent light. This can cause the formation of free radicals and trans fatty acids. Brown glass bottles, black plastic bottles (usually used for flax oil) or other opaque containers are preferable. There is irony in the fact that most manufacturers use clear glass or plastic bottles so the consumer can see how light and clear the oil is. The lightness and clarity are actually signs of a highly processed product, the oil equivalent of white bread, and each processing step carries the risk of damaging chemical changes.

> The clear pale oils sold in the supermarket are the oil equivalent of white bread.

To reduce the damaging risks of light, buy oil from the back of the shelf rather than from the front, as the bottles in the front have been exposed to much more light in the store. Once you get the oil home, put it into well-cleaned dark bottles or cover the bottle with foil to block out light.

Oxygen is necessary for life, but can cause free radical formation in oils and other products. It is theoretically possible to limit contact with oxygen during processing, for example by using a nitrogen flush, but most manufacturers don't bother with this.

What are hydrogenated oils?
Hydrogenation involves filling an unsaturated oil molecule with hydrogen atoms until it is saturated. Saturated fats are usually solid or semisolid.

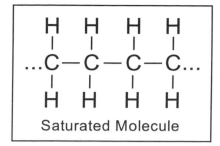
Saturated Molecule

Hydrogenation is the process by which a once-healthy oil is reacted under pressure at high temperatures with hydrogen gas in the presence of a metal catalyst, usually nickel. This process takes six to eight hours. A completely hydrogenated product is saturated, and in theory contains no harmful trans fatty acids, although in actuality some trans fats may be present. It is a dead, useless product that does not spoil on the shelf because even microbes have no use for it. It is preferable to fry with fat (solid) than oil (liquid) as mentioned, but hydrogenated products can contain altered fatty acid molecule fragments from side reactions as well as being contaminated by the metal catalyst. People who are sensitive to the metal nickel may react to the nickel in margarine and hydrogenated fats (see Nickel and Root Canals chapter in *Surviving The Toxic Crisis*).

Is partial hydrogenation better than full hydrogenation?
Partial hydrogenation produces margarine, especially the soft spreadable type, and some shortenings and shortening oils. These are worse than completely hydrogenated products, as they combine the worst characteristics of hydrogenated fats with the toxicity of trans fatty acids.

Margarine contains as much as 35% trans fatty acids [10]. Europe does not even allow the sale of American margarine because it is so high in trans fats.

> **Europe does not allow the sale of American margarine due to its toxicity**

Trans fatty acids in general and margarine in particular have been linked to heart disease and heart attacks [11-17].

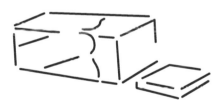

Hydrogenating oils results in an intermediate product that is a dark, malodorous grease. It is then bleached and deodorized chemically to make a pure white, colorless, odorless, tasteless artificial fat. This is then salted and colored and flavored with more chemicals. The result: margarine as we know it.

During World War II when things like margarine were rationed, it came in this white, colorless form and women had to mix in the color to make it look like butter before they served it to their family. They sacrificed for the war effort. Today what you may be sacrificing is your health, which is unnecessary and unwise, since you can have the "real thing", with Vitamin A in the bargain.

Corn oil, egg substitutes and even some "healthy" breads are made with hydrogenated oils. Ironically, margarine and egg substitutes are recommended by cardiologists, the (incorrect) theory being that such products will reduce cholesterol. By saturating oils to make margarine, manufacturers are selling you the very saturated fats they claim to be helping you avoid.

In one study, it was found that eating margarine causes trans fatty acids to be deposited in the heart itself. This blocks the protective oils from the heart muscle [18].

What is the difference between a fat and an oil?
The word "fat" refers to products that are solid at room and body temperature, while an oil is liquid at room or body temperature. As mentioned, trans fatty acids are solid while the cis form is liquid. A bottle of liquid oil, however, can still contain enough trans fatty acids to be more harmful than beneficial, although it will not look or smell different and the amount of trans fatty acids present is not sufficient to cause the oil to solidify.

What kinds of oils should you look for?
In summary:

- Use oils from the list of sources of essential fatty acids. Flax, safflower, and sunflower oils are best.

- Use oils labeled cold-pressed or expeller-pressed, which are usually found in health-food stores.

- Use oils labeled unrefined if you can find them.

- Look for oils in brown glass or opaque containers, preferably refrigerated. Flax oil is most likely to be sold like this.

- Buy in smaller rather than larger quantities so the oil that you have on hand is fresher, i.e. less likely to have undergone oxidative changes.

- Store oils in the refrigerator at home, and keep them from light as much as possible.

- Never fry with or heat oils. Use solid shortening or olive oil if you must fry, but it is better not to fry at all.

- Vitamin E, an oil soluble vitamin which slows down oxygen damage (antioxidant), can be added to oils to prolong their useful life.

What is the optimal ratio of the essential oils?
The optimal ratio of linoleic (omega 6) to linolenic acid (omega 3) is cited by various sources as being anywhere from 1:1 to 1:5. Too much omega 6 oils can increase inflammatory prostaglandin E2 more than protective E1. The optimal ratio for a given individual varies. For example, a woman with premenstrual syndrome (PMS) or a person who is low on steroids and hormones should have proportionately more linoleic acid. A person who is overweight, has a driving type-A personality, or is low on minerals should have more linolenic acid. Flax oil contains a healthful ratio of these oils.

What is a healthy oil combination?
This is a healthy oil recipe which will meet the needs of most people. Use cold- or expeller-pressed oils:

> 1 cup olive oil
> 1/8 cup sesame, safflower, or sunflower oil (or up to 1/2 cup if stomach problems)
> 1/2 cup flaxseed or canola oil
> 1 1/2 cups water
> 1/2 bottle E Gem Oil drops (or 1200 IU Vitamin E oil)
> 1/8 cup liquid lecithin
>
> Coat blender with sesame oil. Add lecithin to bottom. Add all ingredients and mix thoroughly. Keep refrigerated. Texture will be thick. Can be mixed with lemon juice, herbs, mustard, or curry powder. Use plenty of seasoning as oil absorbs flavors. Keeps for one week.

See the *Toxic Immune Syndrome Cookbook* [19] (references, end of this chapter) for healthy dressings and sauces utilizing oils.

This recipe provides both essential amino acids plus oleic acid. The lecithin is beneficial in itself and also makes the oil more digestible and palatable. The vitamin E is an antioxidant that will prevent free radical formation and damage both in the prepared oil and in the body. This prepared oil product will be thick and creamy. It can be used in recipes and in homemade mayonnaise, or salted or seasoned and used as a butter-like spread. Store this oil in a closed container in the refrigerator and away from light.

Can oils actually help you to lose weight?

There is a resistance to eating oils in this weight-conscious society. It may seem hard to believe, but adding several tablespoons per day of essential fatty acids can actually help you to *lose* weight! The usual argument against dieters eating oils is that all fats and oils have nine calories per gram (metric unit of weight, about 1/28 ounce), or 120 calories per tablespoon, and it takes 3500 calories to make a pound of body fat. The picture is much more complex than this, however.

> **Healthy oil can actually help you LOSE weight!**

As discussed in the chapter on Weight Control and Calories, overweight can be caused by either too much wrong or thick fat or too much water in the body, or a combination of both. Water weight is by far the more common type (about 80%). Good oils can aid in weight loss in several ways:

- Essential fatty acids increase the metabolic rate, i.e. the rate at which fats are burned for energy in the fatty acid cycle rather than deposited as fat on the body. Saturated fats, on the other hand, decrease the metabolic rate and make one feel sluggish.

- Essential fatty acids are necessary in producing prostaglandin E1, which helps the kidneys to eliminate excess fluid from the body.

- Water and fat can be held in the body in an attempt to dilute toxins. Oils can dissolve and carry many toxins out of the body, reducing the body's need to retain the excess water or fat.

- Real oils give a satisfying I've-eaten-enough feeling so munching is less likely. Low-fat diets often fail because the dieter usually feels hungry and acts accordingly.

Overweight from both fat deposits and water retention can be less rather than more when sufficient essential fatty acids are part of your diet.

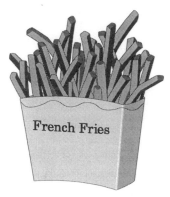

Does eating fat cause you to deposit fat in the body?

If the wrong kind of fat is eaten, the amount not needed for energy in the form of calories is stored as fat. Most people, however, eat far more processed carbohydrates and sugars than they do fats. Excess carbohydrates and sugars are converted to sticky triglycerides, which are then converted to fats for long-term storage. Fat-based overweight (as differentiated from toxic water weight) is therefore more likely to be due to excess carbohydrates than excess fatty food, although fatty food is certainly a contributor.

What causes craving for fatty foods?

A protein in the brain stimulates the craving for good necessary oils when the supply gets low. The person will then eat any kind of fat or oil - fried foods, hamburgers, ice cream, potato chips - to try to ease the craving. If the wrong kind of fat is eaten, the body's needs are still not satisfied and the craving continues and worsens. the use of healthful oils reduces the oil deficiency and thus can ease the craving. In this way the *addition* of oil to the diet can result in the ingestion of *less* oil.

What if you have trouble with oils and fatty foods?

Nausea or gallbladder pain when eating oils and fatty foods can be tied to gallbladder problems, which in turn can be caused by microorganisms such as helicobacter pylori and giardia. Other symptoms of gallbladder problems are tight shoulder muscles, pain in the neck or between the shoulder blades, headaches and head pressure.

What's the real story on cholesterol?

Cholesterol has been in medical news in recent years. It is a sticky substance that can contribute to the formation of plaques and narrowing of blood vessels, with subsequent high blood pressure. This is especially true of low density lipoprotein (LDL, or "bad") cholesterol.

Cholesterol concentration is highest in the brain. The level of cholesterol in the blood influences production of protective hormones such as progesterone. Most of these hormones are contained in the brain [20].

Cholesterol is used by the body to heal injuries to the arterial walls, forming a bandage of sorts over the injury. High density cholesterol (HDL), the good kind, is involved in repair work. Low and very low density cholesterol (LDL and VLDL) are the bad kind that is likely to cause damage.

It is believed by many that high cholesterol levels lead to heart and blood vessel damage because the two are often found together. It is possible that the same process that causes heart problems, such as injury to arteries, also causes an increase in cholesterol to help repair the damage. Cholesterol in this case is not only not the cause of the damage, but an attempt to cure it.

What's the whole truth and nothing but the truth about cholesterol?
There are a number of myths and half-truths surrounding cholesterol.

Myth #1 - **"The lower the cholesterol level, the better."** This would be true if the only cholesterol-related problems were heart and blood vessel diseases. Conventional wisdom is that one's cholesterol level should be 200 mg/dl or below, and that there is no such thing as a too-low level.

> **A lot of what you "know" to be true about cholesterol may not be.**

Studies have shown that some cancers, especially of the colon, lung, and breast, are actually more prevalent among people with lower cholesterol levels (under 130 mg/dl) [21]. While high cholesterol (over 225) has been shown to be a risk factor in heart disease, low cholesterol is more likely to be related to the development of cancer, and high cholesterol even seems to have a protective effect against cancer. In one study, it was found that among men with the lowest cholesterol, 34.5% of deaths were from cancer and 33% of deaths were from heart disease. Among men with the highest cholesterol, 19.4% of deaths were from cancer and 61.6% were from heart disease [22].

In another study, 7000 men and 8262 women in Scotland were followed for 12 years. There were the same number of deaths during this period among the lowest-cholesterol group as among the highest cholesterol group, with more cancer deaths than heart disease deaths in the low cholesterol group and the reverse in the high cholesterol group [23]. It is one author's feeling that when heart disease and cancer statistics as related to cholesterol levels are given equal weight, a total serum cholesterol level of 225 would be ideal [24]. By contrast, the current recommendation, based only on heart disease statistics, is below 200, and the lower the better. One optimal recommendation is a total cholesterol level of 170-180, with an HDL level or 50 or more.

Dry liver, or sclerosis (hardening) of the liver, may also be linked to low cholesterol, and to low levels of the fat soluble vitamins A and E.

Low cholesterol is tied to low oil soluble antioxidants such as vitamins A and E and low oils, which in turn are linked to free radical damage which can lead to cancer. Cod liver oil and vitamins E and C are recommended.

Lowered cholesterol levels have also been linked to higher levels of aggressiveness [25].

Myth #2 - **"Cholesterol level is directly related to intake of cholesterol-containing foods."** This is true only to a limited extent, as the body manufactures its own cholesterol. A number of product manufacturers have jumped on the cholesterol-is-bad bandwagon with labels that proclaim "contains no cholesterol". Strictly speaking, these labels are accurate. However, the body will make cholesterol from such sources as palm oil, saturated fats, and especially sugar, so the no-cholesterol labels won't help you much.

One patient, a man about 50, had cholesterol readings above 400. A low-fat diet brought his reading down to about 380, a negligible improvement. Eliminating sugar brought it down to about 180.

Myth #3 - **"Eggs are bad because they contain cholesterol."** Egg yolks, once thought to be a source of cholesterol, are actually a good source of high-density lipoproteins (HDL), as well as lecithin. HDL is the beneficial kind of cholesterol which helps to thin the blood and fight the detrimental effects of LDL cholesterol. In addition, eggs are one of the most complete proteins and are a beneficial addition to the diet. Eggs should be soft-boiled or poached, as hard-boiling or frying changes the oil in the yolk to the trans form.

> **High cholesterol is usually a sign of arterial inflammation, not the cause.**

Myth #4 - **"Cholesterol is a major cause of heart disease."** About 30-40% of people with atherosclerotic heart disease have elevated serum cholesterol. However, this is about the same percentage as the general population [26], disproving a cause and effect relationship. Most people who die of heart attacks have low or normal cholesterol. Other studies seem to show a relationship between cholesterol and heart disease, so the final word is not yet in. The hydrogenation of oils and rampant heart disease are both relatively recent, and they are likely to be linked. Cholesterol levels may be merely incidental, not cause/effect. Cholesterol buffers inflammation in the blood vessels, and its presence in raised amounts is likely a sign of inflammation, not the cause.

What about cholesterol byproducts?
There is evidence that cholesterol itself is not harmful. It is the formation of oxysterols from the reaction of cholesterol and oxygen which is toxic. The conversion of as little as 0.25% (1/400) of the cholesterol in the body can cause damage. Oxysterols promote accumulation of greasy, sticky lipids (fats) in the blood vessels, and the formation of calcified plaques on blood vessel walls. Oxysterols can also accelerate free radical damage.

When egg yolk and milk are powdered, as is the case with most processed and fast food, many tiny particles are exposed to the air and oxidized to oxysterols. This is not the case with fresh eggs and milk.

Homocysteine is a free radical generator that can oxidize cholesterol to its more harmful form. Vitamins B6, B12 and folic acid dramatically lower homocysteine levels [27,28].

Higher cholesterol usually means more oxysterols, but it is better to control the oxysterols than to limit the necessary cholesterol. Sufficient vitamin B6 (50 mg/day) can prevent oxysterols from getting into arteries. Vitamin C (2-5 grams/day), an antioxidant, and coenzyme Q10 (10-40 mg/day) are also beneficial [29].

Are cholesterol lowering drugs useful?

Cholesterol-lowering drugs may do more harm than good. Drugs to lower the levels of LDL cholesterol may actually raise it in those with very high levels [30]. A study in Finland found that heart attack and stroke deaths were 46% *higher* in those taking cholesterol lowering drugs [31]. Mevacor (lovastatin) lowers not only the cholesterol level but also the level of CoQ10, an antioxidant with a protective effect against heart damage [32].

So is cholesterol bad or good?

Now you must be thoroughly confused. It was easier when you believed that the goal was lower body cholesterol and the method was to avoid eating foods with cholesterol. So now what cholesterol level do you aim for? And what foods will accomplish your goal? If your personal and family medical history is heavy on heart and circulatory disease, aim for the lower cholesterol numbers. If cancer is more of a concern, a higher cholesterol level will be to your benefit.

Your body has a great deal of wisdom. If you eat a balanced, healthy diet, low in sugar and with sufficient essential fatty acids, your body will regulate your cholesterol level just as it did back before we ate processed foods and before anyone even heard of cholesterol. So sit back and enjoy your eggs. Just don't fry them.

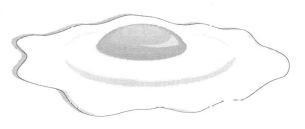

Summary

We need oils for a variety of body structures and functions, including cell membranes and hormones. Deficiency can lead to a number of adverse symptoms.

Fatty acids are the building blocks of oils. There are two essential fatty acids, omega-3 and omega-6. These are obtained from non-rancid, non-heated oils such as flax oil.

Oils can be

• *cis*	*double bonded, bent*	*useful*
• *trans*	*double bonded, straight*	*detrimental*
• *saturated*	*single bonded*	*nonreactive*

Healthful cis oils can become disruptive trans oils if heated or exposed to light or air.

Thinning or emulsifying oils can actually be a weight loss aid.

Cholesterol is not necessarily bad. It is made by the body and a high level is correlated more with sugar consumption, including sweet fruits, than fat intake.

References and Resources

- Bates, C., *Essential Fatty Acids and Immunity in Mental Health*, Life Sciences Press, Tacoma WA, 1987.

- Budwig, Johanna, *Flax Oil as a True Aid Against Arthritis, Heart Infarction, Cancer and Other Diseases*, Apple Publishing, Vancouver BC, 1994.

- Erasmus, Udo, *Fats and Oils*, Alive Books, Vancouver BC Canada, 1986.

- Finnegan, John, *Fats and Oils: A Consumer's Guide*, Elysian Arts, Malibu CA, 1992.

- Kellas, W.R., *Toxic Immune Syndrome Cookbook*, Comprehensive Health Center, Encinitas CA, 2nd ed., 1995.

- Newton, W.L., *Omega-3, The Fish Oil Factor*, Omega-3 Project, San Diego CA, 1986.

- Rudin, Donald O. and Clara Felix, *The Omega-3 Phenomenon*, Avon Books, NY, 1988.

- Rudin, Donald O. and Clara Felix, *Omega 3 Oils: Why You Can't Afford to Live Without Essential Oils*, Avery Publishing Group, Garden City Park, NY, 1996.

VITAMINS

The Regulators That Control How The Body Runs

Things in this chapter that can change your health:

- *Is there a difference between synthetic and natural vitamins?*
- *How do you know what vitamins to take?*
- *What is the best way to take vitamins?*

What are vitamins?

Vitamins and minerals are the micronutrients (micro means small) needed by the body in amounts much smaller than an ounce. If you compare the human body to a car, macronutrients such as carbohydrates are like the gasoline, and micronutrients are like the spark plugs and regulators. Just as the car cannot run without both, neither can your body operate very well without a balance of these vital components. Vitamins regulate our metabolism through our enzyme systems and, like an electrical system regulates the firing of a car's spark plugs, they similarly keep our body systems functioning at peak performance.

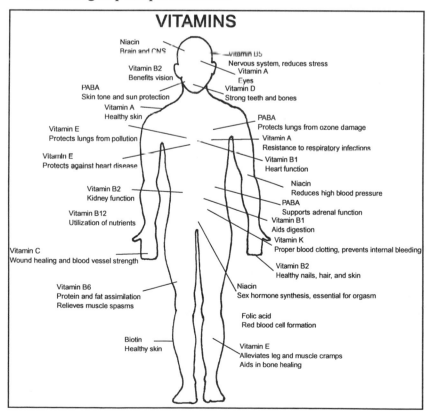

All vitamins are essential to the normal functioning of the body, and a deficiency in even one vitamin (or mineral) is like one missing spark plug - our bodies will not function optimally no matter what other nutrients are present. In fact, each vitamin and mineral is so important that a severe deficiency or lack of any one of them can endanger your life! It is no accident that the word "vitamin" comes from the same word root as "vital", meaning necessary. It cannot be said that one vitamin or mineral is more important than another. Balance and sufficiency is key.

What are vitamins good for?
Although nearly all vitamins are useful to nearly all parts of the body, some vitamins target specific areas, as shown in the picture on the previous page.

What is the difference between vitamins and minerals?
Vitamins are organic in the chemical sense of the word; that is, they contain carbon, while minerals do not. A mineral is a single ion (electrically charged form of an element), while vitamins are compounds, or combinations of atoms.

Do vitamins work alone?
The micronutrients do not work in isolation. They are synergistic, or interdependent. An excess or deficiency of one of them will affect the function of others. For this reason not only the absolute amount but the balance is important. No one nutrient can substitute for another.

Where are vitamins found?
Vitamins are found in food, extracted from food, or synthesized in the laboratory to be chemically identical to naturally occurring vitamins. This chapter and the chapter on Supplements will explore the subject of vitamins, minerals, and amino acids in concentrated, extracted, and synthesized forms. A few vitamins such as vitamin A can be synthesized by the body from certain foods, and biotin and vitamin K can be made in the bowel by friendly bacteria. Most vitamins, however, must be ingested in the form of either food or supplements or they will not be present.

Are synthetic vitamins identical to natural vitamins from food?
Yes and no. With synthetic vitamins, the molecular structure of the vitamin is the same as that of the natural vitamin as far as science knows today, but that isn't the whole story. Natural vitamins from food sources contain cofactors without which the vitamin does not work as it should. For example, a molecule of synthetic ascorbic acid (vitamin C) is identical to a molecule of natural

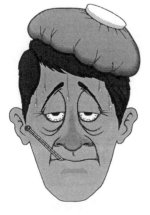

ascorbic acid. However, the natural ascorbic acid has cofactors called bioflavonoids. In addition, vitamin C, a mineral chelator, grabs hold of minerals and metals on its journey through the body.

If you take pure ascorbic acid, especially in large doses, it may deplete the body of essential minerals, especially copper. Food which naturally contains vitamin C usually contains some copper to offset this. If you are taking vitamin C supplements, copper and lysine should also be taken. The copper and lysine form copper lysinate, a chelated compound which is resistant to removal by vitamin C. Large doses (1-6 grams) of vitamin C are sometimes taken to ward off a cold or flu. Although vitamin C has some antihistamine action which reduces the symptoms, vitamin C's removal of copper and virus fighting copper lysinate, can actually worsen the illness unless copper and lysine are also taken.

How should vitamins be taken?
Vitamins are synergistic with food and are meant to be taken as part of your food intake, preferably in the morning. They should usually not be taken with minerals, although there are some exceptions. An adequate intake of healthy oils (discussed in the Oils and Fats chapter) is necessary for the proper assimilation of oil-soluble vitamins.

Do vitamins increase your energy?
Vitamins are not pep pills. They have no caloric or energy value of their own. However, since vitamin deficiencies often show up as fatigue or lack of energy, among other symptoms, a correction of the particular deficiency can increase one's energy and sense of well-being, but only to the extent that the fatigue was caused by the deficiency of vitamins.

What are the two basic types of vitamins?
There are two basic types of vitamins:

- *Oil soluble*   *vitamins A, D, E, and K*
- *Water soluble*   *vitamin C and the B vitamins*

There are other little-known nutrients that either are arguably necessary for life (vitamins B13, B17, or U), are included as part of a better-known vitamin (bioflavonoids as part of vitamin C), go by another name (niacin rather than vitamin B3), or are actually macronutrients (fatty acids are sometimes called Vitamin F). Vitamin D is sometimes considered to be a hormone.

What is the R.D.A.?
The RDA, or Recommended Daily Allowance, came into being in 1941. The diets of healthy, average adults were assessed to determine the minimal amount of each vitamin and mineral needed in the diet to prevent overt deficiency disease such as scurvy (vitamin C deficiency). A bit more is then added as a margin for safety. In this way it was determined that, for example, the RDA of vitamin C is 60 mg per day. Sometimes a dosage range is given. The U.S.R.D.A. (United States Recommended Daily Allowance) is a legal standard for food labeling purposes, and uses the upper end of this range, while the MDR (minimum daily requirement) uses the lower end.

How useful are the RDA figures?
Suppose you were trying to figure out the optimal weight for your particular body, taking into consideration height, gender, bone structure, age, muscle/fat ratio, and heredity. You then come across the statement, "The average adult should weigh 150 pounds". While this statement may (or may not) be statistically correct, it provides little or no useful information for your situation. Similarly, the statement "The average adult needs 60 mg of vitamin C per day" is nearly as useless for your particular situation. The RDA is useful only as a guideline. Many factors can increase (or in rare cases decrease) your needs beyond this figure.

The RDA figures were, in many cases, set over 50 years ago. Times have changed considerably since then, as we are exposed to many more toxins and stressors. Therefore, a food that claims that it provides 100% of the RDA of any nutrient probably doesn't by today's standards.

Who needs more than the RDA of nutrients?

Most of us need more than the RDA for optimal health. Anyone with the following problems has increased nutrient needs:

- *Poor digestion*
- *Smoking, alcohol use, other drugs*
- *Heavy metals such as mercury, nickel, cadmium*
- *Fungus, parasites, worms*
- *Infection of any type*
- *Allergies*
- *Cancer, autoimmune disease, AIDS*
- *Heavy exercise*
- *Chemical toxicity of any kind, which is more likely now than in 1941 when the RDAs were developed.*

The body needs more nutrients under any less than optimal conditions because it has more work to do in healing or detoxifying. This is similar to the way a car going uphill has more work to do than a car on a level surface, and so needs more gas to function.

What form should vitamins be taken in?

Vitamins come in different forms, and these are not created equal. The theory behind the optimal forms for vitamins are discussed in the chapter on Supplements, and the some of the optimal forms themselves are listed later in this chapter.

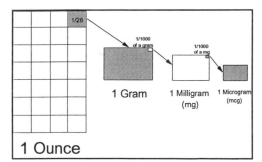

What units are used to measure vitamin dosages?

Vitamin units are expressed in milligrams (mg) or micrograms (mcg) for water soluble vitamins. A microgram is 1/1000 of a milligram. A milligram in turn is 1/1000 of a gram, which itself is 1/28 of an ounce. A microgram is thus one twenty-eight millionth (1/28,000,000) of an ounce, which is a tiny amount indeed.

International Units (IU) are used for oil soluble vitamins. Milligrams and micrograms are units of mass (weight), while IUs are units of activity. For example, two different forms of vitamin E may weigh different amounts but they both have the same activity in the body and so have the same dosage expressed in IUs.

Can vitamins be toxic?

Oil soluble vitamins remain in the body far longer than water soluble vitamins. Although unused vitamin E is excreted after a few days, vitamins A and D can accumulate to the point of causing toxic symptoms if large doses are taken for a long period of time. To put this in perspective, however, vitamins even in excess are far less toxic than most drugs. The toxicity of oil-soluble vitamins lies in their potential for retention and accumulation by the body.

By contrast, unused water soluble vitamins are excreted rapidly. For example, note that vitamin B2 (riboflavin) colors urine bright yellow. If you take vitamin B2 alone or as part of the B complex, you should notice that your urine is bright yellow within an hour after taking it. Several hours later your urine color is back to normal. This shows that the body begins to excrete the excess of vitamin B2 - and by implication all water soluble vitamins - within a very short time, and has completed doing so within a few hours. For this reason, water soluble vitamins are best taken in smaller doses several times a day.

There are a couple of exceptions to the "water soluble vitamins are safe" rule. Niacin (vitamin B3) dilates the blood vessels and can cause a drop in blood pressure if taken in too large a dose (the amount varies, but over 100 mg should not be taken at once unless you have built up a tolerance to it). The drop in blood pressure can be dangerous if you have low blood pressure to begin with and take a large excess. In addition, the histamine effect of niacin cause skin warmth and flushing, and a too-large dose can cause acute discomfort for up to an hour.

Some B vitamins, especially vitamin B6, can cause nerve damage in large excess, so large doses of these are not entirely harmless.

It is nearly impossible to obtain an excess of any vitamin through food sources. Most vitamin overdose symptoms can be reversed when excessive intake is stopped. Many side effects and symptoms are merely unpleasant, not toxic to the body.

Data taken from annual reports of the American Association of Poison Control Centers shows that in the seven year period from 1983 to 1989, there were no deaths at all due to vitamins. By contrast, there were 2069 deaths reported from prescription and non-prescription drugs, excluding suicide attempts and illegal drugs [1].

How is the rest of this chapter set up?
In this chapter - and the minerals chapter is set up the same way - each vitamin is discussed separately, covering the following information:

- *Other names for the nutrient*
- *What it is used for in the body*
- *Dosage (RDA), expressed as daily intake by adults. Most people need more, and most supplement amounts are larger.*
- *The usual amounts used in vitamin preparations*
- *Best natural, or food, sources*
- *Other information on the nutrient*
- *Supplement information - dosages, recommendations*

There are a number of reference books, including those listed in the back of this chapter, that can provide more information on each vitamin.

A table of vitamin deficiency symptoms, listed by symptom rather than by vitamin, follows the discussion of the individual vitamins. Other deficiency symptoms can be inferred from what the vitamin is used for.

Food sources of vitamins are listed, although some of these are not recommended due to other possible problems. For example,

- *Yeast is a fungus*
- *Peanuts can have mold (aflatoxins) and rancid oil*
- *Milk products, wheat, oatmeal, soy, and yeast have high allergic potential.*

Food sources of vitamins include:

Group	Food	A	D	E	K	C	B1	B2	B3	B5	B6	B12	FA	Bi	PA	In	Ch
Vegetables	Vegetables						●			●						●	
	Carrots/yellow veg.	●											●				
	Leafy greens			●	●	●		●		●			●				
	Broccoli			●													
	Alfalfa				●												
	Seaweed				●							●					
	Tomatoes					●											
	Potatoes					●											
Beans/Nuts	Beans/Legumes												●				●
	Soybeans			●													
	Nuts								●				●				
Grains	Whole grains			●						●					●	●	●
	Whole wheat						●		●				●				
	Wheat germ			●							●				●		
	Oats						●										
	Brown rice													●	●		
	Tempeh											●					
Animal Products	Meat								●	●	●	●				●	●
	Liver/kidney							●	●	●	●	●	●	●	●		
	Poultry								●	●							
	Fish		●						●	●							
	Fish liver oil	●	●			●											
	Dairy products	●	●				●	●			●	●			●	●	●
	Yogurt					●											
	Cheese									●				●			
	Eggs	●		●	●					●	●	●	●	●			●
Fruit	Fruit															●	
	Citrus					●											
	Dried fruits								●								
	Apricots													●			
	Cantaloupe										●			●			
Other	Vegetable oils			●	●												
	Yeast						●	●	●	●	●			●	●		
	Molasses									●	●				●		

FA=Folic Acid, Bi=Biotin, PA=PABA, In=Inositol, Ch=Choline

Vitamin A

Used for:

- Powerful immune system stimulant, increases size and function of thymus.
- Correcting night blindness, weak eyesight and some eye disorders.
- Decreases development of epithelial cancers (skin, mucous membrane, lung, intestinal lining).
- Builds resistance to respiratory infections and shortens duration of some diseases.
- Antioxidant to protect against free radical damage, especially as beta-carotene.
- Promotes growth, strong bones, healthy skin, and keeps the outer layers of tissues and organs healthy.
- Aids in the treatment of hyperthyroidism and emphysema.
- Helps to treat acne and open ulcers when applied externally. Birth control pill users may need less.

Sources:

- Fish liver oil, liver, carrots, yellow and green vegetables, eggs, dairy products, yellow fruits. One cup of cooked carrots contains 15,000 IU of vitamin A.

Dosage:

- 4000-5000 IU, although some supplements have up to 25,000 IU.
- Available as water dispersible (mycelized) form, recommended for those who have poor oil digestion.
- Beta carotene, a vitamin A precursor, is also available. Beta carotene is not nearly as toxic as vitamin A, as it is converted to vitamin A only as needed.

Toxicity:

More than 100,000 IU per day over a period of many months can produce toxic symptoms, including hair loss, gastrointestinal upset, scaly skin and rashes, blurred vision, fatigue, headaches and yellow skin.

Of interest:

- Adequate zinc is needed to get vitamin A out of storage in the body.
- Vitamin A help to keep vitamin C from oxidizing.
- Carotene, also called beta-carotene, is found in carrots and other sources, and is the precursor to vitamin A.
- Adequate oil is necessary to convert beta-carotene to vitamin A in the body.
- In a study published in 1932, it was recognized that large doses of vitamin A cut, by more than half, deaths from lung infections that were complications of acute measles [2]. Other studies have shown that vitamin A levels drop considerably during acute viral infections, and a deficiency can develop during infection even in a well-nourished person [3].

- Beta-carotene, the vitamin A precursor, helps protect against cervical cancer [4].

Supplement information:
- Available both as oil and in water dispersible (mycelized) form. The mycelized form is recommended for those with poor oil digestion.
- Beta carotene, the vitamin A precursor, is also available, usually as soft gel capsules.

Vitamin D

Also called: Calciferol

Used for:
- Utilization of calcium and phosphorus for strong bones and teeth. For this reason it is usually added to milk.
- Can help prevent colds in conjunction with vitamins A and C.
- Aids in assimilating vitamin A.
- Prevents rickets, a deficiency disease in which the bones soften and, in children, can grow deformed.

Sources:
- Fish liver oils, oily fish such as sardines and tuna, dairy products; sunlight on skin stimulates its manufacture in the body

Dosage:
- 400 IU, or 5-10 mg of cholecalciferol. May be combined with vitamin A.
- Those who may need more include people who get little sunlight, dark-skinned people, children who don't drink fortified milk, those exposed to mineral oil or smog, and people using anticonvulsant drugs.
- Most people get more than enough, and don't need supplemental vitamin D.

Toxicity:
- More than 25,000 IU daily over an extended period of time can produce toxic effects, including sore eyes, unusual thirst, itching skin, gastrointestinal symptoms, and calcium deposits in the blood.

Of interest:
- Oil in the diet is needed for absorption of vitamin D.
- Sunshine acts on skin oils to produce the vitamin.
- Milk with synthetic vitamin D added can rob the body of magnesium by increasing production of competing calcium.
- Vitamin D has more characteristics of a hormone than a vitamin [5].

Supplement information:
- Usually derived from codfish liver oil and packaged in gel capsules.
- May be combined with vitamin A.

Vitamin E

Also called: Tocopherol

Used for [6,7]:
- Antioxidant which retards cellular aging and harmful changes in body fats due to oxidation and free radical damage.
- Works with vitamin A to protect lungs from air pollution, including damage from cigarette smoking.
- Prevents ozone from oxidizing lung lipids (fats) by being oxidized (sacrificing) itself.
- Prevents and dissolves blood clots.
- Accelerates healing of bones.
- Helps to alleviate leg and muscle cramps
- It can lower blood pressure by acting as a mild diuretic.
- Alleviates fatigue.
- Reduces incidence of atherosclerosis, and protects against ischemic heart disease.
- Increases HDL (beneficial) cholesterol levels while keeping total level the same.
- Increases resistance to and relieves pain from osteoarthritis.
- Relieves restless leg syndrome (leg twitching, especially at night).
- Improves seizure control in epileptics.
- Reduces cystic breast disease and PMS.
- Both oral and topical (on the skin) application can help many skin conditions, including acne.
- Can reduce the gum inflammation of periodontal disease.
- Reduces cells' need for oxygen, which may help to preserve tissues.

Sources:
- Wheat germ, soybeans, leafy greens, broccoli and Brussels sprouts, eggs, whole grains, vegetable oils

Dosage:
- RDA is 8-10 IU, although usually available as 100-400 IU.

- People with a high intake of polyunsaturated oils, women on birth control pills or people taking hormones, and pregnant or lactating women may need more than the RDA.
- Natural mixed tocopherols are the best form.
- Available both as oil or mycelized.

Toxicity:

- Excess vitamin E is excreted much more rapidly than other oil soluble vitamins, and for this reason is less toxic than vitamins A, D or K.

Of interest:

- There are several forms of vitamin E. The alpha tocopherol form is an alcohol and is less stable in oxygen. Vitamin E acetate, phosphate, succinate, and palmitate are esters, which are more stable. The best form overall of vitamin E is natural mixed tocopherols.

- Vitamin E acetate stimulated the immune system of animals in a University of Colorado study. Animals given vitamin E showed a ten-fold increase in B cell performance, and a 3.5-fold increase in T cell activity [5].

- Exposure to pesticides and chemicals can cause brain symptoms which can mimic Alzheimer's disease. Vitamin E stands guard at the cell membrane to keep these toxins out of the cell [6].

- Vitamin E helps the blood use oxygen more efficiently and improves the production of antibodies [10]. It helps prevent an excessive buildup of platelets which can cause blood clots which can lead to heart attack and stroke [11,12]. Vitamin E can also help repair the cells lining the blood vessels [13,14].

- Vitamin E has a significant protective effect on the prevention of heart disease in men and women [15,16]. Two studies done at Harvard Medical School on large populations bear this out. In one study, 87,245 women who took 100 IU - a relatively low dose - of vitamin E daily for more than two years had a 46% lower heart disease risk [17]. In another study, 39,910 male health professionals who took 100 IU of vitamin E had a 37% lower heart disease risk [18].

- Vitamin E can protect against bowel cancer [19].

Supplement information:

- Available both as oil and in water dispersible form.

Vitamin K

Also called: Menadione

Used for:

- Proper blood clotting - prevents internal bleeding and nosebleeds.
- Reduces excessive menstrual flow.

- Supports immune function.

Sources:

- Alfalfa and alfalfa tablets, yogurt, egg yolk, leafy green vegetables, safflower and soybean oils, fish liver oils, kelp.

Dosage:

- No RDA, 300 mcg suggested.
- More than 500 mcg not recommended due to its clotting effect, which can lead to phlebitis, heart attacks and strokes

Of interest:

- Vitamin K can reverse the effect of anticoagulant drugs.
- Vitamin K is made in the bowel by beneficial bacteria.

Supplement information:

- Rarely sold or needed as supplement unless recommended by doctor for specific medical condition.

Vitamin C

Also called: Ascorbic acid

Used for: [8,20]

- Antioxidant which retards the effect of free radical damage. Vitamin C is strongly synergistic with (increases the activity of) other antioxidants.

- Formation of collagen, which is important in the growth and repair of body tissue cells, blood vessels, bones and teeth. Accelerates wound healing.

- Helps the body to absorb iron. As little as 25 to 100 mg of vitamin C can double or triple the absorption of nonheme iron (from sources other than meat) [21].

- Directly toxic to some cancer cells, especially melanoma.

- Helps to decrease blood cholesterol. 500 mg of vitamin C three times a day in athero-sclerotic patients reduced blood cholesterol 35-40% [8].

- Stimulates activity of phagocytes, white blood cells which identify and kill intruders.

- Is important in the production of lymphocytes (white blood cells).

- Aids in preventing and treating viral and bacterial infections, especially colds. It may have a direct killing action on viruses and bacteria in addition to stimulating the immune system. It can suppress transmission of a cold virus [22] and stimulate the immune system, white blood cell production, and the production of interferons (virus fighters) [23]

- Increases efficiency of immune system, both in disease prevention and reduction of allergic symptoms.

- Antihistamine, sometimes used to alleviate cold symptoms for this reason.

- Counteracts formation of nitrosamines, which are carcinogens, from nitrates and nitrites in processed and preserved foods [24,25].

- Acts as a natural laxative.

- Lowers incidence of blood clots in veins.

- Reduces deposits of lipids (fats) in arteries.

- Assists in calcium absorption.

- Reduces body burden of heavy metals such as mercury and lead due to its action as a chelating agent. Recommended during and after mercury removal to remove mercury that newly enters the body. In addition to being a chelator itself, vitamin C raises the levels of glutathione, a metal and chemical chelator [26].

- Helps to fight cancer. In an experiment by Linus Pauling, 1000 controls with cancer who had no vitamin C lived an average of 50 days after the study began and all died of their cancer. 100 experimental patients who took large doses of vitamin C lived an average of 200 days after the study began, and 13 were free of cancer years after treatment [8]. Good results with vitamin C therapy are tied to a lack of immune suppressing chemotherapy, as chemotherapy will decrease the chances that vitamin C will help.

- Prevents destruction of folic acid.

- Can help detoxify drugs such as alcohol, and reduces drug withdrawal symptoms. It offers some protection against the toxic effects of chronic alcohol consumption [27].

- Vitamin C has been shown to have a significant lowering effect on the systolic blood pressure (the first of the two numbers) as compared with a placebo. The amount used in the study was 1000 mg per day for six weeks [28].

- Supplementation of 1000 mg of vitamin C per day has been shown to increase the count, motility and maturity of sperm [29].

- Vitamin C can help protect against the formation of cataracts, most likely because its antioxidant action can help counteract oxidative damage to the lens protein [30-33].

- Vitamin C can help prevent periodontal disease [34].

Sources: Citrus fruits, tomatoes, leafy greens, potatoes

Dosage:

- The RDA is 60 mg, although most people need much more. Excess vitamin C is excreted within 2-3 hours, so intake spread over the day is best. 1-6 grams is sometimes recommended to bowel tolerance (before diarrhea develops), spread throughout day. Should be taken with bioflavonoids and copper.

- Pregnant or lactating women need more, about 80-120 mg.

- Smokers need more, as each cigarette destroys 25-100 mg of vitamin C.
  People who take aspirin, barbiturates or birth control pills need more.

- Cancer patients on chemotherapy should not take supplemental vitamin C.

Toxicity:

- Over 750 mg daily can cause kidney stones, although magnesium and sufficient water can help rectify this.

- Very high doses of over 10 grams daily can cause diarrhea, excess urination, and skin rashes.

- Large doses can deplete the body of essential minerals, especially copper which helps fight viral infections.

- There are no serious or toxic effects known at this time, as excess vitamin C is readily eliminated in the urine.

- Toxicity is more often associated with synthetic vitamin C (ascorbic acid) than with natural vitamin C (ascorbic acid with associated bioflavonoids and cofactors).

Of interest:

- Works best with bioflavonoids, which are found along with vitamin C in natural food sources and some supplements.

- Copper should be taken along with supplemental vitamin C, especially synthetic vitamin C (ascorbic acid), which will leach copper from the body in an attempt to make it more like natural vitamin C.

- Large doses of vitamin C can alter blood sugar and other blood test results. Diabetics who take vitamin C may end up taking too much insulin based on falsely high blood test results.

- Aspirin can triple the rate of vitamin C excretion.

- Severe, prolonged deficiency causes scurvy, which can be fatal. Capillaries and collagen fail. One of the early signs is bleeding of the gums or soft tissue pain and stiffness.

- Vitamin C ascorbate comes from corn, which is a common allergen. The palmitate form from the sego palm is better.

- Vitamin C in water is destroyed after a few hours.

- 33% of severely schizophrenic patients showed definite clinical improvement when given 2-6 grams of vitamin C for at least one month [35]. Many years ago, in 1952, Dr. Abram Hoffer reported the effectiveness of high doses of vitamin C along with niacinamide in the treatment of schizophrenia [36,37].

- Vitamin C deficiency can cause degeneration of the insulin-producing cells of the pancreas [38].

Supplement information:

- One of the most widely taken supplements.
- Vitamin C is available alone or with bioflavonoids (preferred).
- Available in strengths from 60 to 1000 mg (1 gram), in tablets, time-release formulations, powders, and chewable tablets. Powders are usually 5 grams per teaspoon.

Bioflavonoids	
Used for:	Free radical scavenger / antioxidant
Types:	Pycnogenol, rutin, quercetin
Sources:	Citrus fruits, tree bark, seeds
Dosage:	1 mg per pound body weight

The B Vitamins

The common B complex vitamins include B1, B2, B3, B5, B6, B12, folic acid, biotin, and PABA. These vitamins are water soluble and must be replaced daily. They are synergistic and are more potent and effective together. Vitamins B1, B2, and B6 should be equally balanced (e.g. 50 mg of each) to work most efficiently. B complex components may be combined or sold separately.

Vitamin B1

Also called: Thiamine

Used for:

- Promoting growth.
- Aiding digestion, especially of carbohydrates and sugar.
- Keeps nervous system, muscles and heart functioning normally.
- Improves mental attitude.
- Can reduce hangovers the morning after indulging in alcohol.
- Increases stamina and ability to concentrate.
- Essential in Krebs citric acid cycle for energy production.

Sources:

- Yeast, whole wheat, bran and rice husks, oatmeal, peanuts, pork, milk, most vegetables

Dosage:

- 1.0-1.5 mg; more needed by those who smoke, drink alcohol or coffee, or consume a lot of sugar. Physical or emotional stress can also increase the need for vitamin B1.

Toxicity:

- None known officially, although rare symptoms of excess include tremors, edema, nervousness, rapid heartbeat, and allergies.

Of interest:

- Diabetics should avoid B1 supplements, as B1 can inactivate insulin.

Supplement information:

- Dosage sizes are usually 50, 100, or 500 mg.
- Thiamine-5-phosphate is a recommended form.

Vitamin B2

Also called: Riboflavin

Used for:

- Growth and reproduction
- Healthy skin, nails and hair
- Benefits vision and eliminates eye fatigue
- Along with other substances, metabolizes carbohydrates, fats and proteins
- Kidney function

Sources: Milk, liver, kidney, yeast, cheese, leafy greens, fish, eggs

Dosage:

- 1.2-1.7 mg, although more is needed by pregnant or lactating women, people under stress, and vegetarians and those on restricted diets.

Supplement information:

- 100 mg tablets are most common. Riboflavin-5-phosphate is a more easily utilized form.

Of interest:

- Vitamin B2 is America's most common vitamin deficiency.

- Vitamin B2 can increase the effectiveness of some anti-cancer drugs.

- Vitamin B2 often colors the urine bright yellow for a few hours after ingestion. This is not harmful.

Vitamin B3

Also called: Niacin, niacinamide, nicotinamide, or nicotinic acid

Used for:

- Used throughout the body as part of normal metabolism, especially the brain.

- Healthy nervous system and brain function.

- Healthy digestive system; alleviates gastrointestinal disturbances; required for HCl production.

- Healthier-looking skin.

- Reduces migraine headaches.

- Increases circulation and reduces high blood pressure by dilating arteries and veins.

- Helps to remove lipids from arteries.

- Increases energy through proper utilization of food.

- Reduces cholesterol and triglycerides.

- Helps to eliminate canker sores and bad breath.

- Essential for synthesis of sex hormones and some other hormones.

- The histamine release caused by niacin is essential for orgasm. Try niacin 15-20 minutes before sex to increase mucus production and lubrication and to enhance orgasm.

- Niacin in large doses (3 grams per day) can lower serum cholesterol by 25% and triglycerides by 30% in two weeks [8,39].

Sources:
- Liver, lean meat, whole wheat products, brewer's yeast, kidney, fish, poultry, eggs, dried fruits

Dosage:
- 13-19 mg; supplements contain 50 to 1000 mg.
- Start with 100 mg or less and work up as your tolerance increases.
- Niacinamide does not produce the side effects of niacin (flushing, itching) but may not be as effective.

Toxicity:
- Essentially nontoxic in small doses, but can cause burning or itching skin in sensitive individuals. Large doses can reduce the blood pressure too much, causing dizziness.

- The "niacin flush", a feeling of heat caused by histamine release and dilation of blood vessels, can be alleviated by switching to niacinamide.

- Alcoholics, people on drugs, or those who have high chemical toxicity can experience an uncomfortable reaction, including diarrhea.

Of interest:
- Lack of niacin can cause negative personality changes.

- A severe prolonged niacin deficiency can cause pellagra, which can be fatal.

- Some niacin supplements have a buffer such as magnesium stearate, and some are pure. Less of the pure niacin than of the buffered type can be tolerated.

- Niacin in large doses such as 1000 mg is useful in the treatment of schizophrenia [40-44].

- Niacin in one gram doses has been used to treat alcoholism [45-47].

- Niacin has been used by a number of researchers in the treatment and prevention of cancer [48-54].

Vitamin B5

Also called: Pantothenic acid, calcium pantothenate, or panthenol

Used for:
- Cell building, normal growth, nervous system development
- Conversion of fat and sugar to energy via the fatty acid cycle and Krebs cycle.
- Aids in wound healing.
- Fights infection by synthesis of antibodies.
- Utilization of PABA and choline
- Prevention of fatigue.
- Reduces toxic effects of antibiotics.
- Reduces stress, increases stamina.

Sources:
- Meat, whole grains, organ meats, green vegetables, brewer's yeast, nuts, chicken, molasses

Dosage:
- 10 mg; usually found only in B complex formulas in strengths from 10 to 100 mg. May cause insomnia if taken after 2 PM.

Vitamin B6

Also called: Pyridoxine

Used for [55]:
- Amino acid processing.
- Proper assimilation of protein and fat.
- Helps prevent various nervous and skin disorders.
- Production of antibodies and red blood cells.
- Needed for absorption of vitamin B12 and production of hydrochloric acid.
- Alleviates nausea; natural diuretic
- Promotes proper synthesis of antiaging nucleic acids.

- Relieves muscle spasms and cramps.
- Needed for energy metabolism in muscles.

Sources:

- Wheat germ and bran, brewer's yeast, organ meats, cantaloupe, molasses, milk, eggs, beef

Dosage:

- 1.8-2.2 mg; more is needed by those on tricyclic antidepressants, penicillamine (arthritis drug), high protein diets, or those who use a lot of Aspartame (artificial sweetener). B6 supplements should not be taken by Parkinson's disease patients who are taking l-dopa, as B6 will counteract l-dopa and can increase Parkinson's symptoms.

Toxicity:

- 2-10 grams per day can cause neurological disorders. A slight excess of B6 can cause night restlessness.

Of interest:

- B6 can decrease a diabetic's need for insulin.

- The pyridoxyl-5-phosphate form is more easily assimilated than the pyridoxine form, especially if you have poor digestion, low blood pressure, or allergy.

- Inability to remember dreams may be due to a vitamin B6 deficiency.

- Vitamin B6, alone or with magnesium and GLA fatty acids, can help ease premenstrual (PMS) symptoms, as shown in a number of studies [56].

- Vitamin B6 is a cofactor in the formation of dopamine and serotonin, brain neurochemicals which promote a feeling of emotional stability. A B6 deficiency may result in anxiety or depression [57].

- Vitamin B6 deficiency can result in abnormal collagen metabolism which can lead to the development of atherosclerosis. Vitamin B6 also inhibits platelet aggregation and some blood coagulation. Vitamin B6 supplementation can therefore inhibit atherosclerosis, promote healthier arteries and reduce the risk of cardiovascular disease, heart attacks and strokes [58-61].

- Vitamin B6 along with iron and coenzyme Q10 has proven effective in restoring mental function to patients diagnosed with Alzheimer's disease [62].

- Vitamin B6 helps protect against cervical cancer [63].

- 100 mg daily of vitamin B6 has been shown to normalize blood sugar levels in type II diabetics. 50 mg is recommended for maintenance in diabetics [64].

- Vitamin B6 supplementation has been shown to improve [65]:

PMS	depression	carpal tunnel syndrome
exhaustion	arteriosclerosis	kidney stones

schizophrenia   MSG sensitivity   water retention in pregnancy
numbness and tingling in extremities

Supplement information:

- 50-500 mg in supplements.
- Pyridoxyl-5-phosphate (P5P) is a recommended form. Many people have trouble phosphorylating their vitamins, a necessary step for utilization. This is especially true for people with low blood pressure. P5P is already phosphorylated.

Vitamin B12

Also called: Cyanocobalamin, cobalamin

Used for:

- Formation of red blood cells and prevention of anemia.
- Promotes growth and increases appetite in children.
- Increases energy, relieves irritability, improves concentration and balance.
- Maintains a healthy nervous system.
- Needed to properly utilize fats, carbohydrates and proteins.

Sources:

- Liver, beef, pork, eggs, milk, cheese, kidney, tempeh, sea vegetables. The seaweeds arame, wakame and kombu contain 1.4, 43 and 19 mcg of B12 per gram of weight respectively. Tempeh contains 0.5 mcg/g [66].

Dosage:

- 3 mcg. Alcohol users and those who consume a lot of protein need more.
- Sublingual or timed release tablets (50-200 mcg) are recommended as it is not absorbed well through the stomach. Injections are available for severe deficiency.

Of interest:

- A properly functioning thyroid gland aids B12 absorption.

- Lack of vitamin B12 can cause pernicious anemia, in which the red blood cells are too large, rather than being small, efficient and effective. The enlargement is the body's attempt to compensate for poor oxidation. Such cells work about as well as a truck in a sports car's parking space. B12 is a cellular oxidant.

- Pernicious anemia due to a deficiency of vitamin B12 often leads to infertility in men, and is reversible with vitamin B12 injections [67]. In one double-blind study of 375 infertile men whose sperm count was very low, the men responded favorably to injections of mecobalamin, a form of vitamin B12 [68].

- B12 works synergistically with folic acid, and they should be taken together.

- Vegetarians who take in little or no animal protein are often deficient in vitamin B12. Sea vegetables (seaweed), as discussed above, can help remedy this.

- B12 contains the necessary mineral cobalt, as suggested by the name cyano<u>cobala</u>-min.

- Patients with dementia, psychiatric disorders and neurologic symptoms were found to have low serum cobalamin (vitamin B12) levels, even though they had no anemia or enlarged red blood cells, both classical signs of vitamin B12 deficiency. Vitamin B12 supplementation improved the psychiatric/ neurological symptoms in nearly all of the patients studied [69].

Vitamin B15

Also called: Pangamic acid

Used for: Promotes cell oxygenation - used by Russian athletes to prolong performance

Vitamin B17

Also called: Laetrile

Used for: Preventing and treating cancer. Its use for this purpose is controversial.

Folic acid

Also called: Folacin, folate

Used for:

- Formation of red blood cells and, working with vitamin B12, prevention of pernicious anemia.

- Aids in protein metabolism and utilization of sugar and amino acids.

- Production of nucleic acids, division of body cells.

- Improves lactation.

- Protects against intestinal parasites.

- Helps prevent neural tube defects such as spina bifida in a developing embryo [70].

- Helps to clear gout.

Sources:

- Leafy green vegetables, carrots, cantaloupe, apricots, liver, egg yolk, beans, whole wheat.

Dosage:

- 400 mcg; 800 mcg needed by pregnant women. Larger doses are also needed by heavy alcohol drinkers, those taking high doses of vitamin C or aspirin, or taking Dilantin, estrogen, sulfonamides, or phenobarbital.

Of interest:

- May delay hair greying along with vitamin B5, PABA and zinc.

- May reverse some types of skin discoloration.

- Low folate concentrations may be a risk factor for stroke [71].

- Dementia and neurologic deterioration may be partially reversible with folate (folic acid) supplementation [72].

Supplement information:

- Available in 400 and 800 mcg strengths. 100 to 400 mcg are usually found in B complex formulations.

Biotin

Used for:

- Maintaining healthy skin and alleviating eczema and dermatitis.
- Helps keep hair from turning grey.
- Eases muscle pains.
- Helps control fungus overgrowth, but too much can increase fungus growth.
- Biotin works with insulin and helps in the utilization of glucose [73].

Sources: Nuts, fruits, brewer's yeast, liver, kidney, egg yolk, milk, brown rice

Dosage:

- 150-300 mcg; usually found only in B vitamin combinations.
- Biotin can be synthesized in the body.

Of interest:

- Raw egg white contains avidin, a protein which prevents biotin absorption. Even slight cooking inactivates avidin.

- Biotin is made in the bowel by beneficial bacteria, and anything which depletes these bacteria (antibiotics, mercury, fermenting foods) can interfere with biotin production.

Supplement information:

- Usually found only in B complex and multivitamin formulas.

PABA

Also called: para-amino-benzoic acid

Used for:

- Helps form folic acid and is important in the utilization of protein.

- Has sunscreening properties both as a supplement and applied topically (to the skin). Prevents crosslinking of skin and resultant wrinkles due to UV radiation from sunlight.

- Prevents ozone damage to lungs.

- Aids in assimilation of pantothenic acid.

- May prevent hair greying or restore grey hair to its natural color along with pantothenic acid. Can prevent hair loss due to its membrane stabilizing ability.

- Reduces pain of burns.

- Improves skin tone, helps to delay wrinkling.

- Increases energy by supporting adrenal function.

Sources: Liver, brewer's yeast, kidney, whole grains, molasses, rice bran, wheat germ

Dosage:

- No RDA; can be made in the body.
- Those taking penicillin or sulfa drugs (antibiotics) may need more.

Supplement information:

- Usually found in the more expensive brands of B complex and multivitamin formulations in dosages of 30 to 100 mg.
- 30 to 100 mg strengths are available in regular and time-release form.
- Also found in sun protection skin preparations.

Of interest:

- Sulfa drugs work because they resemble PABA. Bacteria try to use sulfa instead of PABA for their metabolic reactions and die of vitamin deficiency.

Inositol

Used for: Hair growth, artery health, fat and cholesterol metabolism

Sources: Fruits, vegetables, whole grains, meat, milk

Choline

- **Used for:**
- Used in phosphatidyl choline, a key ingredient in cell membranes.

- Forms acetylcholine, which is responsible for nerve transmission. A deficiency of this compound has been linked to Alzheimer's disease. When the body doesn't have enough choline, it takes it from the brain, causing destruction of brain tissue [74,75]. Early stages of senility have been reversed with a choline compound, phosphatidyl choline [76].

- Gallbladder and liver function

- Hormone production

Sources: Egg yolks, legumes, meat, milk, whole grains

CoQ$_{10}$

Identity:

- Coenzyme that helps (acts as a catalyst) in oxidation and reduction reactions in the cell, helpful for the heart.

What symptoms correlate with which vitamin deficiencies?
Deficiency symptoms and the associated vitamins that may relieve them include:

Appetite loss	A, B1, C, biotin
Bad breath	Niacin
Body odor	B12
Bruising easily	C and bioflavonoids, E
Cholesterol high	B complex, B3, inositol, choline
Constipation	B complex
Diarrhea	Vitamin K, niacin
Dizziness	B2, B5, B6, PABA
Edema (water retention)	B2, B5, B6, PABA
Eye problems	A, B2
Fatigue	A, B complex, PABA, C, D
Gastrointestinal problems	B1, B2, B3, B5, PABA, C
Hair, dandruff	B6, B12
Hair, dry and dull	B complex, PABA
Hair loss	Biotin, inositol, B complex, C, folic acid
Heart palpitations	B12
High blood pressure	Choline
Infections	A, B5
Insomnia	B complex, biotin
Loss of smell	A
Memory loss	B1, choline
Menstrual problems	B12, folic acid
Mouth sores and cracks	B2, B6
Muscle cramps	B1, B6, biotin, D, E, K
Nervousness	B1, B2, B5, B6, B12, niacin, PABA
Nosebleeds	C and bioflavonoids, K
Retarded growth	B2, B12, folic acid
Skin problems, acne	A, B complex
Skin problems, dermatitis	A, B2, B6

Skin problems, eczema	A, B complex, inositol
Slow healing	A, C
Softening of bones and teeth	D
Vaginal itching	B2, biotin

These symptoms may also be due to deficiencies of minerals, and a similar table of mineral deficiencies appears at the end of the Minerals chapter. Macronutrient deficiencies and a number of toxicities (nutritional and otherwise) can also cause these symptoms. A vitamin deficiency is more likely if little or none of the food sources of that vitamin are consumed regularly, no supplement of the vitamin is being taken, and general nutrition is poor.

A suggestion - a relatively small number of foods reappear in many of the food source lists for these vitamins. A high intake of these foods (e.g. green leafy vegetables, organ meats, whole grains) should cover most or all of your vitamin needs if you are reasonably healthy.

Summary

A deficiency of vitamins is unhealthy, but so is an imbalance.

Natural vitamins from food or taken with food are much better for the body than synthetic.

References and Resources

- The Burton Goldberg Group, *Alternative Medicine: The Definitive Guide*, "Nutritional Supplements", pp. 385-397, Future Medicine Publishing, Puyallup WA, 1994.

- Cheraskin, Emmanuel, *Vitamin C: Who Needs It?*, Arlington Press, Birmingham AL, 1993.

- Ellis, John M., *Vitamin B6, The Doctor's Report*, Harper and Row, NY, 1973.

- Goodman, Sandra, *Vitamin C: The Master Nutrient*, Keats Publishing Inc., New Canaan CT, 1991.

- Lesser, M., *Nutrition and Vitamin Therapy*, Grove Press Inc., New York, 1980.

- Lieberman, Shari, and Nancy P. Bruning, *The Real Vitamin and Mineral Book*, Avery Publishing Group, Garden City Park NY, 1990.

- Mindell, Earl, *Vitamin Bible*, Warner Books, New York, 1985.

- Mindell, Earl, *Shaping Up With Vitamins*, Warner Books, New York, 1985.

- Passwater, Richard, *Supernutrition, Megavitamin Revolution*, Pocket Books / Simon and Schuster Inc., New York, 1975.

- Pauling, Linus C., *Vitamin C and the Common Cold*, WH Freeman and Co., San Francisco CA, 1970.

- Pearson, Durk, and Sandy Shaw, *Life Extension*, Warner Books, NY, 1982.

- Rogers, Sherry A., *Tired or Toxic?*, Prestige Publishing, Syracuse NY, 1990.

- Shute, Wilfred, *Dr. Wilfred E. Shute's Complete Updated Vitamin E Book*, Keats Publishing, New Canaan CT, 1975.

MINERALS

Batteries For The Body

Things in this chapter that can change your health:

- *How do you know what minerals to take?*
- *What is the best way to take minerals?*
- *Not all minerals are created equal.*

What are minerals?

Minerals are the ionic, or charged, form of metals and other elements. They are of comparatively low molecular weight, and are located near the top of the periodic table. The periodic table and definitions of terms such as ionic and molecular are found in the chapter on Basic Chemical Concepts in *Surviving The Toxic Crisis*.

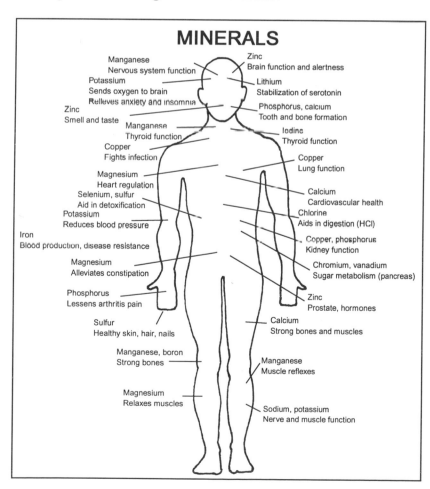

MINERALS

Manganese
Nervous system function

Potassium
Sends oxygen to brain
Relieves anxiety and insomnia

Zinc
Smell and taste

Manganese
Thyroid function

Copper
Fights infection

Magnesium
Heart regulation

Selenium, sulfur
Aid in detoxification

Potassium
Reduces blood pressure

Iron
Blood production, disease resistance

Magnesium
Alleviates constipation

Phosphorus
Lessens arthritis pain

Sulfur
Healthy skin, hair, nails

Manganese, boron
Strong bones

Magnesium
Relaxes muscles

Zinc
Brain function and alertness

Lithium
Stabilization of serotonin

Phosphorus, calcium
Tooth and bone formation

Iodine
Thyroid function

Copper
Lung function

Calcium
Cardiovascular health

Chlorine
Aids in digestion (HCl)

Copper, phosphorus
Kidney function

Chromium, vanadium
Sugar metabolism (pancreas)

Zinc
Prostate, hormones

Calcium
Strong bones and muscles

Manganese
Muscle reflexes

Sodium, potassium
Nerve and muscle function

Like vitamins, all of the minerals are necessary, and many of them work synergistically with other minerals, vitamins, and macronutrients. The balance between them is often more important than the presence of an absolute amount.

Where are minerals used in the body?

Although most minerals are needed throughout the body, certain minerals target certain areas:

What are the major minerals?

The major minerals are those which are needed in larger amounts than the others. The major minerals are calcium, magnesium, phosphorus, sodium, and potassium.

What are trace minerals?

Some minerals are called trace minerals, in reference to the smaller amounts needed. They are no less important than the major minerals. They generally work synergystically with the major minerals.

What forms of minerals are there?

If you read the labels on supplements which contain minerals, you may notice that minerals are expressed as two words rather than simply calcium, chromium, or potassium. The second word in the mineral's name refers to the form (molecular structure) of the mineral. Some examples are chromium picolinate, calcium citrate, and magnesium oxide. Although minerals themselves (calcium, potassium) are not organic (carbon containing), the complete form may be organic or inorganic.

> **Not all forms of minerals are created equal.**

What forms of minerals are best?

Not all forms of minerals are created equal. Some are better absorbed, some are better utilized, some are cheaper, and some have a greater potential for side effects.

Minerals which are acidified are more water soluble and would therefore stand a greater chance of being absorbed and utilized by the body, which is 83% water. The opposite of acid is alkaline, and alkaline mineral forms stand much less chance of being absorbed and used, especially if your stomach is low in HCl.

Some of the most effective acidic mineral forms are citrates and malates, which are used in the Krebs citric acid cycle which converts sugar to energy.

Aspartates are not as desirable if you have little body fat. Aspartates convert fat to sugar for energy, and if there is not much body fat the fatty myelin sheath of nerves can be attacked. Symptoms resembling multiple sclerosis (MS) can result.

Picolinates are also not as desirable, as picolinate is a waste product for the body. An exception is chromium picolinate, which should be taken with chromium nicotinate for balance. Chromium picolinate is better for quick energy and weight loss, but nicotinate is also recommended.

Carbonates and lactates are alkaline and so are not very well absorbed. Bone meal, oyster shell, and dolomite are hard, insoluble alkaline forms of calcium which do little good as they pass through the body without being absorbed. These forms may also contain lead, a toxic metal.

Orotates are good, but have been banned from sale in this country.

Iron fumarate and citrate are the best-absorbed forms of iron. Iron is usually difficult to absorb and can cause constipation, and these forms minimize these problems. Free radical damage can occur if too much iron is taken.

Magnesium has a tendency to loosen the stool (hence the use of Milk of Magnesia to relieve constipation). Magnesium glycinate is a form of magnesium that will not loosen stool, i.e. cause diarrhea. Magnesium citrate and other forms of magnesium, on the other hand, will generally loosen stool; this is sometimes desired.

Glycinates such as magnesium glycinate are good. The glycinate pulls the magnesium into the body. Only 20% of the magnesium ingested is used, but side effects such as diarrhea are avoided.

Be aware that balance is the key in taking magnesium. If you take high levels of magnesium without calcium, you can lower your calcium levels until myocardial infarction occurs, i.e. the heart just stops under stress.

A new product, Kona Gold (see Sources section in the back of the book) takes minerals from deep undersea to avoid contaminants such as cadmium. The resulting product is a pure source of necessary minerals which are essentially predigested so they can be taken any time, rather than just on an empty stomach.

What are chelated minerals?

Chelation refers to the process of binding a mineral (or metal) to a molecular group which holds it tightly. Chelating minerals - the label will say "chelated" - causes the mineral to be more easily absorbed into the body. However, the chelator may bind so tightly to the mineral that it will not release the mineral for use by the body. Acidifying chelated minerals facilitates absorption.

Acidified minerals or acidic forms of minerals are best, followed by chelated minerals. Alkaline forms are the most useless, especially if there is low HCl such as may be caused by allergy.

A very effective form of chelated minerals is dipeptide chelates. Dipeptides are formed from two amino acids and can pass easily through the intestinal wall into the bloodstream by design. Chemically hitching a mineral to a dipeptide facilitates its passage into the bloodstream. Since the mineral-dipeptide complex is pulled across the gut wall rather than simply passively diffusing through, these preparations are better for people with weakened digestive systems. Some dipeptide chelates are made by Metagenics Inc. - see Product Sources section near the back of the book.

Buyer Beware! Many manufacturers of "chelated" minerals simply put the chelating agent and the mineral together in the mixing drum rather than chemically combining them (the difference between a mixture and a compound is discussed in the chapter on Basic Chemical Concepts in *Surviving The Toxic Crisis*). The chelating agent is essentially worthless and any advantage of chelation of minerals is lost.

At what time of day should minerals be taken?

If minerals with the same charge, usually +2, are taken at the same time, they may fight for binding sites. Ideally minerals should be taken several hours apart, but this is not always practical. Most minerals, especially the calming mineral calcium, should be taken before bed on an empty stomach. An empty stomach contains more HCl, which will acidify the mineral to enhance absorption. However, calcium should be taken in the morning before exercise if you have a tendency to form arterial plaques. Copper should be taken in the morning, both to avoid competition with the other +2 minerals (refer to Periodic Table in Basic Chemical Concepts chapter in *Surviving The Toxic Crisis* for +2 minerals) and to work with vitamin C and lysine.

What is this chart, and how is it read?

This chart illustrates the antagonist relationships between the different minerals and metals. The relationship A → B means that A is an antagonist to B, i.e. A interferes with the absorption or action of B. If there is no directional arrow, this means that they antagonize each other. This chart can both be read to see specific mineral relationships, or can be seen as a whole to illustrate the sometime complexity of mineral balancing.

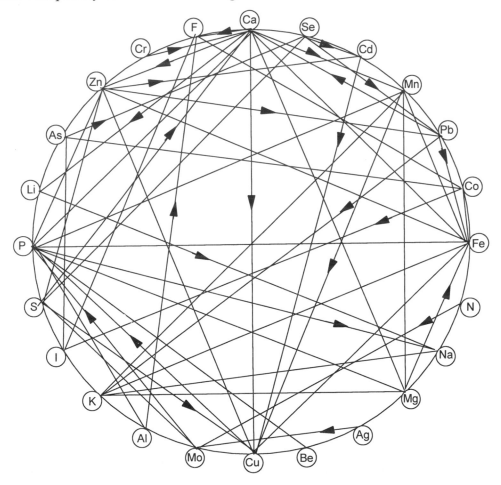

What are the minerals, their uses, their sources, and dosages?

As with the vitamins, the USRDA dosages of minerals tend to be low, and are not meant to be prescriptive. While vitamins may need to be taken daily for up to a month before deficiency symptoms are alleviated, some mineral deficiency symptoms can be relieved by the appropriate mineral within a half hour of taking the mineral! Examples are magnesium for menstrual

> **Some mineral deficiency symptoms can be relieved by the appropriate mineral within a half hour of taking the mineral!**

cramps or potassium for insomnia, if these conditions are caused by a mineral imbalance. An amount of these minerals that is not much larger than the RDA can provide dramatic relief.

How is the rest of this chapter set up?

This chapter is structured in the same way as the vitamin chapter. The essential minerals, both major and trace, are listed alphabetically. There are a number of reference books, including those listed in the back of this chapter, that can provide more information on each mineral.

The major minerals and their principal sources are:

		Ca	Cl	Co	Cu	I	Fe	Mg	Mn	Mo	P	K	Se	Na	S	Zn
Vegetables	Vegetables	●														
	Leafy greens						●	●	●			●				
	Onions				●								●			
	Spinach						●	●								
	Seaweed		●			●										
	Corn							●								
	Beets								●							
	Tomatoes											●	●			
	Potatoes											●				
	Broccoli												●			
	Celery													●		
	Cabbage														●	
Beans/ Nuts	Soybeans	●														
	Nuts / Seeds	●					●	●	●		●	●				●
	Beans / Legumes	●			●		●		●	●				●		
Grains	Whole grains				●				●		●					
	Whole wheat / germ							●					●			●
	Oatmeal						●									
Animal Products	Meat			●			●				●				●	●
	Liver / kidney			●	●		●						●			
	Fish	●		●	●						●		●		●	
	Shellfish			●	●	●	●						●			
	Poultry										●					
	Eggs / yolks						●			●	●				●	●
	Dairy products	●		●							●					
Fruit	Dried fruits						●	●								
	Prunes				●											
	Citrus						●					●				
	Apples						●									
	Bananas											●				
	Cantaloupe											●				
	Persimmons											●				
Other	Salt (Iodized)		●			●								●		
	Molasses						●									
	Yeast															●

Calcium (Ca)

Used for:

- Strong bones and muscles and healthy teeth, in combination with phosphorus.
- Cardiovascular health, in combination with magnesium.
- Alleviating insomnia.
- Aids nervous system, especially impulse transmission.

Sources:

- Green vegetables, milk and dairy products (not a good source because they contain too much competing phosphorus), soybeans, sardines, nuts, seeds, salmon, beans

Dosage:

- 800-1200 mg. A 2:1 ratio of calcium to magnesium and a ratio of 2.5:1 of calcium to phosphorus is optimal, although 1:1 ratios (equal parts calcium and magnesium or phosphorus) are available. Citrates, malates and orotates are best.

If deficiency:

- Fatigue, inability to stay asleep, pain in elbow, knee, shoulder, hip, or long bones. Deficiency can be caused by increased urination or diarrhea.

Of interest:

- There is more calcium in the body than any other mineral - 2-3 pounds, mostly in the bones and teeth. Calcium comprises 20% of bone.

- Calcium is one of the two minerals most deficient in the diet of American women (iron is the other). Supplementation is often recommended.

- 20% of an adult's bone calcium is reabsorbed and replaced every year.

- Too much phosphorus, found in milk and cheese, can deplete calcium. Ironically these products are considered to be a good source of calcium, based on laboratory tests which measure only calcium. Calcium and phosphorus must be in a 2.5 to 1 ratio. If there is too much calcium relative to phosphorus, as when calcium supplements are taken, the excess calcium can contribute to arthritis, bone spurs, calcium deposits in the arteries, kidney stones and gallstones. If the phosphorus is too high relative to calcium, as when cheese or phosphoric acid containing soft drinks such as colas are consumed, the body, sensing a deficiency of calcium, may pull it out of the bones which can lead to osteoporosis [1]. A significant association was found between the weekly consumption of at least 1.5 liters (about four 12-ounce cans) of phosphoric-acid-containing soft drinks (primarily colas) and calcium deficiency. Low serum calcium in children, who commonly drink sodas, can lead to subnormal intelligence, muscle spasm seizures, intestinal malabsorption and cardiovascular problems. In adults, phosphoric acid can promote kidney stones and osteoporosis [2].

- If there is arterial inflammation, too much calcium can cause plaques to form on the arteries. This is a particular problem for those with high blood pressure. Calcium should be taken in the morning before exercise by those with high blood pressure.

- Spinach has high levels of calcium as assayed in the laboratory. However, oxalic acid, found in spinach and some other greens, and phytates found in grains can interfere with calcium absorption [3].

- Estrogen stores calcium for childbirth contractions, but too much calcium can cause cramps. Magnesium, which replaces calcium on binding sites, is recommended for menstrual cramps.

- Calcium has a calming effect, necessary for the stress of childraising. Women's estrogen helps to keep up the calcium stores needed for this.

- Wisconsin has soil heavy in natural calcium, which is best for docile animals such as cows. Not surprisingly, Wisconsin is well-known for its dairy products.

- Too much calcium may cause a relative magnesium deficiency, and thus constipation and other magnesium deficiency symptoms.

- Calcium is used by the body to buffer inflammation. This can have deleterious effects by causing arterial plaques, bone spurs, cataracts, and bursitis.

- Weight bearing exercise can help put calcium back in bone.

- Although calcium is needed to build bone and prevent osteoporosis, other nutrients are needed to allow the body to incorporate calcium into the bone matrix. Especially needed are boron, magnesium, zinc, silicon and copper [4].

- Calcium can protect against bone cancer and colon cancer [5].

- 1000 mg of calcium daily has been shown to lower blood pressure [6-8].

- Supplementation with both calcium and manganese can help relieve PMS symptoms, especially those relating to mood, concentration, pain, and water retention [9,10].

Supplement information:

- Calcium is included in most multimineral supplements.

- Available as 100 and 500 mg tablets and in combination with magnesium.

- Orotates, citrates, malates and aspartates are best absorbed and utilized; chelated calcium is less desirable.

- Bone meal and dolomite, sources of calcium, are difficult to digest and may contain toxic lead. One patient, a 70 year old woman, took bone meal, which not only did not help her osteoporosis but caused constipation.

- Carbonates are also not recommended because they are alkaline and difficult to absorb.

Chloride (Cl)

Used for:

- Digestion (hydrochloric acid)
- Works with sodium and potassium
- Aids in detoxification by helping liver function.
- Helps regulate the blood's acid-alkaline balance.

Sources: Salt, kelp. Rarely needed as supplement. No RDA.

If deficiency:

- Fatigue, nausea, loss of appetite. Chloride can be lost through sweating or vomiting.

Chromium (Cr)

Used for:

- Sugar metabolism, in combination with insulin; deters diabetes. Chromium and insulin convert glucose to glycogen for storage. Chromium is also known as glucose tolerance factor (GTF).

- Protein transport. Aids growth.

- Deterrent for arteriosclerosis by keeping triglycerides out of blood.

Sources: Meat, shellfish, chicken, brewer's yeast, corn oil

Dosage: No RDA; average intake is 50 to 200 mcg.

If deficiency: Hypoglycemia or diabetes; low energy and weight gain

Of interest:

- Zinc can substitute for deficient chromium.

- Inadequate chromium levels increase the risk for cardiovascular disease. It may help prevent buildup of plaque in arteries by lowering the LDL (harmful) cholesterol and increasing HDL (beneficial) cholesterol [11]. Cardiovascular disease incidence is lowest in Thailand, where natural chromium levels are the highest.

- Patients with coronary artery disease have significantly lower chromium levels than controls with normal arteries [12]. Several other studies link chromium deficiency and heart disease [13,14].

- Hair analysis showed that 64% of the population (of 1000 samples analyzed) is low in chromium [15]. This is not surprising since most of our food is chromium deficient.

- Since chromium is involved in sugar metabolism, the body actually loses chromium when refined sugar is ingested. Thus a person who eats a lot of sugar is likely to have both a greater need for and a lesser supply of chromium [16,17].

- 70% of people over age 77 are chromium deficient [4].

- 40% of people over age 40 who don't have diabetes have abnormal glucose tolerance tests. 50% of these improved with chromium supplementation [4].

- While whole wheat has 1.75 mcg/g of chromium, white flour has only 0.23 mcg/g (less that 1/7 as much), and white bread contains 0.14 mcg/g [4].

- Diabetic children have significantly lower levels of chromium found by hair analysis than non-diabetic children [18]. One implication of this: Might chromium supplementation reduce the incidence or severity of childhood diabetes? It was found that experimental chromium deficiency in animals can bring on diabetes, which is then reversible with chromium supplementation [19]. In a study done 30 years ago, chromium supplements given to diabetics brought glucose tolerance tests back to normal within 4 months in 50% of patients [20].

- Exercise increases the amount of chromium in the tissues [21]. Chromium can restore normal insulin function in type II diabetics [22]. Daily doses of 150 mcg of trivalent (biologically active) chromium help to normalize glucose tolerance in type II diabetics [23].

Supplement information:
- Available in the more expensive multimineral formulations.

- Chromium is also available as chromium picolinate or as GTF (glucose tolerance factor) chromium, which is recommended. The nicotinate form is even better.

Cobalt (Co)

Used for: Red blood cells; can deter pernicious and other anemias

Sources: Meat, milk, shellfish, kidney, liver

Dosage: No RDA, no more than 8 mcg recommended

If deficiency: Pernicious anemia

Of interest:

- Cobalt is a major part of cyanocobalamin, or vitamin B12.

- Strict vegetarians may be deficient in cobalt.

Copper (Cu)

Used for:

- Increases the effectiveness of the immune system.

- Converting the body's iron into hemoglobin, thereby keeping energy up.

- Works with the amino acid tyrosine to pigment hair and skin.

- Used with zinc to convert thyroxin (T4) to T3, a necessary part of thyroid function. If your T4 on a blood panel test is normal or high but your T3 is low and you have symptoms of low thyroid (sluggishness, weight gain), you may be deficient in copper and/or iodine.

- Involved in fructose metabolism. Use of large quantities of high fructose corn sweeteners may deplete copper levels.

Sources:

- Beans and peas, whole wheat and other whole grains, prunes, liver, seafood

Dosage:

- No RDA, 2-3 mg suggested. Copper supplements can be taken after meals to reduce nausea. Copper should be taken when large doses of vitamin C are concurrently being taken.

If deficiency:

- Frequent colds and infections, fatigue, acid indigestion, anemia

Of interest:

- The amino acid lysine when taken with copper forms copper lysinate, a virus fighter.

- Used with zinc to convert thyroxin (T4) to T3, a necessary part of thyroid function. If your T4 on a blood panel test is normal or high but your T3 is low and you have symptoms of low thyroid (sluggishness, weight gain), you may be deficient in copper and/or iodine.

- Essential for utilization of vitamin C, and is found in natural vitamin C as a cofactor.

- Excess copper can lower zinc level due to the fight for binding sites in the body.

- If copper is depleted, it can disarm the immune system. Large amounts of vitamin C, a metal chelator, can grab onto copper and other minerals ad remove them from the body. Cold symptoms may improve when vitamin C is taken partly because there is not enough copper to continue the battle. Supplementation with copper and other minerals is recommended if large amounts of vitamin C are taken. The amino acid lysine when taken with copper forms copper lysinate, which keeps vitamin C from flushing copper out of the body.

- Lower copper leads to lower bone mineral content.

- People with too high a copper level may be sociopathic.

- In animal experiments, pregnant rats with insufficient copper had an increased incidence of fetal neural and cardiac abnormalities [24]. It follows that supplementation with copper during pregnancy may lower the incidence of certain birth defects.

- Insufficient copper can cause signs of aging, such as loss of skin elasticity and depigmentation of skin and hair. Copper supplements restores natural color to white hair in an animal study [25].

- Copper makes mucus turn from yellow to green during a sinus infection.

- Copper supplements should be taken after meals to reduce nausea.

Supplement information:

- Usually in multimineral supplements in 2 mg doses.

- Should be taken when large doses of vitamin C are taken.

Iodine (I)

Used for:

- Optimal thyroid function, leading to greater energy and weight control.
- Promotes proper growth, and healthy hair, skin, teeth and nails.

Sources:

- Sea vegetables and kelp, seafood, food grown in iodine-rich soil, iodized salt, onions

Dosage:

- 50-150 mcg. This is an amount so tiny you could hardly see it on the head of a pin [3]. Should be taken with zinc and copper. Liquid dulse (seaweed extract) is a natural and preferred form of iodine. More than the minimum may be needed by people with poor thyroid function and/or goiter.

If deficiency:

- Poor thyroid function, fatigue, weight gain, goiter (swollen thyroid)

Toxicity: An excess of iodine can adversely affect thyroid function.

Of interest:

- Used with zinc to convert thyroxin (T4) to T3, a necessary part of thyroid function. If your T4 on a blood panel test is normal or high but your T3 is low and you have symptoms of low thyroid (sluggishness, weight gain), you may be deficient in iodine and/or copper.

- Chlorine and fluorine (as fluoride) are in the same row of the Periodic Table as iodine, and thus have similar binding characteristics in the body, i.e. can replace iodine. Chlorine (from tap water, including showers) and fluoride (some tap water, toothpaste) can block receptors in the thyroid, resulting in symptoms of low thyroid function.

- Iodine protects against breast cancer [26].

- One patient, a woman in her 40s, had throat hoarseness due to iodine deficiency, which itself was caused by mercury dental fillings. Her hoarseness went away when she was given iodine, calcium, copper and zinc. And after she had the mercury amalgams removed and replaced with a safe composite, it went away, never to return.

Iron (Fe)

Used for:

- Production of hemoglobin and certain enzymes
- Can cure and prevent iron deficiency anemia and accompanying fatigue
- Proper metabolization of B vitamins
- Disease resistance
- Good skin tone

Sources:

- Muscle and organ meats, oatmeal and farina, shellfish, dried peaches, egg yolks, nuts, beans, molasses, asparagus, spinach

Dosage:

- 10-18 mg (higher figure is for premenopausal women due to monthly blood loss). Pregnant and lactating women need 30-60 mg. Some iron tablets contain over 300 mg of iron in the hope that 10-15 mg will be absorbed. The remainder can cause constipation. Inorganic forms of iron such as ferrous chloride and ferrous sulfate is poorly absorbed [27]. Fumarate and citrate are the best forms of iron supplements.

If deficiency: Anemia

Toxicity:

- Iron is very toxic to children in overdose. Excess iron taken by a pregnant woman can be dangerous to the fetus.

Of interest:

- Too much iron can lead to free radical damage, which includes heart attack due to damage to the heart muscle lining. Premenopausal women are nearly immune to heart attack, in part because they lose iron every month due to menstrual bleeding. Donating blood regularly might impart the same protection to men [28].

- People with parasitic infestations often need more iron, as the parasites take some of the person's iron stores.

- People with sickle-cell anemia, hemochromatosis, or thalassemia should not take iron supplements.

- Phosphoproteins in eggs and phytates in whole wheat can bind iron, making it biologically unavailable.

- Iron is one of two major dietary deficiencies for women (calcium is the other).

- Only about 8% of ingested iron is absorbed and utilized. Vitamin C can increase iron absorption.

- Excess sugar, white flour, and fat can lead to iron deficiency.

- Iron supplementation should be avoided if you have a bacterial infection, as bacteria need iron for growth.

- If you have an iron deficiency which resists correction by iron supplementation, check magnesium, copper, zinc, manganese and vitamin C, a deficiency of which can interfere with iron utilization [4]. Mercury from dental fillings or other sources can contribute to mineral deficiencies.

- Iron overload in the tissues has been associated with Sudden Infant Death Syndrome (SIDS). Baby foods, vitamins and formula are often fortified with iron. Babies were designed to be fed exclusively on mother's milk for the first 4-6 months of life, and human milk is very low in iron, an indication that babies were not meant to have or need supplemental iron until after the 4-6 month period [29].

Supplement information:
- Inorganic iron preparations such as ferrous sulfate can destroy vitamin E, and may cause stomach upset.
- Organic iron forms such as ferrous gluconate and ferrous citrate, and hydrolyzed protein iron fumarate are more easily assimilated and do not destroy vitamin E.
- Organic dosage sizes are available up to 320 mg.

Lithium (Li)

Used for:

- Stabilization of serotonin neurotransmitters. Lithium carbonate is given to manic-depressive patients for this reason.

- Sodium and potassium increase the effectiveness of lithium carbonate and lower the need for it. Mercury suppresses all three minerals.

Magnesium (Mg)

Used for:
- Metabolism of calcium, vitamin C, phosphorus, sodium and potassium.
- Effective nerve and muscle functioning.
- Helps muscles to relax, relieves muscle and menstrual cramps.

- Converts blood sugar into energy.

- Relieves indigestion.

- Important in bone and tooth formation, even though magnesium is only 0.1% of bone.

- Plays key role in cellular metabolism, many enzyme systems, protein formation, and control of cellular energy through ATP and ADP (biochemical energy pathways). Magnesium is in over 300 enzymes and metabolic pathways [4].

- Fights depression and stress.

- Helps to prevent calcium deposits, kidney stones, and gallstones.

- Acts as natural tranquilizer when combined with calcium.

- Clears up constipation in most forms other than magnesium glycinate. Magnesium is the main ingredient in Milk of Magnesia for this reason.

- Regulates heartbeat. Irregular heartbeat (PVCs, fibrillations) may be due to magnesium deficiency, especially if no organic heart problem can be found.

- Magnesium has been shown to reduce the death rate from myocardial infarction by 70-82% [30]. In many cases the magnesium level determined whether the heart attack victim lived or died. In one study, *all* heart attack victims with low magnesium levels died [31]. Magnesium administered in emergency rooms to heart attack victims may well be more beneficial and much safer than (or in addition to) the drugs and procedures currently in use.

- Magnesium has the potential to reverse osteoporosis. In a study in Israel, 75% of postmenopausal women taking 250-750 mg of magnesium for two years experienced a 1-8% increase in bone density. Controls without magnesium had bone density *losses* of 1-3% during the same period [32].

Sources:
- Nuts, seeds, corn, citrus, dark green vegetables, wheat, figs, apples, wheat germ and bran

Dosage:
- 300-450 mg. People with kidney disease , those on diuretics, and alcohol drinkers [33] may need more.

If deficiency:
- Constipation, menstrual cramps, heart palpitations, heart disease. Low levels of intracellular magnesium are common in those with chronic fatigue syndrome. Magnesium transports calcium to bones - if deficient in magnesium, calcium may not get to its destination.

Of interest:
- Nearly half the population is deficient in magnesium according to hair analysis [15]. In another study, the JAMA reported that in blood tests of 1033 patients, 51% were

deficient [34]. In yet another study, it was estimated that 80% of the population is magnesium deficient [35]. 90% of doctors do not do magnesium testing, i.e. 90% of the patients deficient in magnesium were missed.

- Low levels of intracellular magnesium are common in those with chronic fatigue.

- Aspirin was tested and found to be effective for the prevention of myocardial infarction (MI), or heart attack in this country. Aspirin studies in England showed very little effect. The difference? Buffered aspirin containing magnesium was used only in the U.S. study, so it was very likely the magnesium and not the aspirin which had the protective effect [28].

- A 12 ounce can of soda has about 30 mg of phosphorus, causing the elimination of about that amount of magnesium from the body. A diet rich in sugar, fat, and phosphate increases the need for magnesium [36].

- Magnesium deficiency is related to high blood pressure, stroke, sensitivity to noise, arthritis, asthma, insomnia, irritability, and depression.

- Protein, vitamin C, and calcium are all needed for proper magnesium absorption.

- Premenstrual syndrome (PMS), with bloating, mood swings, and other symptoms, has been linked to low magnesium levels in the blood [37,38]. Taking magnesium in levels only slightly above the RDA can dramatically improve symptoms in as little as 30 minutes. Also, since it is the magnesium:calcium balance that is at least as important as the absolute amount of magnesium, it is possible that taking calcium supplements without magnesium may increase PMS symptoms as well as the other magnesium-deficiency symptoms discussed here.

- Magnesium has been shown to help migraine headaches [39].

- Blood tests for magnesium may not be very accurate. One of the best ways to determine magnesium deficiency is by IV (intravenous) magnesium challenge. When magnesium is given by this route - although oral ingestion will also work - any easing of symptoms indicates that the person was indeed magnesium deficient [40].

- Brain fog may be due in part to magnesium deficiency since the synthesis and breakdown of many brain chemicals and hormones are magnesium dependent. Aluminum and mercury fight magnesium, so a toxic excess of these metals can contribute to a magnesium deficiency.

- Magnesium deficiency can cause mast cells to release more histamine, which can cause or worsen allergy symptoms.

- Since magnesium relaxes muscles, any spastic condition of the muscles (cramps, tremors, twitches, back pain), colon (colitis), blood vessels (hypertension, migraines), heart (arrhythmias) or elsewhere in the body may be related to magnesium deficiency.

- Diuretic drugs increase both the flow of urine and the amount of minerals lost in the urine. Magnesium loss creates a particular problem - magnesium controls the sodium pump in a way that diuretics mimic. As magnesium is depleted, more water is retained, leading to the use of more diuretics in a vicious cycle [41].

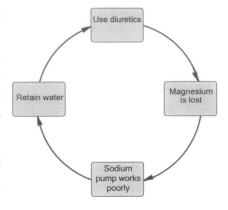

- Of 33 patients admitted to the intensive care unit for chronic obstructive pulmonary (lung) disease, 47% had low muscle magnesium [42].

- Low levels of magnesium are linked to the development of Alzheimer's disease [43]. Decreased levels of magnesium and calcium enhance the accumulation of aluminum in the brain [44]; aluminum accumulation is linked to Alzheimer's disease.

- When taking magnesium alone, it is very important to balance it with calcium. A 50 year old man was taking magnesium for muscle cramps. His heart stopped while swimming because he didn't have enough calcium to support the magnesium. Magnesium helps muscles to relax by transporting out potassium and lowering calcium. His heart, a muscle, apparently relaxed too much.

Supplement information:
- An organic form of magnesium such as magnesium glycinate or citrate is recommended over an inorganic form such as magnesium oxide. Magnesium glycinate or citrate are recommended because they are organic, acidic, and magnesium glycinate rarely causes diarrhea.

Manganese (Mn)

Used for:
- Activates enzymes for proper use of biotin, vitamin B1 and vitamin C.
- Formation of thyroxin by the thyroid gland.
- Digestion and utilization of food.
- Reproduction.
- Aids in muscle reflexes.
- Can eliminate fatigue.
- Normal central nervous system function, memory.
- Reduce nervous irritability and dizziness.
- Manufacture of synovial fluid to keep joints lubricated.
- Helps prevent bone loss [45].
- Necessary for the function of an enzyme that lets the body make detoxifying glutathione.

Sources: Nuts, leafy green vegetables, egg yolks, whole grains, peas, beets

Dosage:

- No RDA, 2.5-5 mg recommended.
- Heavy milk drinkers and meat eaters may need more.
- Large amounts of calcium and phosphorus can inhibit absorption.

If deficiency:

- Low levels can set up conditions for Alzheimer's disease.
- Manganese can affect synovial fluid in the joints, with resulting stiffness if deficiency. Manganese deficiency can lead to bone, cartilage and disk degeneration.

Of interest:

- Long lived people such as the Hunzas and Vilcabambans have higher manganese levels.
- Most of manganese (10-20 mg) is concentrated in the bone, liver and kidney [12].
- The action of manganese on certain brain neurotransmitters accounts for the calming effect often seen when a manganese deficiency is corrected [46].
- Over half the manganese is lost in refining wheat to white flour [47].

Molybdenum (Mo)

Used for:

- Necessary to utilize sulfur based amino acids such as glutathione, methionine and cysteine, which help clear the body of metals and toxins.
- Aldehyde oxidase is a molybdenum dependent enzyme that helps detoxify acetaldehyde from beverage alcohol as well as formaldehyde.

Sources: Beans

Phosphorus (P)

Used for:

- Nearly all physiological biochemical reactions.
- Normal bone and tooth structure, and healthy gums.
- Niacin assimilation.
- Lessens arthritis pain.
- Transference of nerve impulses.
- Normal kidney functioning.
- Heartbeat regularity.
- Aids in growth and body repair.
- Aids in metabolism of fats and starches.

Sources: Milk, cheese, fish, poultry, meat, grains, eggs, nuts and seeds

Dosage: 800-1200 mg. Deficiency is rare in modern meat-eating society

Of interest:

- If the diet is high in phosphorus (e.g. soft drinks, meat, dairy), body tries to maintain Ca:P ratio (2.5:1 ratio optimal) by pulling calcium from bones, possibly leading to osteoporosis.

- Vitamin D and calcium are essential to proper phosphorus function.

- Excess phosphorus is more common now due to a diet richer in animal foods. Fish, for example, contains phosphorus in a 26:1 ratio with calcium (1:2.5 ratio recommended).

- High phosphorus can lead to loss of bone calcium, then to absorption of toxic aluminum which can contribute to premature aging and Alzheimer's disease.

- Heavy concentrations of natural phosphorus are found in Kentucky's soil, making it a good place to breed race horses and a poor place to breed docile cows (The opposite is true of Wisconsin's high calcium environment).

- Vitamin D can help the assimilation of phosphorus.

Potassium (K)

Used for:

- Works with sodium to regulate water balance and heart rhythms.
- Aids in clear thinking by sending oxygen to the brain.
- Aids in excretion of body wastes.
- Helps in allergy treatment.
- Reduces blood pressure.
- Reduces cramps
- Relieves anxiety and insomnia.
- Relieves fatigue.

Sources:

- Citrus fruits, bananas, cantaloupe, tomatoes, watercress, leafy green vegetables, sunflower seeds, potatoes, persimmons

Dosage:

- 1875-5625 mg (unofficial).
- More may be needed by those with diarrhea, mental and physical stress, hypoglycemics, those who are on diuretics or fasting or on a low carbohydrate diet, drinkers of alcohol or coffee, those who have a heavy consumption of sugar, heavy exercisers.

If deficiency:

- Inability to fall asleep or get back to sleep with mind racing, fatigue, rapid or pounding heartbeat, muscle cramps, tightness or pain, kidney pain, twitching, muscle pain, anxiety, difficulty breathing deeply.

- Loose stools, laxatives and frequent urination can deplete potassium.

Toxicity: Side effects may be found at levels above 25 grams (25,000 mg).

Of interest:

- About 1/3 of the population is deficient in potassium according to the hair analysis of 1000 people [12].

- Potassium must be in balance with sodium, otherwise nerve and muscle functions suffer.

- if you are tired but can't get to sleep, especially if accompanied by mind racing, tossing and turning, this may be due to potassium deficiency. A potassium supplement can help you sleep within 20-30 minutes of ingestion if your insomnia is due to this cause.

- Potassium is a major useful ingredient in sports drinks, as much exercise fatigue is due to mineral loss from sweating. A potassium supplement would have essentially the same effect without the ingestion of harmful and expensive flavors, sweeteners and artificial colors.

- Potassium supplements, or the maintenance of high potassium relative to sodium, can help reduce blood pressure and reduce the need for antihypertensive or diuretic drugs [48-51]. It is possible that the antihypertensive effects of a low sodium diet is actually attributable to the more favorable potassium/sodium ratio rather than to an absolute lower amount of sodium. The use of "Lite" salts to season food, which contain potassium chloride rather than sodium chloride, probably also contributes to the beneficial effects attributed to the low sodium diet.

Supplement information:

- Available in inorganic (sulfate, chloride, oxide, carbonate) and organic (gluconate, citrate, fumarate) forms. Organic is recommended.
- Dosages are available up to 600 mg, which is the equivalent of 99 mg of elemental potassium.

Selenium (Se)

Used for:

- Antioxidant properties, especially in combination with vitamin E.
- Works with detoxifying sulfur-based amino acids such as glutathione.
- Helps alleviate hot flashes and other menopausal symptoms.

- Treats and prevents dandruff both as dietary supplement and topical application.
- May neutralize certain carcinogens.
- Increases stamina.
- Reduces incidence of cancers of the breast, colon, pancreas, prostate, bladder and lung. Selenium can protect against cervical cancer [52].

Sources: Wheat germ and bran, tuna, onions, tomatoes, broccoli

Dosage:

- 50-200 mcg (unofficial); exceeding 200 mcg not recommended.
- Men need more than women due to loss in semen.

If deficiency: Colon cancer, heart disease.

Of interest:

- If too much selenium is taken, garlic breath and body odor may result.

- There is a link between low serum selenium levels and cardiovascular disease. The link may be due to selenium's antioxidant effects [53]. Selenium also reduces platelet aggregation [54].

Supplement information:

- Selenium is sometimes combined with vitamin E and other antioxidants such as vitamins A and C.

Sodium (Na)

Used for:

- Helps nerves and muscles function properly in balance with potassium.
- Aids in carbohydrate digestion.
- Helps keep calcium and other minerals soluble in the blood.
- Raises blood pressure
- Prevents heat prostration and sunstroke - this is why salt tablets are sometimes given to athletes and runners.

Sources: Salt, kelp, shellfish, celery, organ meats

Dosage:

- The unofficial allowance is 1100-3300 mg, although those who exercise vigorously, sweat heavily, or have a high potassium intake may need more.
- Excess intake is more common than deficiency in the U.S. due to large amounts of salt in most processed and restaurant foods.
- Deficiency, however, is possible among those on strict diets or those who consume very little pre-prepared food. Deficiency is not uncommon in less developed parts of the world, especially those that are miles from the sea.

If deficiency:

- Heavy fatigue, low blood pressure, nausea, depressed appetite, cold hands and feet, thirst even after drinking water. A glass of salt water can relieve these symptoms within 10-30 minutes.
- Vomiting or heavy sweating can rapidly deplete sodium.

Of interest:

- Excess salt can raise blood pressure in hypertensives (those with blood pressure over 130/85). This is generally undesirable. Salt can also raise low blood pressure, as from shock, or in many people (especially women) who have chronic illness. However, salt has little or no effect on normotensive people, or those whose blood pressure is in the normal range of around 120/80.

- Low blood pressure (below 110/75) may be a symptom of sodium deficiency. Other symptoms are cold extremities, fatigue and nausea.

- Salt deficiency fatigue, in which one can barely move but can't sleep, can come on quickly. It can be relieved as quickly (10 to 30 minutes) with a small glass of salt water (1 tsp. of mineral or sea salt in a glass of water).

- High salt intake can lead to symptoms of potassium depletion - see listing under Potassium.

Sulfur (S)

Used for:

- Healthy hair, skin, nails
- Maintaining oxygen balance for proper brain function.
- Works with B complex vitamins for basic body metabolism.
- Aids the liver in bile secretion.
- Helps fight bacterial infections.
- Used topically for skin problems and dandruff.
- Is part of some amino acids, such as methionine, cysteine and glutathione. These help detoxify the body of metals and other toxins.

Sources: Beef, beans, fish, eggs, cabbage

Dosage: No RDA. A diet sufficient in protein is generally sufficient in sulfur.

If deficiency: Poor detoxification of metals and chemicals

Of interest: Smells like rotten egg in many forms and while the body is detoxifying.

Works best with:

- Vitamins B6, B12, C, folate, magnesium and molybdenum are needed for detoxifying system to work properly.

Supplement information:
- Rarely found as food supplement except in sulfur based amino acids such as glutathione. Available in topical form.

Vanadium (V)

Used for: Sugar metabolism and regulation; can help with hypoglycemia and diabetes.

If deficiency: Hypoglycemia, diabetes

Zinc (Zn)

Used for:
- Directing efficient flow of body processes.
- Maintenance of cells and enzyme systems.
- Needed along with copper to convert thyroxin (T4) to T3 so it can be used by the body.
- Required for the liver to move vitamin A from storage.
- Blood stability and acid-base balance.
- Normalizes reproductive organ function, protects the prostate gland, and raises progesterone and testosterone (sex hormone) levels.
- Zinc is part of superoxide dismutase (SOD), which controls oxygen free radicals which form carcinogenic peroxides.
- Essential for sense of taste and smell.
- Decreases cholesterol deposits, helps prevent arteriosclerosis and treat atherosclerosis [55,56].
- Useful in treatment of mental disorders, especially schizophrenia.
- Required for the body's natural chelation processes.
- Acne in teenagers responds favorably to zinc supplements.
- Can help reduce body odor.
- Needed for digestion of protein and insulin production [57]. There is a high incidence of maturity onset diabetes among alcoholics, possibly due in part to zinc depletion.
- Essential for protein synthesis.
- Contractibility of muscles.
- Brain function and mental alertness.

- Accelerates healing time.

- Helps prevent bone loss [58]

Sources: Meat, wheat germ, brewer's yeast, eggs, pumpkin seeds

Dosage:

- 15 mg.
- Alcoholics, diabetics, the elderly, women with menstrual irregularities, and men with prostate problems may need more.

Toxicity:

- Zinc is rarely toxic, although it can cause nausea in women.
- Doses over 150 mg/day can lead to an otherwise unusual condition called sideroblastic anemia, which has the symptoms of fatigue, anorexia, dizziness, pale skin, and heart and liver failure [59].

Of interest:

- White lines and spots on nails are an early deficiency symptom.

- To determine whether zinc deficiency exists, taste a weak (0.1%) solution of zinc sulfate (available commercially as Zinc Tally). A strong unpleasant or metallic taste indicates sufficient zinc. A slight taste that increases as the solution is held in the mouth may indicate a slight deficiency. A severe deficiency may well exist if very little or no taste is detected.

- Are you seasoning your food more now than you used to, or more than most people? Do you use a lot of salt, hot sauce, ketchup, sugar, soy sauce or other flavoring to try to get your food to have some flavor? This may be a sign that your sense of taste is adversely affected by zinc deficiency.

- An increase of zinc in the diet increases the need for vitamin A.

- Zinc together with vitamin B6, vitamin E, and GLA fatty acids can help relieve impotence.

- Zinc deficiency has been linked to low sperm counts, motility, and seminal volume, which can be reversed with zinc supplementation [60-63].

- Milling, or refining, of wheat causes an 80% loss of zinc.

- The highest concentration of zinc in the body is found in semen. Sexually active men risk greater zinc loss than women, and this may lead to prostate problems in older men.

- Zinc deficiency is common among anorexics, and by suppressing taste and appetite probably exacerbates the disease. Zinc deficiency can cause alternate bingeing and lack of interest in food, or bulimia.

- Although zinc is important for immune system function, daily amounts over 100 mg can impair the immune response.

- In one study only 13% of randomly selected patients had normal zinc levels, and 68% ingested less than 2/3 of the RDA for zinc [64].

- Zinc deficiency is linked to dyslexia [65].

- Mercury (from dental fillings) and cadmium (as from cigarettes) can contribute to zinc deficiency due to fight-for-site. This is part of the reason that those who are quitting smoking rediscover their appetite. Zinc supplementation can reduce the cravings that are usually part of quitting smoking because of the relationship between zinc and cadmium.

- Zinc supplementation has been shown to slow the accumulation of toxic aluminum in the brain [66,67].

- Children who have repeated ear infections are likely to be zinc deficient [68].

Supplement information:
- Zinc picolinate or zinc gluconate is recommended.
- Also available as 0.1% liquid.
- Tablet dosages range from 15 to over 300 mg.

What symptoms correlate with which mineral deficiencies?
Deficiency symptoms and their associated minerals include:

Acne	Cu, Fe, Mn, Zn
Anemia	Fe, also most minerals
Appetite loss	P, Na, Zn
Arthritis	Ca, Cu, Fe, I, Mg, Mo, Se
Body odor	Zn, I
Brittle bones	Ca (primarily) and others
Cold sensitivity	Na
Dandruff	Se
Decreased fertility	Cu, Fe, Mn, Zn, I
Dental cavities	Ca, Cu, Fe, Na, P
Dizziness	Mn, Ca, Cu, Fe, I, K, Na
Drowsiness	Ca, Cu, Se
Dull dry hair	I
Ear noises	Mn, K
Eczema	Cu, I
Edema	I, K, Na, P
Frequent colds	Cu, Zn
Gastrointestinal	Cl
Hair loss	Cl, Ca, Cu, I, Se, Mo
Headaches	Ca, Cu, Fe, I, Se, Zn
Heart arrhythmias	Ca, Cu, Fe, K, Mg, Na, P

Hyperactivity	Ca, Fe, Na, P
Hypoglycemia	Ca, Fe, I, Na
Insomnia	K, Ca, Cu, Fe, I
Leukemia	Cu
Loss of smell, taste	Zn
Mental fog	Cu, K, Ca, Fe, Mg, Na
Mental retardation	Fe
Muscle cramps	Cl, Na
Nervousness	Mg
Pallor	Fe, I
Periodontal disease	Ca, Mg, Fe
Psychosis	Ca, Cu, Fe, I
Retarded growth	Zn, Co
Seizures	Ca, Fe, K, Na, P
Sinus problems	Ca, Fe
Soft bones, teeth	Ca
Tremors	Mg, Ca, Cu, Fe, Na, P
Ulcers	Ca, Fe

General symptoms caused by a deficiency in nearly any mineral(s) include: fatigue, excess bleeding, abdominal pain, diarrhea or constipation, lack of stamina, emotional disturbance, muscle weakness and pain, and increase in allergies.

References and Resources

- The Burton Goldberg Group, *Alternative Medicine: The Definitive Guide*, "Nutritional Supplements", pp. 385-397, Future Medicine Publishing, Puyallup WA, 1994.

- Colgan, Michael, *The New Nutrition: Medicine For The New Millennium*, Apple Publishing Co. Ltd., Vancouver BC, Canada, 1995.

- Garland, Cedric and Frank Garland, *The Calcium Connection*, Putnam and Sons, NY, 1988.

- Mindell, Earl, *Vitamin Bible*, Warner Books, New York, 1985.

- Moore, Richard, *The High Blood Pressure Solution: Natural Prevention and Cure with the 'K' Factor*, Healing Arts Press, Rochester VT, 1993. *Controlling blood pressure through balancing potassium (K) and sodium.*

- Pfeiffer, Carl, *Zinc and Other Micro-Nutrients*, Keats Publishing, New Canaan CT, 1978.

- Rogers, Sherry, *Tired or Toxic?*, Prestige Publishing, Syracuse NY, 1990.

- Underwood, EJ, *Trace Elements in Human and Animal Nutrition*, Academic Press, Orlando FL, 1987.

SUPPLEMENTS

It's All In The Packaging

Things in this chapter that can change your health:

- *Are supplements necessary?*
- *What are the different types of supplements, and what forms should you take?*

What are supplements?

Supplements are nutritional components supplied in a form other than natural food. These can be supplied in capsule, tablet, powder, or liquid form. Supplements include the following, alone or in combination:

- *Vitamins*
- *Minerals*
- *Beneficial bacteria*
- *Enzymes*
- *Amino acids*
- *Food extracts such as garlic*
- *Oils*
- *Cofactors (go-withs)*

Are supplements necessary? - Pros and Cons

There is considerable debate regarding the necessity of vitamin, mineral, and amino acid supplements. One school of thought is that supplements are unnecessary, that a healthy, balanced diet rich in unadulterated foods contains all of the nutrition the body needs. This makes sense, since our species would have died out long ago if a natural unsupplemented diet had been inadequate.

The opposite position is taken by many doctors, scientists and, not surprisingly, supplement manufacturers. They contend that times have changed to the point where supplements are now necessary:

- Food plants and animals are bred for size, appearance, tenderness, and shelf life rather than for nutrition.

- Plants grown for human and animal food are grown in depleted or artificially augmented soil. Nutrients can't be in the plants if they are not in the soil.

- Too many calories would accompany the amounts of food that provide all of the nutrients we need, as we are now too inactive to burn off all of those calories.

- Problems in digesting, absorbing and utilizing food nutrients are common, especially as one grows older.

- Even if natural foods were sufficient for a healthy person, most of us are not healthy as healthy may have been defined 100 years ago, since most of us carry around toxic chemical and metal burdens and/or suffer from degenerative changes that increase our nutrient needs.

Do most people need supplements?

There is truth in both schools of thought, pro and con. The Standard American Diet (which appropriately forms the acronym SAD), with its fast foods, refined foods, processed foods, and nonfoods, is quite deficient. The same is true for many weight loss or other strict dietary regimens, some of which have ironically been undertaken for health reasons. A person who stays on one of these diets for a long period of time passes from diseases of excess to relative good health and then eventually to diseases of deficiency. Supplementation is virtually a necessity in these cases to prevent and correct deficiency. Supplemental is the key word here. Supplements do not fully take the place of nutrition derived directly from food. Supplementation, not substitution, is the key.

> **Supplement, not substitute**.

Think of it this way. One can build up financial health by saving $5 a week, but this is not sufficient if severely in debt and paying interest to start with. If you are nutrient deficient, you may have a nutrient debt that nutrients in food can't correct alone.

Even if an optimal diet is followed, as described in this and other books, supplementation may still be needed or at least useful. A healthful diet can provide adequate nutrition, barring unusual circumstances. However, there is a difference between adequate and optimal, and supplements, used judiciously, can help to bridge that gap.

The distinction should be made between therapeutic and maintenance supplementation. Therapeutic supplementation is intended to be relatively short term to remedy a particular deficiency. Maintenance supplementation generally refers to a lower dose over a longer period of time to maintain an optimum state of nutrition.

What nutrients should you take in supplement form?

The chapters on Vitamins, Minerals, and the macronutrients list indications for additional nutrients. Once you and/or your doctor have determined that you should take supplements, and which supplements you should take, there are still questions to be answered. These questions and their answers form the basis for this chapter.

What other supplement questions are there?

Supplements are not created equal, even though the labels on any two products specify the same type and dosage. Some important questions addressed in this chapter and in the chapters on Vitamins and Minerals are:

- *Tablets, capsules, powders, gels, or oils?*
- *Immediate or timed-release?*
- *Coated or uncoated?*

- *Synthetic or natural?*
- *Organic or inorganic forms?*
- *What does chelated mean, and is it necessary?*
- *Acidified, enzyme supported?*
- *Single vitamins and minerals, or combinations?*
- *What dosage is adequate, optimal, toxic?*
- *Taken with food, or on an empty stomach?*
- *What supplements should be taken together, or separately?*
- *Should they be taken in the morning or at night?*

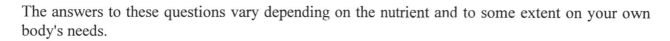

The answers to these questions vary depending on the nutrient and to some extent on your own body's needs.

What form of supplement should be taken?

The form of the supplement - pill, capsule, powder, liquid - is usually simply a matter of convenience or personal choice, although some forms are better absorbed or have fewer additives. Capsules are better than tablets for product delivery, and liquids are the best form for electrolytes. Both tablets and capsules are convenient, pre-measured, easy to store, and have a long shelf life. A tablet may be larger than the equivalent capsule because binders are usually necessary to hold the tablet together, and capsules are usually easier to swallow. These are important considerations if swallowing pills is a problem for you. Capsules may also be larger than the dose needed because the empty gel capsules come in standardized sizes. If mixing the medication with food is desired, it is easier to open a capsule than to grind up a tablet. Powders and liquids also allow easy mixing with food, as well as being a more convenient way to take higher dosages; however, the taste and texture may be objectionable.

Oil soluble vitamins A, D, and E often come in a soft gel capsule. These vitamins can also be mycelized, a process that renders them water soluble and easier to digest. Oil based vitamins are fat soluble and more stable and last longer in the body, but the mycelized form is more readily absorbed since it is water soluble if oil digestion is a problem. Mycelized vitamins are liquid and are taken with a dropper or plastic squeeze bottle.

Summary of advantages:

Capsule	Tablet	Liquid	Powder	Gel capsule
No binders	Convenient	Good for	Better for	Easy to
Better product delivery	Pre-measured	electrolytes	large	swallow
Convenient	Easy to store	Mycelized	amounts	
Pre-measured	Long shelf life	easier to		
Easy to store		absorb		
Long shelf life				
Easier to swallow than tablet				
No unpleasant taste				

What are some problems with tablets?

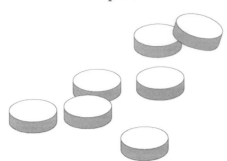

Tablets, as mentioned, have binders to hold them together when pressed into tablet form. After tablets are made, they are tested, and one of the tests is dissolution testing. Dissolution testing involves monitoring the time it takes the tablet to dissolve in simulated gastric juice, usually a hydrochloric acid solution of pH 2, which is considered normal stomach acidity. However, as discussed in the chapter on Digestion, many people have stomach juices which are not as acidic as the norm for a variety of reasons such as allergy, fungus, mercury, parasites, and fermentation of food. Tablets which dissolve properly in the laboratory may not as readily dissolve in your stomach, and may be excreted virtually unchanged.

Additives such as binders, fillers, coatings, colors, and waxes all have their advantages but may be of concern to people with allergies. These products are more likely to be found in tablets than in capsules.

- Binders hold a tablet together but are not found in capsules.

- Fillers are necessary when the dosage is so low that a tablet or capsule without fillers would be impossibly tiny. Fillers are also used to fill up capsules, which only come in standard sizes.

- Coated tablets have a longer shelf life, are easier to swallow, and mask unpleasant flavors. However, the coating also makes them harder to dissolve.

- Algins are used to help tablets disintegrate after swallowing.

- Colored tablet coatings and colored capsules are used for product identification but are otherwise useless and the chemical colorant may be harmful.

- Flavors and sweeteners are used in chewable tablets.

- Waxes are sometimes used to make the coating smooth and shiny, and are also used in timed-release formulations.

What about timed release formulations?

Timed-release formulations, which contain wax or a similar product to allow the tablet to dissolve slowly, are good for water soluble vitamins where the excess is excreted within a few hours rather than being saved for later in the day. A less convenient alternative is taking supplements several times a day.

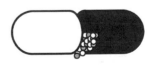

Which are better, synthetic or natural vitamins?

Natural vitamins are extracted from naturally occurring substances, such as vitamin C (ascorbic acid) from rose hips, while synthetic vitamins are made in the laboratory from other ingredients. Although ascorbic acid is ascorbic acid regardless of where it comes from, natural vitamin C is accompanied by bioflavonoids and copper to make up the more easily utilized vitamin C complex. Synthetic vitamins are more likely to cause allergic and toxic reactions and gastrointestinal distress. On the other hand, synthetics are much cheaper, if this is a consideration.

Many products labeled as natural actually contain mostly synthetic ingredients. The small percentage of natural ingredients - as little as 5% - legally qualifies the preparation to be called "natural". This is reasonable in many cases. A single 500 mg tablet of vitamin C extracted along with bioflavonoids entirely from rose hips would be far too large to swallow and prohibitively expensive.

What do organic and inorganic mean?- probably not what you think

The terms inorganic vs. organic vitamins and minerals are not synonymous with synthetic vs. natural, a common misconception. Organic in this case means carbon-containing, and thus would include all vitamins. Minerals can be present in either the inorganic (salt) form, such as potassium sulfate or carbonate, or the organic form, such as potassium malate or citrate. Organic forms are usually more readily utilized by our bodies, which are of course also organic. In addition, salt forms are usually alkaline, while organic forms are more often acidic. Acidic forms are more easily broken down and utilized by the body. If there is insufficient hydrochloric acid present in the stomach, acidic vitamin preparations are a must.

What are chelated minerals, and are they better?

Chelation (pronounced key-lation) refers to the process by which minerals are changed into a more absorbable form by binding with a chelating agent. A certain amount of chelation occurs in the body, but it is inefficient and most of the unchelated mineral is excreted unused. For example, only two to ten percent of ingested inorganic iron is actually absorbed. The lower figure is more likely if fungus, parasites, campylobacter, or heavy metals are present. Chelation, usually by binding with amino acids, causes minerals to be assimilated three to ten times more readily. Chelated minerals appear more expensive than their nonchelated counterparts, but are actually cheaper after considering the greater amount of mineral actually utilized.

Minerals are chelated to more easily pull them into the body. One disadvantage of chelated minerals is that the mineral may bind so tightly to the chelator that it is not released in the body and is therefore unavailable. Minerals chelated with dipeptides, discussed in the chapter on Minerals, are one of the best forms.

Chelated minerals are better than nonchelated forms such as oyster shell and bone meal, but acidified minerals are even better as they are in a form that is more completely utilized.

Colloidal minerals, a very fine suspension of minerals in a water base, are an excellent way to get minerals in an easily absorbable form.

Should nutrients be taken singly or in combination?

Vitamins and minerals are sold either singly or in combination. Combinations include:

- *Multivitamins*
- *Multi-minerals*

- *Multivitamins plus minerals*
- *Vitamins and go-withs such as vitamin C and bioflavonoids*
- *B complex vitamins in balance*
- *Complementary minerals in balance such as calcium and magnesium*
- *Nearly any combination of vitamins, minerals, go-withs, herbs and botanicals, and amino acids*

It is nearly impossible to make any blanket recommendations since nutrient and dosage needs are highly individualized, depending on age, health, gender, or use of drugs such as alcohol or tobacco. Multinutrient supplements are cheaper and more convenient if your needs match the amounts and combinations available, or if you are taking a low dosage multinutrient supplement simply for insurance - a practice of questionable value given the individuality of nutrient needs but usually harmless.

Should supplements be taken with food?

> **Vitamins should be taken in the morning with food.**

Vitamins should be taken in the morning with food, as they are synergistic with food and are found along with food in nature. Minerals are better taken in the evening on an empty stomach for better absorption, as there is more hydrochloric acid in an empty stomach.

What is the U.S.R.D.A.?

The U.S.R.D.A. (United States Recommended Daily Allowance), also called the RDA, provides adequate dosages of vitamins and minerals, provided you don't have any special needs, severe deficiencies, allergies, heavy metals, or digestive problems. Adequate is defined as the amount needed to prevent overt deficiency symptoms, such as scurvy from too little vitamin C. Unfortunately, this amount is insufficient for most of us to achieve optimal health.

How can you figure out the optimal supplement dosage?

The optimal dosage for each nutrient can be calculated approximately by looking at the RDA, adding (or in rare cases subtracting) for your special needs, adding extra for insurance without approaching toxic limits, and subtracting that which you get from your typical diet or other supplements. It is important to make sure everything is in balance where balance is important, as with some B vitamins (B-12, folic acid) and some minerals such as calcium and magnesium. Exhausted yet from pushing calculator buttons? Relax - there is a large margin for error and a wide variety of supplement regimens which will give you some benefit. In most cases - with oil soluble vitamins A, D, E, and K and the mineral iron being the major exceptions - the body will use what it needs and excrete the rest.

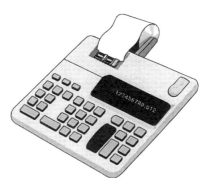

You don't have to figure out your needs alone. There are clinical nutritionists and other specialists who can help you figure out your particular nutrient needs, without your playing "vitamin roulette".

Does the government protect our interests?
Don't count on it. The 1992 FDA's *Dietary Supplements Task Force Final Report* has as one of its stated objectives, taking "...what steps are necessary to ensure that the existence of dietary supplements on the market does not act as a disincentive for drug development" [1]. This is the same taxpayer-funded government agency that is presumably looking out for our best health interests.

Is megavitamin therapy beneficial or harmful?
Megavitamin therapy, also called orthomolecular therapy, has been used for certain conditions and its use has been controversial. In megavitamin therapy doses of 20, 50, or 100 times the RDA are taken for treatment of a particular condition. Large doses of one to six grams of vitamin C (1000 to 6000 mg as compared with the RDA of 60 mg) to ward off or treat a cold may be beneficial and are considered harmless due to the body's ability to quickly excrete the excess unless certain conditions are present such as the tendency to form kidney stones. Megavitamin therapy has been shown to help delay tumor recurrence in bladder cancer, and possibly of other cancers as well [2].

> **As a general rule, megavitamin regimens are best left to the discretion of a health care professional with the expertise to understand nutrition and the biochemistry of the body**.

Megavitamin therapy, also called orthomolecular medicine, can be of considerable benefit if used appropriately. However, huge vitamin doses can act more like drugs than like nutrients, with the potential for toxicity and creating an imbalance of other nutrients. Application of this type of therapy is best left to a professional.

If large doses of nutrients are taken, it is better to build up or taper off the dosage slowly to give the body time to adjust.

What forms and dosages are available for each nutrient?
Individual supplement information is provided in the chapters on Vitamins, Minerals, and Amino Acids and Protein. Nearly all vitamins and minerals, and some amino acids, are available in multinutrient combinations as well.

Are all supplements created equal?
If you compare two or more brands of supplements that, according to the label, are the same, the contents may not be identical. "Chelated" minerals **Buyer Beware!** may not really be chemically chelated, as discussed. Also, it was found that about 80% of brands of beneficial bacteria such as acidophilus did not match their label claims.

Recommended brands and suppliers of supplements are found in the Product Sources listing near the end of the book.

References and Resources

- The Burton Goldberg Group, *Alternative Medicine: The Definitive Guide*, Future Medicine Publishing, Puyallup WA, 1994. *The following chapters deal with nutritional supplements:*
  "Nutritional Supplements", pp. 385-397
  "Orthomolecular Medicine", pp. 398-404

- Hoffer, Abram, and Morton Walker, *Orthomolecular Nutrition*, Keats Publishing Inc., New Canaan CT, 1978.

- Huemer, Richard P., *The Roots of Molecular Medicine: A Tribute To Linus Pauling*, W.H. Freeman and Co., NY, 1986.

- Mindell, Earl, *Vitamin Bible*, Warner Books, New York, 1985.

- Pearson, Durk and Sandy Shaw, *Freedom of Informed Choice: FDA Versus Nutrient Supplements*, Common Sense Press, Neptune NJ, 1993.

- Rosenbaum, M.E. and D. Bosco, *Super Fitness Beyond Vitamins: The Bible of Super Supplements*, New American Library, NY, 1987.

DIGESTION

The Little Things That Make A Big Difference

Things in this chapter that can have an impact on your health:

- *How poor digestion can affect your nutrition and health.*
- *Antacids can be the worst thing for "acid stomach".*
- *What are some digestive problems and what can be done for them.*
- *Natural digestive aids.*
- *Microwaved, overcooked, and irradiated food = dead food.*

What is digestion?

Digestion is the process by which proteins, carbohydrates, and fats are broken down to the amino acids, glucose, and fatty acids that can be utilized by the body. Vitamins and minerals are also extracted by this process. Even if your diet is good, poor digestion can lead to malnutrition since nutrients are not broken down into usable molecules.

It is important to understand how digestion occurs and why it is so important in order to recognize and treat digestive problems.

What are the problems of poor digestion?

Poor digestion can lead to:

- A waste of nutrients taken into the body from the diet.

- Fatigue due to poor nutrition, especially deficiencies of B vitamins, minerals, and glucose to form stored glycogen.

- Food allergies, especially to proteins such as casein from milk and gluten from grains, since the immune sys-

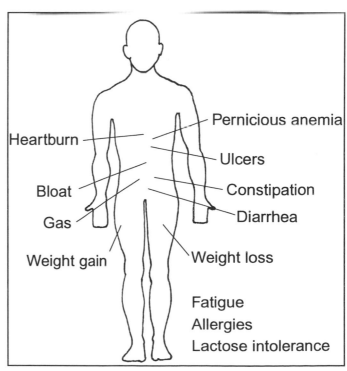

tem can react to undigested food.

- Physical symptoms such as heartburn, gas, bloating, diarrhea and constipation.

The Digestive System

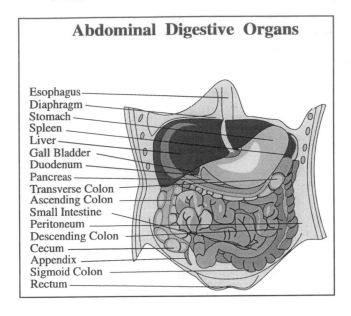

Abdominal Digestive Organs

Esophagus
Diaphragm
Stomach
Spleen
Liver
Gall Bladder
Duodenum
Pancreas
Transverse Colon
Ascending Colon
Small Intestine
Peritoneum
Descending Colon
Cecum
Appendix
Sigmoid Colon
Rectum

Where does digestion start?

Digestion begins in the mouth. Chewing breaks down food mechanically into small pieces, exposing more surface area for digestive enzymes to act upon. Chewing also stimulates the release of hydrochloric acid (HCl) in the stomach. The water and mucus in saliva moistens food and allows it to be swallowed easily. Saliva also contains an enzyme, amylase, which starts the breakdown of carbohydrates to simple sugars.

Once swallowed, food moves through the throat and esophagus into the stomach. Mucus produced in the esophagus helps the food to move towards the stomach by providing lubrication. A downward muscular contraction of the entire digestive system called peristalsis, in combination with one-way valves, keeps the food flowing in the right direction.

Although food proceeds on a downward path, from the mouth through the intestinal system and final processing, gravity has little to do with food reaching its ultimate destination. Digestion can proceed while lying down or even in zero-gravity space. The one-way valves include the valve between the esophagus and the stomach that, when functioning properly, keeps acid and food from splashing back up from the stomach into the esophagus. If the valve is not functioning properly, the splashing, or reflux, of acid can lead to the familiar symptoms of "heartburn". Another valve is the one in the throat that blocks the trachea and prevents food and liquids from entering the lungs. To see how this works, swallow while exhaling. The flow of air stops until swallowing is complete.

What happens when food gets to the stomach?

The stomach is a tough, thick-walled muscular organ located just above the intestines. In the stomach, food is mixed with gastric juices containing water, hydrochloric acid, and enzymes. Alkaline mucus, which coats the inside of the stomach, protects the cells of the stomach wall from being digested themselves.

Hydrochloric acid (HCl) in the stomach, released about 30 to 60 minutes after chewing, activates pepsinogen, a proenzyme, to become the enzyme pepsin. Both pepsin and HCl begin the process of digesting protein by breaking the peptide bonds linking the amino acids together. This process is called denaturing the protein. If you have ever added vinegar or lemon juice (acid) to milk (protein), the resulting curds that you observed are denatured protein.

The stomach also produces a substance called intrinsic factor, which transports vitamin B12 through the wall of the small intestine into the blood.

Once in the stomach, the food and gastric juices form a milky white liquid mixture called chyme, which is physically mixed and further broken down by stomach contractions. The stomach takes from two to six hours to empty, depending on the amount and composition of the food. Stomach emptying time also depends on physical activity, which slows the digestive process by diverting energy elsewhere.

How fast does food leave the stomach?

Simple sugars, complex carbohydrates, proteins, and fats are emptied from the stomach in that order of rapidity (sugars fastest, fats slowest) if only one of these foods makes up most or all of the stomach contents. If a mixture of foods is present, stomach emptying time is determined by the presence of protein and fat. Fruit along with protein can speed stomach emptying time as compared with protein alone, but fruit will then ferment in the process because its passage is slowed by the protein. Whole grains will go through the digestive system in about 4-7 hours; the fiber in the grains speeds digestive time. White flour tends to clump on the intestinal walls, which slows digestion. The faster the digestion time, the better, since food will have less time to ferment and putrefy.

What happens after the food leaves the stomach?

Most of the digestive process occurs in the small intestine, especially in the duodenum, which is a C-shaped tube located directly after the stomach. Digestive enzymes are secreted by the pancreas and liver. These digestive enzymes are:

- *Protease (pronounced pro-tee-ace), which digests protein*
- *Amylase, which digests carbohydrates*
- *Lipase, which digests fats. Bile also digests fats.*

These enzymes depend on an alkaline pH for their activity. Stomach acid triggers the pancreas to produce bicarbonate ions (HCO_3^-), which neutralize the acidity of the chyme and produce alkaline conditions for digestion.

By the time the chyme leaves the duodenum, most of the breakdown from foods to simple nutrients has taken place. The billions of cells that line the small intestine complete the breakdown to the basic nutrients - amino acids, fatty acids, glucose, vitamins, and minerals - and assimilate them.

What happens at the end of the line?

If a nutrient is not broken down sufficiently, or if it is not recognized and assimilated through the wall of the small intestine into the bloodstream, it joins other unusable material in its journey through the five feet of large intestine. The material in the large intestine also includes

- *Fiber*
- *Bile*
- *Water*
- *Living and dead bacteria, mostly beneficial ones (99%)*
- *Minerals*

The large intestine secretes no digestive enzymes. A few vitamins such as biotin and vitamin K are produced by the beneficial bacteria in the large intestine, and these vitamins, sodium, and water are absorbed through the walls. The food residue is pushed into the colon via peristalsis about three or four times a day. After 12 to 14 hours in the colon, during which time water is absorbed or added as needed and thoroughly mixed by the kneading and churning actions of the colon, peristaltic action propels the colon contents into the rectum, which is then expelled as stool.

What are the accessory organs to the digestive system?

The liver, gallbladder, and pancreas, although they are not part of the digestive tract, play an important role in digestion. The liver produces bile, which digests fats. Bile is concentrated and stored in the gallbladder and released from there to the duodenum when stimulated by fat-containing foods. Bile also splits fats into smaller particles so the pancreatic enzyme lipase can break them down to fatty acids. The pancreas also secretes the two other major digestive enzymes, protease and amylase [1,2].

The liver also produces bicarbonate, which neutralizes stomach acid so that reactions can take place in the intestines more efficiently.

Enzymes

What are enzymes and why are they so important?

Enzymes are specialized proteins which are vital for digestion and for all biochemical reactions in the body. There are about 2000 enzymes in the body. Most enzymes are attached to proteins, but some are attached to trace minerals.

A person who is ill and has a high fever can die if the fever goes to 108 degrees. This is due in part because the heat inactivates certain enzymes vital to life [3]. Muscular dystrophy is thought to be due to an enzyme deficiency, and this may be true of other diseases and conditions as well. The liver makes most regulating enzymes, so lowered liver function, as from toxins, can reduce enzyme levels and may lead to enzyme deficiency diseases.

In addition to being produced by the body, enzymes are also supplied by food - but only certain foods, under certain conditions. It is possible to digest food and survive without taking in food enzymes - many people on the Standard American Diet (SAD) do just that - but this is far from optimal. For one thing, if the body is busy making digestive enzymes that could otherwise be supplied by food, there will be less energy and raw material (amino acids) available to make enzymes for other body processes. In addition, pancreatic enzymes work only in the duodenum; nature intended that enzymes begin working in the upper portion of the stomach before being deactivated by HCl. These enzymes can be supplied only by food. Food enzymes can be responsible for up to 75% of the digestive process before the body's enzymes kick in.

What kinds of foods supply enzymes?

Enzymes are present only in live foods that are very close to their original source:

- *Raw vegetables and fruits*
- *Nuts and seeds*
- *Sprouts*
- *Whole grains*
- *Raw milk products; also yogurt and cheese*

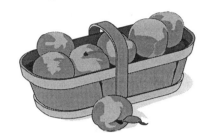

If vegetables and fruits are juiced, however, they can lose much of their enzyme content within an hour after juicing. Raw meat also contains beneficial enzymes. Animals on a combination diet of raw and cooked foods are generally healthier than animals eating only cooked and processed foods. However, it is not recommended that humans eat raw meat due to difficulty in digestion and risk of parasites and salmonella bacteria.

Enzymes are very temperature sensitive and are destroyed if heated over 118 degrees F (only 20 degrees above body temperature). Cooking, roasting, steaming, pasteurizing, microwave cooking, canning, and most processing techniques will kill the enzymes, and once dead they cannot be recovered. Slow cooking at a lower temperature can preserve some enzyme activity. Stomach acid will deactivate most food enzymes, but only temporarily - once in the alkaline environment of the intestines, they regain their activity.

When nuts, seeds, and grains are sprouted, both the sprouts and the water used to soak them are rich in beneficial enzymes. Plain good-quality yogurt, even though it is made from pasteurized milk as required by law in many states, becomes yogurt through the actions of the beneficial bacteria lactobacillus acidophilus. This process results in an enzyme-rich product. Similarly, the process of making cheese utilizes enzymes which are present in the final product, provided it is real cheese and not a processed cheese (non)food.

Signs of enzyme deficiency include:

- *Enlarged pancreas*
- *Increased white blood cell count 30 minutes after eating cooked foods*
- *Food sensitivity*
- *High urinary indican level. Indicans are toxic byproducts from undigested protein that is putrefying (rotting) in the colon [4].*

Hormones

What hormones are involved in digestion?

Several gastrointestinal hormones contribute to the digestive process. These respond to different types of food by stimulating or inhibiting substances needed for digestion. Some of these hormones are [5]:

- The stomach produces gastrin, which responds to protein fragments (polypeptides) and distension from food bulk, and stimulates release of HCl.

- The small intestine produces secretin, which responds to acid in the small intestine, and stimulates bicarbonate, bile, and enzyme release.

- Cholecystokinin (CCK), also made in the small intestine, responds to fatty acids and amino acids in the intestine. It stimulates enzyme release and gallbladder contraction.

- Gastric inhibitory peptide inhibits gastric acid (HCl) production.

Bacteria

Why is the bacterial content of the digestive tract so important?

The digestive tract is home to a variety of beneficial bacteria which are vital to our life and health. There are several trillion protective bacteria of about 400 different species in the human body, most of which live in the digestive tract. About a third of the dry weight of fecal matter is made up of dead or living bacteria. About four pounds of your total weight consists of these bacteria [6].

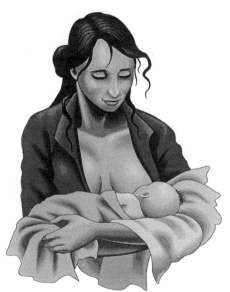

Bifidus sets up colonies on the intestinal wall, and is a home and support of sorts for acidophilus bacteria. Bifidus and acidophilus keep fungus and harmful microorganisms under control. Bifidus is supplied to babies through breastfeeding. A baby who is not breastfed will not have as much protection against fungus and pathogenic (unhealthful) bacteria.

Acidophilus works with bifidus to control fungus and pathogenic bacteria. In addition to being found naturally in the body, it is supplied by such foods as yogurt, cabbage, and Jerusalem artichoke (not related to regular artichoke). Both bifidus and acidophilus are available in supplement form. Biotin, butyrates and lactic acid are byproducts of acidophilus. These make the colon more acid and therefore more inhospitable to fungus, thus the name <u>acid</u>ophilus.

Bacteria in the large intestine produce vitamin K and biotin, aid final digestion, and keep urine pH to a healthful level of around 6.0 via lactic acid to keep fungus in check. These bacteria are so numerous that a substantial part of fecal matter is composed of these dead bacteria.

Protective intestinal bacteria have purposes other than digestion and keeping yeast and fungus under control. Protective bacteria have many functions in the body, including [7]:

- Manufacture of B vitamins, including biotin, niacin, vitamin B6 and folic acid [8].

- Manufacture of lactase, the milk digesting enzyme [9].

- Produce substances that kill or control invading bacteria and yeasts [10,11].

- Anticarcinogenic action [12].

- Digestive tract and bowel efficiency [13].

- Help reduce high cholesterol levels [14].

- Bifidus from breast milk helps the baby's digestive and immune systems function properly, making allergies and malabsorption problems less likely [15].

- Protect against damage from radiation and toxins [16].

- Recycle estrogen, helping to prevent osteoporosis and menopausal symptoms [17].

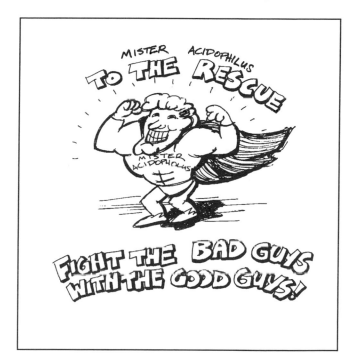

- As a supplement they are useful in treating a wide variety of health conditions, including allergies, arthritis, irritable bowel syndrome, and some forms of cancer [18].

At least a half-dozen different detoxification reactions are carried out by gut flora [19].

pH

Why is pH important?
The term pH refers to the acidity or alkalinity of liquids, including body fluids. A pH of 7.0 is considered neutral, with acidity defined as a pH of less than 7 and alkalinity being a pH of more

than 7. The farther away from 7.0 a pH reading is, the more acid or alkaline the fluid is. pH is discussed in detail in the chapter on Basic Chemical Concepts in *Surviving The Toxic Crisis*.

Since pH is extremely important nearly everywhere in the body, slight pH changes in the blood, urine, stomach juices, and other fluids can cause or signify a drastic change in function. pH var-•ies considerably depending on where it is measured.

- Blood should be about 7.35-7.4. Not coincidentally, this pH is also recommended for pools and hot tubs. In both cases this pH is optimal for discouraging fungus and bacterial overgrowth.

- Urine should be 6.0 to 6.2. A pH which is too alkaline can encourage or be caused by bacterial and fungal fermentation and growth. A person with a bladder infection is sometimes encouraged to drink cranberry juice, which will acidify the urine and coat the kidneys. A pH reading below 5.5 can be indicative of heavy metals and chemicals.

- Stomach juices should be 1.8 to 2.0, a corrosive level but one which is necessary for proper digestion, especially of protein. Stomach pH is often too high, and therefore ineffective, but very rarely too low in spite of the prevalence of so-called acid indigestion, which is normally caused by allergy or helicobacter.

- The intestinal tract is alkaline, and the actual pH varies in different parts of the intestine.

There are a number of mechanisms, backup mechanisms, and feedback loops to keep pH in body fluids within a narrow optimal or at least acceptable range.

In a procedure called the Heidelberg test, a transmitter which can detect and send pH readings is swallowed. This gives a readout of the pH in the stomach and intestines as it passes through. A similar test uses a string coated with a solution that changes color according to the pH. The string is in a capsule which is swallowed while the end of the string is held. After the capsule dissolves the string is withdrawn and the color of it is compared to a color chart.

What happens if there is not enough HCl in the stomach?

The pH of gastric juice should be 2.0 or lower. A pH of over 2.0 is an indication of hypochlorhydria, or too little hydrochloric acid in the stomach. Many people are deficient in HCl because of allergy, including nickel allergy, since allergy triggers the sympathetic fight-or-flight part of the nervous system rather than the parasympathetic digest-repair-and-restore part. The body then prepares for danger rather than working on digestion.

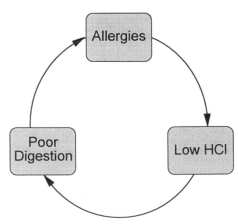

One indicator of low HCl is a high chloride reading on a

standard blood panel test. High may not mean out of range but rather high relative to the mid-point of the range (usually about 102). If chloride is high while sodium is low or normal, this could mean that the chloride is not being used to make sufficient HCl. Low HCl can be due to low niacin or copper intake, or to allergies as discussed above.

It has been known for over 20 years that gastric (stomach) HCl decreases with age [20], and helicobacter pylori tends to increase with age.

If hypochlorhydria is present, it will interfere with digestion by preventing the conversion of pepsinogen to pepsin for protein digestion. Insufficient HCl will not trigger the bicarbonate mechanism to make the duodenum alkaline and therefore hospitable for digestive enzymes. Hypochlorhydria therefore severely compromises one's nutrition even if sufficient nutrients are present in the diet.

Hydrochloric acid also has the function of killing harmful bacteria and parasites that are almost invariably ingested along with food. Many Americans are deficient in stomach acid, and this may explain the high incidence of the "tourist trots" - the gastrointestinal infections with resultant pain and diarrhea that result from contaminated food and water ingested in less-developed countries. Sufficient stomach acid, present in the natives who habitually consume less processed food than we do, protects them from these same bacteria and parasites.

How can stress interfere with digestion?

When you are stressed, whether physical or mental, the body tends to remain in sympathetic-dominant mode rather than in parasympathetic digest mode. When stressed, the body senses that it has more important things to do than digest. HCl and digestive efficiency as a whole may suffer.

How can chewing gum interfere with digestion?

Chewing triggers the release of HCl. Constant chewing, as of gum, causes HCl to be released in greater quantities than are needed, and over a longer period of time. After a while, there is not enough HCl left to be available when it is needed.

What can be done for insufficient HCl?

While chewing gum can deplete HCl, chewing food thoroughly can start the digestive process before the food reaches the stomach, making up for low HCl levels to a certain extent.

Betaine hydrochloride is sometimes recommended to increase the stomach's acidity (decrease pH). For optimal digestive assistance, enzymes should be taken at the beginning of the meal and HCl at the end. While supplemental HCl can be useful when properly applied, there are some cautions associated with its use:

- In the infrequent cases where the digestive problem is not due to insufficient stomach acid, the additional acid will not only not remedy the problem but can create a new one.

- If too much acid is taken, the body's entire acid-base balance can be thrown off. Blood becomes too acid, and the body has to work harder to correct the imbalance. Heavy metals, some chemicals, and vinegar from fermentation can also cause a condition of over-acidity.

- A too-high stomach acid content will spill over into the duodenum, preventing digestive enzymes from working optimally.

- Normal acid production in the stomach can be affected adversely if acid is supplied by ingestion rather than by the body. Herbal bitters can be a gentler way to supply HCl.

Insufficient stomach acid is a symptom of a system imbalance rather than a primary problem, and it would be better to assist the body in producing HCl as it was designed to. This can be accomplished with sufficient food enzymes, beneficial bacteria such as acidophilus, and vitamins and minerals.

Is there such a thing as too much stomach acid?

Sometimes too much acid is present, or is suspected due to heartburn (also called sour stomach).

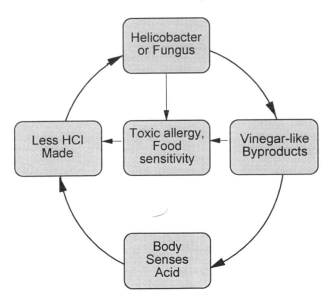

This is rarely due to too much HCl, as is commonly believed. In fact, too little HCl sets up the conditions for too much stomach acid of another sort.

When helicobacter pylori (discussed in the Bacteria chapter in **Surviving The Toxic Crisis**) or fungus are present, and insufficient HCl is available to kill these organisms, then they grow out of control. They then produce vinegar-like acidic byproducts from their metabolic processes. In addition, these organisms cause fermentation, which first makes intestinal fluids and urine more alkaline (pH about 8.2), and then acidic (pH about 4.5) as the body tries to correct the problem. While HCl is made in response to chewing, the symptom-causing acid is produced continuously, causing discomfort. In a vicious cycle, the body senses that enough acidity is present, makes even less HCl, and the microorganisms proliferate even more.

One patient, a man in his 60's, had helicobacter which caused stomach acidity. He had his mercury fillings removed, was treated for helicobacter and fungus, and was given acidophilus. His urine pH stabilized at about 6.2, and he felt much better; no more acid indigestion and as a bonus, his allergies went away!

What evidence is there that the problem is not always too much HCl?

When it was believed that too much HCl (which is rare) was the problem, antacids were given to counteract the acid. These gave temporary relief, but worsened the problem in the long run. However, when more HCl was given in the form of supplements, symptoms were alleviated long-term. If there had been too much HCl present already, more HCl would have worsened the problem, but this was not the case.

Both insufficient HCl and too much HCl can cause indigestion. To determine which, if either, is your problem, try taking a tablespoon of cider vinegar or lemon juice, which are both acids, in a glass of water. If it helps relieve the indigestion, you may need HCl supplementation. If it makes your symptoms worse, you probably already have too much. It is also possible that you have a raw stomach caused by years of turning carbohydrates to vinegar, and you aren't ready for HCl in pill form.

Gentian herbal bitters help control helicobacter and stimulate HCl production.

What happens when antacids are taken for sour stomach?

In a misguided attempt at self medication, antacids are sometimes taken. Antacids are symptom suppressing drugs, and are not a good idea for several reasons:

- By suppressing HCl, microorganisms grow even more out of control and, in the cycle described previously, produce even more harmful acid.

- The symptoms may not be due to excess acid of any kind, so that antacids will not correct the problem and may make it worse in the long run.

- The digestive distress, if due to an ulcer, may be alleviated by the antacid just enough to delay seeking needed professional help. Ulcers are not caused by too much acid, but can be made worse or more uncomfortable in the long run by it.

- Rebound hyperacidity is possible - the stomach may simply send in another blast of HCl when the pH gets too high from the antacid. More likely, fermentation and the waste byproducts of microorganisms that thrive in a more alkaline environment produce a vinegar-like acid that can add to the "acid indigestion" problem.

- If gastric juice is made too alkaline, digestion will be impaired.

- The blood and urine can become too alkaline, leading to decreased mineral absorption - minerals such as calcium must be in the ionic state to be absorbed, and acidity favors the ionic state.

Digestive Problems

What are some digestive problems?

Symptoms include

- *Heartburn*
- *Gas*
- *Allergies*
- *Bloat*
- *Ulcers*
- *Constipation*
- *Diarrhea*
- *Weight gain or loss*
- *Pernicious anemia*
- *Lactose intolerance*

Heartburn does not involve the heart. Sometimes called sour stomach, it is a burning sensation, often caused by the reflux of acid back into the esophagus from the stomach.

Ulcers can have a number of causes, including

- *Giardia*
- *Fungus*
- *Antibiotics*
- *Non-steroidal anti-inflammatory drugs (NSAIDs)*
- *Helicobacter pylori*
- *Allergy, especially nickel allergy*
- *Mercury from metal fillings*

All of these set up conditions of microorganism growth and keep the body in sympathetic, or attack, mode. Insufficient HCl is then made and the problem worsens as too much of the wrong kind of acid is made.

Ulcers can occur when too much acid (from fermentation or rarely from too much HCl), too little protective alkaline mucus, and/or low omega 6 oils causes the acid to eat a hole in or thin out the stomach lining. The stomach is literally digesting itself in that spot. Ulcers can perforate and bleed and be life-threatening, or they may just be painful and inconvenient. Stress can worsen them by increasing sympathetic dominance and decreasing HCl production and parasympathetic repair-and-restore functions.

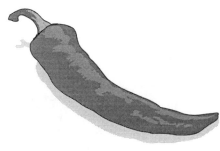

Spicy foods and pepper appear to aggravate ulcers but can be healing over time. Cayenne, a type of hot pepper, is sometimes taken in capsules to increase protective mucus thus helping to heal digestive problems. Milk and antacids can feel soothing in the short run but can aggravate the problem in the long run. Vitamin A has a protective effect on the stomach lining. Licorice (the herbal extract, not the candy) is useful in ulcer treatment and prevention of relapses. Cabbage juice, a good source of acidophilus, is also healing.

Flatulence (gas) can be caused by putrefaction in the large intestine. Putrefaction often occurs when undigested protein is broken down by bacteria. Certain foods such as beans and cabbage can be gas-producers. While it is a good idea to avoid these foods if they cause trouble for you, on a more basic level a properly functioning digestive system should be able to handle these foods without incident. Putrefaction often occurs when food stays in the intestines too long. Sufficient dietary fiber will speed up the di-

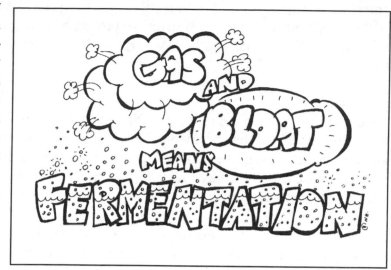

gestive and elimination process. Ironically, too much fiber, or fiber introduced into the diet or increased too quickly, can also cause gas. Supplemental digestive enzymes, pantothenic acid and lemon juice may help. Apple cider vinegar is recommended by some, but it can worsen the fermentation problem so it is best avoided. Activated charcoal tablets may be useful in severe cases.

Constipation can be caused by insufficient fiber in the diet. Fiber increases stool bulk and softens the stool as discussed in the chapter on Carbohydrates. Fermentation in the small intestine draws water from the bowel, leading to hard stools and constipation. Other causes are:

- *Low bile*
- *Low silica*
- *Too little water*
- *High calcium*
- *Low oils*
- *Low levels of good bacteria*
- *Low peristaltic action*
- *Low magnesium*
- *Too much iron*
- *Low digestive enzyme levels*
- *Pinched lumbar nerve that controls the colon*

Overuse of laxatives often makes the problem worse by interfering with proper peristaltic action. Increasing fluid intake may help. Magnesium in most forms can loosen the stool. If stool loosening is not desired, Mag Glycinate (magnesium glycinate), made by Ethical Nutrients should be taken when magnesium is needed for other reasons such as irregular heartbeat. Note that magnesium should be taken in balance with calcium; the ideal dosage schedule is more magnesium in the morning and more calcium before bed to avoid competition for binding sites.

Constipation can result from the use of medications, including some antibiotics, anti-inflammatories, muscle relaxants, opiates / narcotics, analgesics, antacids, antidepressants, blood pressure medication, and diuretics. Toxic metals such as mercury, iron, lead, arsenic and bismuth can also contribute to constipation [21].

Diarrhea is often a sign of an infectious or toxic process within the gastrointestinal system. It can be dangerous in a baby or if severe or prolonged due to dehydration and electrolyte (mineral) imbalance. Minerals help to hold water, so a lowered mineral level can increase or prolong the diarrhea.

If the diarrhea is not severe, resist the temptation to treat it symptomatically with medication because you may worsen the problem. Diarrhea is the body's way of clearing out the disease process or toxic overload, and you won't be doing yourself any favors by artificially suppressing this protective mechanism. Acidophilus, taken orally or rectally, can help correct the problem causing the diarrhea. Two ounces rectally by syringe is recommended. Colonics can also help by assisting the cleansing process.

Diarrhea that lasts for months or years can be symptoms of the potentially serious conditions of colitis and ileitis (Crohn's disease). Other causes of diarrhea are parasites, fungus, klebsiella bacteria, and diverticulitis. Too much magnesium relative to calcium can also lead to diarrhea.

Allergies to foods are often caused by a problem nicknamed "leaky gut". In a healthy digestive system, only glucose, amino acids, fatty acids, and micronutrients are absorbed into the bloodstream through the walls of the small intestine. If digestion is incomplete for whatever reason, undigested food is usually excreted. However, small molecules of undigested food sometimes cross the intestinal barrier and enter the bloodstream. These food molecules, which are non-self protein, do not belong in the bloodstream. This fact is recognized by the immune system, which attacks them.

Once sensitized in this way, a person can experience an allergic reaction whenever the offending food is eaten. These allergies may be obvious and traceable to a particular food, or they may cause vague symptoms such as fatigue, headache, and asthma. Improving your digestion will often alleviate food allergies. Grinding grains in a coffee grinder can make them easier to digest.

Digestive distress of any type often has an allergic component. Be aware of what types of foods bring on your symptoms, such as beans (gas) or tomatoes (heartburn) and avoid them.

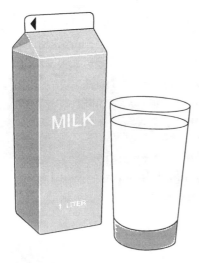

Lactose intolerance affects many people who cannot drink milk or eat milk products without digestive distress such as pain or diarrhea. It is caused by a deficiency of the enzyme lactase, which digests lactose (milk sugar). Avoiding milk products is one solution. Acidophilus, a beneficial bacteria found in good quality plain yogurt, in capsules, or in commercial products such as Lact-Aid and acidophilus milk, can aid in the digestion of lactose, increasing one's tolerance to milk.

The casein protein in milk was meant to be digested by calves, not humans. Cows have four stomachs to assist in digestion, while we have only one, and our one stomach often does not break casein up completely into single amino acids. The resulting polypeptides (groups of amino acids) can become allergens, creating milk intolerance.

Due in part to lactase deficiency, milk is one of the most common allergens. Others are wheat, corn, soy, citrus fruits, and tomatoes. The protein in these foods is usually the allergen.

Why is a diet of both protein and vegetables important?
Pernicious anemia, as discussed earlier in this chapter, can be caused by either insufficient vitamin B12 in the diet or by lack of intrinsic factor necessary for its absorption. Pernicious anemia is sometimes a problem for vegetarians, since vitamin B12 is found in animal products. Heavy meat eaters who consume few vegetables can also suffer from pernicious anemia due to lack of folic acid, usually found in vegetables.

What is the connection between digestion and the nervous system?
Digestion is a function of the parasympathetic nervous system, which is also responsible for repairing and restoring tissues. If you are physically (toxins etc.) or emotionally stressed, you are in sympathetic mode and it is difficult for the parasympathetic mode to kick in, resulting in poor digestion.

Another aspect of the parasympathetic / digestion connection is that if you eat too late in the evening, your body, in parasympathetic mode, will try to handle both digestion and repair while you sleep. Both functions can suffer.

The nerves from the lower spine help in digestion. A problem with this part of the spine can adversely affect digestion, and vice-versa.

Promoting Healthy Digestion

How can you promote healthy digestion?
Healthy digestion can be achieved in a number of ways:

- Good nutrition in general is important, as described throughout this section of the book. Complete fresh non-processed proteins such as eggs, fish, chicken and lamb, and vitamins C, E, and the B complex specifically aid digestion.

- Sufficient hydrochloric acid production is assisted by raw food enzymes, complete proteins, copper, and vitamin A, niacin, and B complex. The herb gentian triggers the release of stomach acid by suppressing helicobacter.

- Get sufficient enzymes, provided by raw foods and acidophilus.

- Chew food thoroughly to mechanically break it up, to stimulate HCl production, and to get maximum benefit from salivary amylase.

- Eat slowly to avoid swallowing air and to avoid eating too much.

- Dietary lecithin helps to digest fats, and with vitamin C helps to prevent gall-stones.

- Relax while eating to turn off the sympathetic mode and stimulate the healing parasympathetic mode.

Beyond Food Combining

How can food combining be of benefit?

Judicious food combining helps to prevent fermentation, discussed in the chapter on Carbohydrates. Fermentation and putrefaction are lessened if food is sped through the digestive tract as quickly as possible, and if certain food combinations are avoided at the same time. There are several basic rules based on these principles [22]. These rules may appear to conflict with advice given elsewhere in this book section. As before when there is an apparent conflict, follow the advice that best fits your body, situation, or problem. Food combining suggestions that are useful if fermentation is a problem for you - urine pH over 6 or 6.5 is a sign of this - include:

- **Protein rotting** - Proteins, especially meat proteins, and starches eaten together can putrefy (rot) in the stomach. The combination will ferment and putrefy faster than either one separately, and the protein will retard the transit time to digest while the starch ferments. To determine transit time, eat something that will usually show up in the stool such as corn kernels, and note how long after eating they are seen in the stool. Increased body odor, caused by putrefaction, is sometimes noticed after eating meat with starch.

- **Proper ratio** - You can eat either proteins or starches (complex carbohydrates) at a meal along with vegetables or salad until you get to a 30/40/30 ratio of protein/starch/vegetables.

- **Fermentation, high urine pH** - Fruit is especially prone to fermentation - consider how wine is made. For this reason, eat fruit alone on an empty stomach so it can speed through the intestines before it has time to ferment. Optimally, fruit should be the first thing you eat in the morning if you eat it at all, followed by protein to modulate blood sugar spikes. Allow a half hour after eating fruit before eating other foods, and three hours should elapse after eating other foods before eating fruit. Sweet fruit such as bananas, dates, dried fruits, and grapes should be eaten after other fruits. **Caution**: Many people can't tolerate fruit, and fruit should not be eaten at all unless urine pH can hold steady at pH 6.2. Other people are prone to hypoglycemia, insulin spikes, and sugar/energy surges and crashes. Such people, if they eat fruit at all, might be better off combining it with protein.

- Vegetables combine well with any one of: fruits, protein, or carbohydrates.

- Starches combine well with oils, which slow sugar uptake, while protein and oils are a poor combination.

- Grains should be cooked fresh to avoid fermentation, and cooked only until chewy, not soggy.

- Grains should be ground in a coffee mill or spice grinder before cooking if they are not being digested, i.e. if whole grains are showing up in the stool.

Food combining is only for those with allergies and poor digestion and is to be used only until the patient's health and urine pH are stable.

What kinds of herbs can aid digestion?

Various plants and herbs and their extracts can also be used to support healthy digestion and to relieve minor digestive problems. These herbs and the conditions they help relieve include [23]:

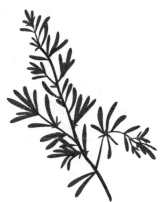

- **Digestive enzyme activity** - Allspice, cloves, and similar aromatic herbs contain eugenol, which promotes digestive enzyme activity. Cinnamon has a similar effect.

- **Digestive aids** - Anise, valerian, and bitters, taken after meals, are digestive aids.

- **Unsettled stomach** - Coriander and comfrey can settle the stomach. Marjoram settles the stomach, and can be helpful for motion sickness.

- **Bile and fat digestion** - Dandelion may trigger bile flow, aiding fat digestion. Goldenseal, turmeric and peppermint trigger the release of bile or stimulate its flow.

- **Gas** - Dill, fennel and savory may help prevent, treat, or expel gas.

- **Diarrhea** - Fennel may treat diarrhea by killing bacteria. Dill may also help with infectious diarrhea

- **Ulcers** - Licorice and peppermint help to heal and prevent stomach ulcers. Red pepper (cayenne), contains capsaicin, which triggers the flow of saliva and stomach fluids. It has some use in healing ulcers.

- **Fungus** - Myrrh helps to control fungus.

- **Worms** - Oregano may help to expel intestinal worms.

- **Protein digestion** - Papaya contains papain, an enzyme which is similar to pepsin. It helps to digest protein. Ginger helps to break down proteins, and can be used to relieve abdominal cramping and nausea.

While severe digestive distress such as colitis, ileitis, or bleeding ulcers may require professional aid, most people should benefit by these suggestions.

References and Resources

General

- The Burton Goldberg Group, *Alternative Medicine: The Definitive Guide*, "Enzyme Therapy", pp. 215-223, and "Constipation", pp. 640-5, Future Medicine Publishing, Puyallup WA, 1994.

- Rogers, Sherry A., *Tired or Toxic?*, Prestige Publishing, Syracuse NY, 1990.

Enzymes

- Cichoke, Anthony, *Enzymes and Enzyme Therapy: How to Jump Start Your Way to Lifelong Good Health*, Keats Publishing Inc., New Canaan CT, 1994.

- Howell, Edward, *Food Enzymes for Health and Longevity*, Omangod Press, Woodstock Valley CT, 1980.

- Howell, Edward, *Enzyme Nutrition: The Food Enzyme Concept*, Avery Publishing Group, Wayne NJ, 1987.

- Santillo, Humbart, *Food Enzymes*, Hohm Press, Prescott AZ, 1987.

- Wolf, Max and Karl Ransberger, *Enzyme Therapy*, Vantage Press, NY, 1972.

Bacteria

- Chaitow, Leon and N. Trenev, *Probiotics*, Harper Collins, NY, 1990.

Digestive Problems

- Castleman, Michael, *The Healing Herbs*, Rodale Press, Emmaus PA, 1991. *A guide to herbs, including those for digestive problems.*

- Hoffman, Ronald, *Seven Weeks to a Healthy Stomach*, Pocket Books, NY, 1990.

- Perkin, Steven, *Gastrointestinal Health*, Harper Perennial, NY, 1992.

- Scala, James, *Eating Right For A Bad Gut*, Plume Books, NY, 1992.

- Trickett, Shirley, *Irritable Bowel Syndrome and Diverticulosis*, Thorson's / Harper Collins, London England, 1992.

OTHER NEEDS

More Than Just Bit Parts

The body has needs other than the obvious nutrients. Water, air, exercise, sleep and light are also crucial to life and well-being.

Water

Why is water so important?
Water makes up about 70% of our bodies. Interestingly, water also makes up about 70% of this planet's surface. The electrolyte balance in sea water is about the same as in our bodies, only more concentrated [1], an example of our connection to our planet.

Water is necessary for all bodily processes as both an active participant and as a solvent. It is sometimes called the universal solvent, as it will dissolve (break into ionic components) nearly anything given enough time. Water can erode stone yet it is safe enough to bathe a baby in. Water is so important that the average person, deprived of water in any form (including food), will die after about three days with no water.

What exactly is water?
Water is written chemically as H_2O. This means that each water molecule consists of two hydrogen atoms bound to one oxygen atom. The configuration is slightly bent, accounting for some of its solvent characteristics.

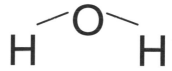

Why water = life:
Water has a number of functions in the body. These include:

- Water is a solvent for all substances and nutrients in the body. Without water thousands of processes would not happen. For example, blood, lymph, kidney function, digestion and adrenal function are dependent on water.

- Water helps to carry nutrients and other substances to where they are needed in the body.

- Water is a major constituent of every cell, and of blood plasma, cerebrospinal fluid, and every other body liquid. Water is in every body part. Water is even in teeth (10%) and bones (13%) [2].

- Water helps to carry out wastes from the body in the form of urine, feces, and sweat.

- Water helps to regulate body temperature like the water in a car radiator.

How much water do we need to drink?

Many people do not drink water directly at all, preferring to get their liquid from beverages with a more interesting taste. Most people who follow the guidelines of thirst will get an adequate level of water in whatever form. However, adequate is not the same as optimal. In addition, water in any form other than plain H_2O has drawbacks, as explained shortly.

Eight glasses of water per day, or about 1/2 gallon, is often recommended. Most of this should be taken in relatively early in the day, as bodily processes requiring water are most active in the daytime.

Asthma, pain, arthritis, ulcers and high blood pressure can all result from chronic dehydration. Increasing the intake of water can help relieve these ailments [3,4].

Is it possible to drink too much water?

Unless one drinks prodigious amounts or has some sort of rare kidney or other disorder, the general rule is: the more, the better. It is nearly impossible to get too much, since the body will quickly eliminate any excess. This rule assumes that good quality water, discussed later in this chapter, is used.

How do you know if you are getting enough water?

A blood test, blood urea nitrogen (BUN), measures the concentration of protein in the blood. If the BUN or BUN/creatinine (creatinine is a protein waste product) ratio is high (above 20), this may indicate that the protein in the body is not sufficiently diluted, i.e. that not enough liquid is taken in.

Are other liquids as beneficial as water?

Other liquids supply water, and as a source of water are nearly as good as drinking plain water. However, nearly all liquids other than plain water have disadvantages:

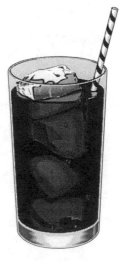

- Artificially sweetened or sugar sweetened beverages with artificial colors and flavors are definitely to be avoided, as they are nothing but a combination of harmful chemicals dissolved in water.

- Coffee and non-herb tea are diuretics, which means that they increase water elimination and carry water and electrolytes out of the body.

- Caffeinated beverages make the body more alkaline, promoting fungus growth.

- Alcohol is a diuretic, and in addition pulls water out of cells and into intercellular spaces, accounting for the water bloat seen in alcoholics. Caffeinated beverages and alcohol are also drugs with other harmful effects such as vasoconstriction and adrenal exhaustion.

- Juices contain water, beneficial enzymes, and nutrients. Fruit juices and juices from sweet vegetables such as carrots also contain sugar, and the harm from too much natural sugar can more than negate the benefits of drinking the juice. Juice from non-sweet vegetables such as cucumbers or celery is comparatively healthful in moderation, but can still grow fungus over a long period.

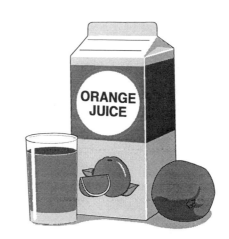

- Milk contains casein protein and lactose, which are both common allergens.

Does the temperature of the water matter?

Many people have a water temperature preference - cold, hot, or room temperature. Cold water quenches thirst faster, but as a result a person may tend to drink less of it. Cold water also slows down digestion. Hot or warm water opens the gut so allergens can permeate it, a condition called leaky gut. Room temperature water is best tolerated and utilized by the body.

If you have ever gone to a person practicing energy medicine, such as an acupuncturist or homeopath, the practitioner may have asked you whether you prefer warm, cold, or room temperature water. The answer to the question gives the doctor useful information about the presence and type of disharmony in your body. It is not uncommon to change your preference to room temperature water after treatment.

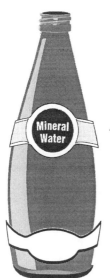

What about carbonated water?

Carbonated water gets its name from carbon dioxide (CO_2), which is forced into the water by pressure from machinery or sometimes by natural processes. The colder the water, the more carbon dioxide can be dissolved in it.

Both you and your cells take in oxygen and breathe out carbon dioxide. The fact that the body considers carbon dioxide to be a waste product should be an indication that taking in more carbon dioxide in the form of carbonated beverages or otherwise would be undesirable.

Carbonated beverages, even natural ones, tend to make the body too alkaline, a condition which fosters fungus growth. Your body must then expend energy better used elsewhere to correct this alkaline condition. The phosphorus in carbonated beverages tends to leach calcium out of the body, causing a person to be jittery, have trouble sleeping, or eventually develop osteoporosis (bone loss).

Carbonated beverages with sweetening, colors, and flavors are even worse because all of these chemicals are harmful.

Is all water the same?
Technically, all water is H$_2$O and is therefore the same. However, there is a great difference in what may be in the water, depending on source, filtration, and treatment.

What contaminants might be in water?
Many contaminants can be found in water, as discussed in the chapter on Water Pollution, Fluoride and Chlorine in *Surviving The Toxic Crisis*. These include:

- *chlorine*
- *dirt*
- *metals*
- *fluoride*
- *pesticides*
- *organic compounds*
- *microorganisms*

Is there a legal limit to the amount of harmful substances in the water?
The Environmental Protection Agency (EPA) sets guidelines limiting the amounts of the above contaminants which can be found in any water that is used for drinking, including tap water and bottled water. However, even if you have municipal water which passes inspection, the water can pick up an unacceptable level of contaminants from the piping in your house.

How can you tell if your water is acceptable?

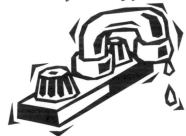

If you have a private well or an older house, it may be wise to have your water tested at your tap, rather than at the source, to pick up contamination from household pipes. There are private companies which do this for a fee. It may be possible to have your water tested free by a company that would like to sell you an expensive water treatment system. However, their results may be biased towards finding problems - correctable, of course, by their product.

The best testing laboratory is one that is independent and state certified. State or local health departments sometimes test for bacteria free of charge. The American Council of Independent Laboratories (phone 202-887-5872) and The American Association for Laboratory Accreditation (phone 301-670-1377) can direct you to testing labs in your area [5].

What are some of the other problems with tap water?
Green stains in the sink are usually from copper salts leaching from copper pipes in older homes. This may not be harmful, although copper stains can be an indirect indication of harmful lead contamination from the lead which was often used to solder copper pipes.

Water with a **reddish brown stain** is usually rusty from iron deposits from your pipes. Let it run until clear before using it.

Odors - If your water smells like rotten eggs, this is the gas hydrogen sulfide, which is a product of bacterial growth. The bacteria involved rarely cause anything more serious than diarrhea.

Cloudy water can be due to dirt, iron particles, or bacteria, or to something as harmless as tiny air bubbles that dissipate quickly. Cloudiness is most likely to be a problem when it appears suddenly, such as contamination from flooding or a broken pipe.

What are your options other than tap water?

If your tap water has an unpleasant taste or odor, or a water assay indicates unsafe levels of contaminants, you have two main options:

- *Install a home water treatment system*
- *Buy bottled water*

What types of water treatment systems are there?

The water treatment system you buy depends on several factors:

- *What types of contaminants need to be removed*
- *How much of the water needs to be treated (faucet, whole house)*
- *Budget considerations*

There are three main types of home water treatment systems, which can be used alone or in combination:

- *Activated carbon filter*
- *Reverse osmosis / membrane*
- *Distillation*

Carbon filters work through absorption of pollutant molecules, which are chemically attracted to the carbon and stick to it. Carbon filters arc good for removing organic chemicals and unpleasant tastes and odors, but they do not remove heavy metals. Prices range from a small $25-$35 device that screws onto a faucet and is not very effective to about $1000 for the whole house [5,6]. Carbon filters need to be replaced every 6-12 months and cost about $40 per year. Most carbon filter systems can be reverse-flushed, which is important for cleaning the system.

Reverse osmosis units force pressurized water through a membrane that rejects contaminants, and the treated water is sent to a holding tank. A reverse osmosis unit can remove many organics, metals, and microorganisms, but may miss small organic molecules such as trichloroethylene (TCE). Costs range from $100 for a faucet mounted unit to $500-$1500 for an under-sink unit. Reverse osmosis for the whole house is about $2000 to $5000. Filters need to be changed periodically; if this is not done they can become contaminated with bacteria and will actually worsen water quality.

Distillation involves heating water to the point of steaming, and it then recondenses. Distillation removes bacteria, minerals, metals, and some chemicals although not most organics. Distillation costs $100-$1000 for a single faucet, and $800-$4000 for the whole house.

Once the bacteria-killing chlorine is removed from the pipes, however, bacteria can grow between the water cleaning unit and the faucet. Water cleaners of whatever type may be better for this reason if installed to serve a particular faucet or showerhead.

What are some other water treatment methods?
Other methods include:

- Magnets, which supposedly remove metals but only work on elemental iron. They are essentially useless.

- Silver salts kill microorganisms. However, when exposed to chlorinated water, the kind most of us have, toxic silver chloride ($AgCl$) is formed. Silver chloride can cause arthritis or joint pain and a bluish skin discoloration.

- Copper kills microorganisms. High altitude streams tend to be both blue-green from copper salts and crystal clear from a lack of microorganisms. Copper salts are okay for pools but not for the water you ingest into your system.

- Ultraviolet (UV) light is effective against microorganisms. It is sometimes used as part of a home water treatment system. However, UV only kills bacteria present at the time of the UV treatment. It does nothing to prevent the introduction and growth of more bacteria. It also kills bacteria at the point of treatment, and as is the case of the treatments that remove chlorine, nothing is done to keep bacteria from multiplying between the treatment point and the faucet.

- Ozone, also used to kill microorganisms, is used in much of Europe and in Los Angeles as a less toxic alternative to chlorine. Although the ozone is toxic while actually in use, the treated water contains no residue and is safe. Ozonation is also recommended to keep pool and hot tub water clean.

- Enzymes to clean water, especially in hot tubs and pools. An example for hot tubs is Spa Magic by CDE Research, Oceanside CA.

Can we summarize these methods?

To remove:	Use:
• Microorganisms	Reverse osmosis, distillation, UV, ozone
• Heavy metals	Reverse osmosis, distillation
• Chlorine	Carbon, reverse osmosis
• Organics	Carbon, distillation (only some organics)
• Minerals	Water softener, distillation

Is it only your drinking water that needs to be treated?

Chlorine and other contaminants are absorbed into the body through the skin during bathing or showering. If you are unwilling to drink your tap water, you should not be showering in it either. Filters which attach to your shower nozzle can be installed for under $50.

> **If you are unwilling to drink your tap water, you should not be showering in it either.**

What about water softeners?

Minerals such as calcium and magnesium make the water "hard", meaning that a whitish crust or soap scum may be deposited on the sides of the tub, and your hair probably won't feel as clean. Hard water causes more wear on water-using appliances such as water heaters and washing machines due to mineral buildup.

A water softener puts sodium chloride (salt) in the water, and the water soluble sodium chemically replaces the less water soluble minerals. A water softener treats the whole house and costs $1000- $3500. Water softeners make the water taste slightly salty and the treated water is not desirable for drinking for this reason. New installations of water softeners are banned in some communities, especially in California, for environmental reasons.

What about bottled water?

Bottled water can be purchased in one or two gallon plastic bottles at the supermarket, or empty bottles can be filled with filtered tap water from vending machines. Bottled water can be delivered to your home, but you pay more for the convenience. A caution: before you upend the large bottle on your water dispenser, clean the tap and be sure the bottle isn't dusty. Otherwise, the dust that collects on the top of the bottle will drift down into the water reservoir when the bottle is upended.

Bottles made of hard clear plastic outgas toxins less than the soft, cloudy bottles and so the clear bottles are more the more desirable of the two, although glass is best.

A caution on refilling plastic bottles from vending machines is in order. If you toss empty plastic bottles into the car for filling and let them bake in the heat for a while, the small amount of water in the bottom of the bottle can be contaminated with plasticizer from the bottle that is liberated by the heat. Bacteria and algae can also proliferate in the warm water, and all of these contaminants are mixed with the new water.

With all of these options, which are best?

All bottled water must meet EPA guidelines for drinking water. The guidelines are no more stringent than for the water that comes out of your faucet, although it may taste better. There is no one answer to the question of which water is best. Contaminant levels will rarely be a problem, so the choice is left up to the individual based on taste, cost, and convenience.

Should you drink distilled or "drinking" water?

Water in bottles is often labeled as being distilled water or drinking water. The difference lies in the mineral content. Distilled water has the minerals removed, and drinking water either does not have them all removed or is made up of distilled water with some minerals added. There is some difference in taste, and the drinking water has the taste that most people are used to.

Health-wise, distilled water tends to flush both beneficial minerals and harmful metals from the body to a slightly greater extent than drinking water, if this is a consideration. Otherwise, let taste be your guide.

Air

What is air made of?

Air in theory is composed of about 78% nitrogen (N_2), 21% oxygen (O_2), and 1% everything else. In many polluted areas of the country, air contains considerably less than 21% oxygen and considerably more "everything else".

Air Composition

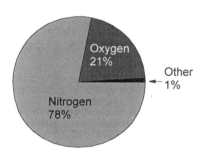

How much air do we take in?

We take about 10,000 breaths of air per day, inhaling about 1.5 pounds of oxygen and exhaling one pound of carbon dioxide and about 200 chemicals.

Why is air so important?

The constituent of air that we need for life is oxygen. Oxygen is needed for the processes of all cells, and without it they, and we, will die. The brain is an especially avid consumer of oxygen. Irreversible death of brain cells can occur after as little as four minutes without oxygen.

How can you get the most out of the air you breathe?

To get the most out of the air you breathe, there are two considerations:

- *Maximize oxygen consumption*
- *Minimize harmful contaminants*

What happens if you don't get enough oxygen?

People who fly or climb to high altitudes without supplemental oxygen often experience muddled thinking, not surprising considering the brain's huge need for oxygen, and less energy. If the oxygen level gets low enough, a state of no energy will be reached, a condition known as death. On a daily level, getting less than the optimum amount of oxygen can lead to brain fog and lowered energy.

Some conditions such as toxins and allergies can cause red blood cells to clump up, lowering their ability to transport oxygen. The end results, often fatigue and brain fog, are due to oxygen starvation of the organs and tissues.

Does nitrogen do anything?
The amount of oxygen is much more important than the amount of nitrogen, which is an inert (not biologically active) gas which serves to carry the necessary oxygen.

How can you maximize oxygen consumption?
Oxygen consumption can be maximized in three ways:

- *Increase the amount of oxygen in the air*
- *Increase the amount and depth of your breathing*
- *If your blood is clumped, identify and treat the cause to maximize oxygen transport*

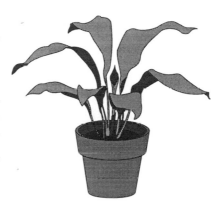

The amount of oxygen in the air can be increased by living in a less polluted area. If moving is impractical, green plants can be used in the house and yard. Plants take in carbon dioxide, our waste product, put out oxygen, and absorb pollutants on either a household level (houseplants) or global level (rainforests).

How can you improve your breathing?
Most of us do not use our full lung capacity. A natural response to breathing bad air is to breathe more shallowly, as most people do when near a diesel-belching truck or a fire. Since the air quality in most areas is less than optimal, many of us do not breathe as deeply as we should. Poor posture contributes to shallow breathing by compressing the lungs to the point where they do not expand fully.

Try the following: Sit upright without slumping. Inhale slowly as deeply as you can, expanding your abdomen as you do so to the greatest extent possible. A small amount of discomfort may be normal, as you expand parts of your body which have not been used in a while. If there is pain on deep inhalation, or you start coughing, the cause of this should be checked out - you may have roundworm, an infection, or lung tissue scarring. Once you have inhaled deeply, exhale as thoroughly as possible. Your abdomen should contract inward on the exhale.

By inhaling more deeply, you bring more oxygen to the alveoli in deeper parts of your lung, and from there to the blood, which carries it throughout the body. Exhaling completely gets rid of carbon dioxide and other wastes, some of which stays pooled in the lungs indefinitely when you are only breathing shallowly.

How often should you do this breathing exercise?
The more you breathe this way, the better. Ideally, you will reach a point where your breathing is deeper than it had been, even when you are not consciously doing breathing exercises. You will probably find that your respiration rate (number of breaths per minute) decreases as you get

more out of each breath. After making a sustained improvement in your breathing, you will probably notice increased energy and clearer thinking.

How does air pollution affect us?
Air pollution in general lowers the amount of oxygen available, and the specific pollutants have many toxic effects of their own.

How can you lower the level of air pollutants in your home?
As discussed in the Air Pollution chapter in **Surviving The Toxic Crisis**, indoor air is frequently more polluted than outdoor air. One simple way of improving indoor air quality is to open as many windows as is possible.

A second way is to lower to the greatest extent possible the amount of pollution entering your indoor air. Ways to do this include:

- *Ban cigarette smoking*
- *Reduce or eliminate the use of sprays (hairspray, insecticide, cleaners, paint)*
- *Vent cooking odors to the outside with a fan*
- *Wash bedding in hot water to reduce dust mites*

What about air cleaners?
Another way to reduce pollution is to use an indoor air cleaner. The main types of air cleaners use filters, electrical attraction, electron/ion generator or ozone. Some cleaners use a combination.

Filters will trap particulates such as dust, pollen, bacteria, and smoke, but they will not trap gases, and odors are caused primarily by gases. The finer the filter, the smaller the particles that will be trapped, but finer filters get clogged sooner and need to be cleaned or replaced more frequently. The highest quality High Efficiency Particulate Arresting (HEPA) filters trap up to 99.97 percent of particles, while a pleated filter traps up to 95 percent of particles. Filters have a major drawback, however: they will only filter the air that actually reaches them, so that only the air within a few feet of a filter may actually be cleaned.

> **A major drawback of air filters is that they only filter the air that actually reaches them, not all the air in the room.**

In an **electrostatic air cleaner**, a high voltage wire charges particles, which in theory collect in a filter. In actual use, many of the particles tend to collect instead on walls and furnishings, which is still preferable to having them collect in your lungs. Electrical filters have little effect on gases and their odors.

Negative ion generators, as the name implies, give off negatively charged particles such as are found by the ocean, rivers and waterfalls. Negatively charged air is presumably more natural and is said to improve mood and health.

In an **ozonation** type filter, an ozone generator uses a high voltage electric charge to convert oxygen in the air to ozone, which destroys gas particles and microorganisms. The clear fresh smell that you may have noticed around waterfalls is caused in part by ozone.

The Alpine Air Purifier (Alpine Air, Blaine MN) combines the benefits of ozone, negative ions and a filter, and is one of the most effective devices tested.

Is ozonation safe and effective?
Ozone can be toxic in concentrations higher than that found in nature, but it is so reactive that it is usually only a hazard when the ozonator is on at high levels and not afterward.

Ozonators can be used in two ways:

- Some ozonators produce high quantities of ozone and are meant to be used only when a room or building is not inhabited and then turned off.

- Some ozonators produce lower levels of ozone and are meant to be run more or less continuously.

Ozone (O_3) breaks down to O_2 (regular molecular oxygen) and O (singlet oxygen). Singlet oxygen is very reactive against bacteria, fungi and chemicals. For example, ozone reacts with toxic formaldehyde (found in paneling, cabinets and home furnishings) to form harmless byproducts:

$$HCHO \text{ (formaldehyde)} + 2O_3 \rightarrow CO_2 \text{ (carbon dioxide)} + H_2O \text{ (water)} + 2O_2 \text{ (oxygen)}$$

It reacts similarly to convert many other toxic chemicals such as solvents, ammonia, and plastics. By reacting with and deactivating chemicals ozonation can also reduce odors around the house.

Low levels of ozone are not toxic in an acute (short-term) sense to most people. However, with prolonged exposure there is the potential for long-term free radical damage which is linked to cancer and other degenerative diseases. This risk should be weighed against the benefit of having other hazardous substances removed from the air. Optimally an ozone generator should be turned up when nobody is home, and down when people are in the room.

How well do these cleaners work on smoke?
Tobacco smoke consists of very tiny particles and gases, and is harder to remove from the air than dust. Many air cleaners will change a strong fresh-tobacco-smoke smell to a faint stale-ashtray smell, which some people find even more objectionable.

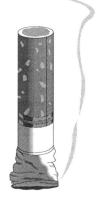

Vacuum your troubles away?
Use a central vacuum or water-filtered vacuum cleaner to pull out pollutants without redistributing them. Meile and Rainbow are two brands that work well for this purpose.

How do you know what type of air cleaner to get?
The best type of air cleaner for you depends on what your major pollution problems are - dust, smoke, gases, dust mites, etc. Another major consideration is financial.

Most air cleaners are rated with a CADR number. CADR stands for clean air delivery rate, which is the number of cubic feet of clean air a unit delivers each minute. The higher the CADR rate, all else being equal, the better the unit is at cleaning your air. The more effective units, not surprisingly, cost more. Other factors to consider is noise level, as even the quietest cleaners tend to drone. A certain amount of maintenance is needed for most types of cleaners, consisting of cleaning or replacing filters [7].

Exercise

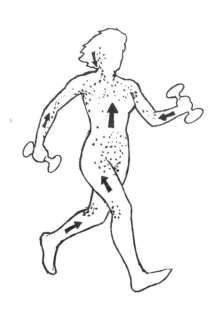

Why is exercise so important?
We are designed to move. Use of the body leads to growth and repair, while underuse leads to atrophy, or withering of the muscles. Those of us who don't exercise much or at all become less physically functional and we lose our strength and endurance over time.

Other systems of the body are linked to the assumption that we will move regularly. The lymph nodes, especially dense in areas such as the neck, under the arms, in the groin, and behind the knees, are designed to be pumped to move toxins out of the body. These areas are the ones that are moved during walking and other exercise.

Lymph is pumped when you run - as the heel goes up, lactic and uric acids enter the bloodstream and acidify the blood, keeping the pH at the desired 7.35-7.4, which also discourages fungus growth.

What are the benefits of exercise?
There are a wealth of exercise benefits. These include [8]:

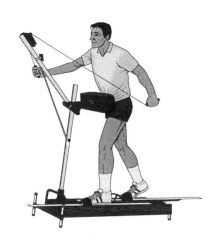

- *Increase energy and stamina*
- *Maintain proper weight, redistribute weight*
- *Increase suppleness and flexibility*
- *Strengthen heart and stimulate circulation*
- *Sleep more soundly, need less sleep*
- *Relieve stress and tension*
- *Learn self-discipline, increase self-esteem*
- *Strengthen the immune system*

- *Detoxify by working the lymph system*

- *Breathe better, use lungs more fully, get more oxygen to cells and tissues*

- *Firm and tone muscles, increase muscle strength and endurance*

- *Exercise releases brain chemicals called endorphins, which act as a natural tranquilizer.*

- *In women, exercise increases progesterone and reduces estrogen, potentially easing PMS and cramps.*

Exercise has been proven to help one live longer. Going from a sedentary (non-active) state to a physically trained state can reduce a person's biological age by ten to twenty years. In a Stanford University study, 16,936 Harvard alumni, ages 35 to 74, were followed for 12 to 16 years. They found that death rates were a third lower in those who burned at least 2000 calories a week exercising [9].

The muscle fiber of people who don't exercise becomes marbled with fat, like the muscle meat of a steer that has been penned up [10].

Many native tribespeople of Africa and other continents think little of walking or running thirty or more miles a day. Although some of them, such as the Masai of East Africa, eat a diet high in meat and milk products, they have a very low rate of cardiovascular disease [11]. Such a diet would be a significant risk factor in the average sedentary American male. Other native tribespeople exercise and eat as their bodies were designed to, and have a very low rate of nearly all chronic illnesses compared to Americans.

Exercise has been shown to reduce the intraocular pressure of glaucoma by 20%, in a study involving sedentary glaucoma patients doing 40-minute exercise sessions four times a week for 12 weeks. However, intraocular pressure returned to pretraining levels three weeks after stopping the exercise [12].

Help your flame burn brighter

There are three types of exercise, and the best one or ones for you depends on what you are trying to accomplish.

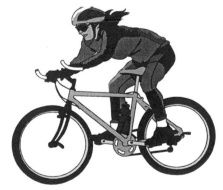

- *:Aerobic, or oxygen-using*
- *Anaerobic, or weight-bearing*
- *Slow-movement*

Exercise can be aerobic or anaerobic. Aerobic refers to oxygen-using, and takes oxygen from the body and therefore from the cells. In so doing it starves the cells to a certain extent, which helps them to build larger, more numerous, and more effective mitochondria, the power plants of the cell. The more mitochondria you have, the more energy you will have and the more fat you will burn. Since the heart is a muscle, cardiovascular health is also increased with aerobic exercise.

Aerobic exercise provides more oxygen to the cells and organs of your body. Oxygen causes a flame to burn brighter and cleaner, and in your body can increase your metabolic rate so food is converted to energy more efficiently (cleaner burning).

Aerobic exercises are those which can cause you to be short of breath after a while, including:

- *walking*
- *running*
- *bicycling*
- *jogging*
- *rowing*
- *skiing*
- *fast dancing*
- *jumping rope*
- *skating*

A steady sustained motion for at least 15-20 minutes is necessary for the aerobic effect to kick in.

Do weight training and sports also have benefit?

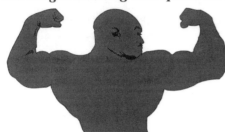

Anaerobic exercises are those which do not involve sustained motion and will usually not cause you to be out of breath. Although they do not build mitochondria, they have other benefits, such as toning and strengthening muscles and strengthening bones. Anaerobic exercises include weight lifting, most sports (motion is not sustained), and exercises on most types of gym equipment. One type of anaerobic exercises are those that focus on building up or toning a specific group of muscles, such as the pectoral (chest) muscles, arm biceps, or legs.

Weight bearing (anaerobic) exercise in one's 20s and 30s and beyond can lessen the damage from osteoporosis, or bone loss. Osteoporosis is associated with aging, especially in women, but it may well be a disease more of inactivity than of aging [13].

How can you keep your joints flexible and stabilize your structure safely and effectively?

Slow movement exercise such as Tai Chi is discussed in the Structural chapter in *Surviving The Toxic Crisis*. Its goal is to recruit muscle spindle bundle fibers and maximize range of motion. Muscle fibers are to the body what suspension cables are to a bridge. They stabilize your body's structure. Slow movement exercise also works the lymph glands, which help in detoxification. They also work the capillaries, getting circulation to muscles and cells, and even helping to bring back atrophied muscles.

Yoga and some forms of dance are also slow-motion-type exercises. These types of exercises can be done by almost anyone, even without a prior physical exam.

What type of exercise is best?

The answer to this question depends on your exercise goals. No one plan is best for everyone. A combination of the two is best; aerobic is better for overall health if you want to choose. It is important to find something you like to do, or you are unlikely to stick with it for very long.

How much exercise is desirable?

If you are basically sedentary (not very active), then even small amounts of exercise will have some benefit. There is no one magic number of minutes which is optimal for everyone.

Is it possible to exercise too much?

Yes, one can overdo it. Overexercising can lead to loss of too much body fat. A certain amount of body fat is necessary for optimal body functioning, especially for women. If a woman's body fat level drops too low, she can stop menstruating and become infertile, since the body senses famine conditions and decides that procreation could result in the loss of both mother and baby.

Exercise raises metabolic rate, the rate at which food is burned for energy, but only up to a point. Overexercising, with the resulting drop in body fat, alerts the body to famine conditions and the need to conserve fuel. The metabolic rate then drops.

Too much exercise can also cause stress on joints and bones. If you are in pain, rest; don't push yourself too far or you may cause injury.

Exercise can contribute to stress if the exercise is regarded as a grim duty.

What should you do before starting an exercise program?

It is advisable to get a physical checkup before starting a major change in behavior, such as a strict diet or exercise program. It is especially crucial to check cardiovascular health using a stress test, in which heart rate and blood pressure are monitored while exercising on a treadmill. Check also for structural problems, which can be worsened by the wrong type of exercise.

It is important to learn how to exercise properly to minimize harm to the body. A sports medicine practitioner or gym instructor can give this advice, or there are many books and magazine articles on the subject. Manufacturers of exercise equipment can steer you in the right direction, but be aware that their primary purpose is to sell their product, and the salesperson may not be sufficiently knowledgeable to help you with your health concerns.

Stretching to warm up before exercise, and to cool down after exercise, are important to avoid injury and shock to the body. Proper equipment is necessary to maximize benefits and avoid injury. This equipment includes good shoes which absorb 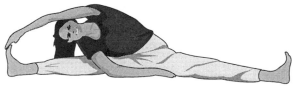 shock from pounding, and specialized gear such as bicycle helmets or shin guards depending on the type of exercise.

Drink plenty of water, although cold water can cause stomach cramps. A body that is working hard and sweating needs more water than one at rest. Electrolytes such as sodium and chloride (salt), potassium, magnesium, and calcium are also lost through sweat and need to be replaced.

How can you increase your motivation to exercise?

Many people are convinced of the benefits of exercise, but have a hard time sticking with a program. They join health clubs that they stop attending after a few weeks. They make New Year's resolutions that don't last. They buy expensive exercise equipment that soon gathers dust in the garage. Sound familiar?

What's wrong with the logic here?

> *1. Health is my first priority.*
> *2. Exercise is an important part of staying healthy ... but*
> *3. I don't have time to exercise because of my other priorities.*

Is it time to rearrange your priorities?

What can you do to stay on an exercise program? There are a number of things you can do to increase your chances of success [8].

- Evaluate your goals - weight loss, strength, appearance, energy - and choose an exercise program appropriately.

- When you think about exercise, you make a choice: exercise or excuse. Only action, not intentions, gets results. Be aware of this if excuses are your pattern. Accept full responsibility for your behavior, rather than blaming circumstances.

- Choose an exercise that you like to do, or you are not as likely to stick with it.

- Write down specific daily exercise goals, and check them off when done.

- Remind yourself of positive associations with exercise, such as feelings of well-being, taking in the scenery while running, or the weight you have lost so far. This is especially important when negative thoughts threaten your success.

- An exercise partner or group can supply some of the willpower you may be lacking. A commitment to someone else is often taken more seriously than a commitment to yourself.

- Past history, such as the many previous failed attempts, need not have any bearing on the present - unless you let it.

- Focus on the benefits, not the activity.

- Use music with a beat, a video, or reading when exercising (when appropriate) to keep your mind busy and help set a pace to keep you going.

- Picture yourself in a body that looks, feels, and works as you want it to.

These suggestions can also be applied, with slight modification, to the other programs in this and other books.

Sleep

Why is sleep necessary?

The active energy producing functions are in use during the day, or more accurately during periods of wakefulness. Repair, restoration, rebuilding, and healing take place primarily during sleep.

What happens if you don't get enough sleep?

Sleep deprivation can occur as an occasional event such as a late night party, or can build up over time as many busy people get slightly less sleep, or poorer quality sleep, than they need. Insufficient sleep can cause a number of symptoms, many of which have been shown by clinical experiments. Some symptoms of sleep deprivation are:

- Daytime fatigue and sleepiness, although fatigue has an almost infinite number of possible causes.

- Reaction time is slowed considerably after sleep deprivation, important when driving or operating dangerous machinery.

- Irritability, or a lessened ability to cope with the stresses of daily life.

- Disorientation and a spacey feeling.

- Severe sleep deprivation can lead to hallucinations and psychoses. It is as if the mind were so intent on dreaming that a pseudo-dream state occurs when awake.

- Fibromyalgia, or generalized body pain, can occur with sleep deprivation, since the body's repair and restore functions which occur during sleep may be deficient.

Interestingly, these are also symptoms of chronic fatigue/ chemical sensitivity, although sufferers get plenty of sleep. There may very well be a connection. A person who is dealing with toxins and allergies is sympathetic-dominant and doesn't spend enough time in parasympathetic rebuild-and-restore mode. Since the parasympathetic mode is accessed mostly during sleep, a sleep-deprived person may have many of the same symptoms of parasympathetic deprivation.

What is the connection between sleep and the immune system?

Chemicals originating in normal intestinal bacteria cause certain body cells to produce substances called interleukin-1 and cytokines. These have two functions - they stimulate the immune system and make people sleepy [14]. This may be why people who are ill usually feel more sleepy than usual, at least during the day.

Why is this significant? The immune system may help us to sleep, and sleep enhances the immune system. Conversely, too little sleep may result in immune system dysfunction, or a faulty immune system may be one of the many causes of insomnia.

Is sleep deficit common?
In this busy world, many people are shortchanged on both quantity and quality of sleep, and the deficit is usually cumulative. With so many obligations, many of us view sleep as something expendable, and get used to cutting back. Teenagers and mothers with young children are most likely to be getting less sleep than they need.

How can you tell if you are getting enough sleep?
You may not be getting enough sleep if you experience one or more of the following:

- You don't wake up naturally around sunrise.

- You regularly need an alarm clock to get up.

- You don't feel refreshed when you awaken, and you feel even worse if you go back to sleep.

- You nod off during the day, especially if you're bored.

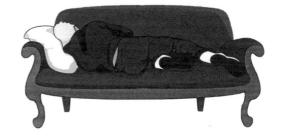

- You feel like you must have a nap to get through the day.

- You sleep less than seven hours a night for five or more continuous nights.

- You have trouble concentrating, or are often irritable or impatient.

- You are dependent on external substances such as coffee or alcohol to wake you or help you sleep.

Any of these symptoms can be due to poor sleep rather than to sleep deficit, or to factors other than sleep.

Is it possible to get too much sleep?
Yes, an adult should not need more than nine hours of sleep. Paradoxically, too much sleep can cause drowsiness and fatigue because spending too much time in bed can lead to lighter sleep levels and more fragmented sleep.

A person may sleep too much because of depression or avoidance of an unpleasant task. Such a person will often experience a strong desire for a nap or early bedtime, thus allowing postponement of the task.

How much sleep do you need?

The amount of sleep needed varies greatly by age. The older one gets, the less sleep is needed. Some sleep needs by age are [15]:

- *Infant*   *14 to 16 hours*
- *Two to ten years*   *10 to 12 hours*
- *Teen*   *9 to 10 hours*
- *Adult*   *7 to 8 hours*
- *Elderly*   *5 to 6 hours*

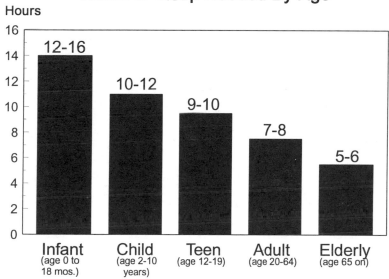

What are the different levels of sleep?

There are five sleep levels in an adult. Four of these are called alpha, beta, theta, and delta, the first four letters of the Greek alphabet. The levels get progressively deeper from alpha to delta [16]. Delta sleep is the stage in which physical restoration occurs, including increased protein synthesis and growth hormone production.

The fifth level is called REM sleep. REM stands for Rapid Eye Movement, and was so named when sleep researchers in the 1950s found that this stage was when dreams occur.

What is the purpose of dreaming?

Dreams are believed to have beneficial, in fact necessary, effects. Experiments with rats have led to the theory that the animal integrates what it has learned during the day with what it already knows to increase its survival chances [17,18]. The application of this theory in humans suggests that we also integrate the day's events into memory to improve our functioning.

How important is dreaming?

Experiments done as early as the 1950s involved waking people whenever they entered REM sleep, although they were otherwise allowed to sleep as much as they wanted. By the next night they increased the number of periods of REM sleep as if to make up for lost time. These subjects soon became irritable, less coherent in speech, and their reaction time decreased. Control subjects were wakened an equivalent number of times during non-REM periods, and their waking behavior was that of people who were well rested.

Subjects deprived of REM sleep but who could otherwise sleep as much as desired closely resembled those who were sleep deprived overall. Both sets of deprived subjects started hallucinating after several days of deprivation, suggesting that they were dreaming while awake. Results of these studies suggest that dreaming is perhaps the most important part of sleep.

What can cause insomnia?

Many things can cause lack of sleep or poor sleep, known as insomnia. These include:

- Vitamin and mineral deficiencies, especially calcium and potassium

- Amino acid deficiencies, especially tryptophan and tyrosine. Tryptophan converts to melatonin, enabling you to go to sleep. Tyrosine converts to norepinephrine, allowing you to stay asleep.

> **Deficiencies of potassium, tryptophan, tyrosine and melatonin can all contribute to insomnia.**

- Adrenal malfunction, causing disturbance of the circadian (day/night) rhythm.

- Night work, which also upsets the day/night rhythm

- Heavy meals late in the day put a load on the digestive system just when the body's systems need to wind down for the night.

- Hypoglycemia (low blood sugar) can cause one to awake with cravings.

- Anemia

- Sugar eaten before bedtime can cause a rise in the level of blood sugar and a temporary energy lift which becomes sleeplessness at night. It can also cause nightmares.

- Allergies can cause many symptoms, including sleeplessness.

- Drugs such as alcohol, sleeping pills, caffeine, and smoking

- Chemical toxicity, like allergy, can be responsible for insomnia. Toxins can adversely affect neurotransmitters, and detoxification procedures can help.

- Pinworms come out of the anus to lay their eggs at night, and the resultant itching can be a cause of nighttime restlessness.

- Toxic emotions such as anger and guilt can keep one awake.

- Too little exercise during the day, or exercise too late in the evening

- A depressed immune system

- Fungal or bacterial infection

- Sunglasses during the day or bright lights at night can confuse the brain's normal day/night cycles and behavior.

> **Sunglasses during the day or bright lights at night can confuse the brain's day/night cycles.**

- Poor sleep can be caused by electromagnetic interference such as that from electric blankets, heated waterbeds, and electric clocks near the head [19].

- Insomnia in infants is often due to cows' milk allergy. This may be a possible factor even in breastfed infants if the mother drinks cows' milk [20].

Can't sleeping pills and alcohol enable one to sleep better?

Sleeping pills cause a person to fall into a state that resembles sleep but does not go through the stages that characterize recuperative sleep. The REM stage is particularly affected, and people on sleeping pills do not dream as much as they need to. Eventually they develop symptoms similar to those in sleep-deprived people. After a long period on sleeping pills (as little as a few weeks), tolerance (lack of effect and a need for more) develops, then rebound insomnia.

Alcohol is a depressant drug which helps one to fall asleep but actually causes wakefulness later at night. Alcohol taken with sleeping pills or other depressant drugs such as barbiturates can form a dangerous or even lethal combination.

What nutrients can relieve insomnia?

Useful mineral supplements, which should be taken before bedtime, include:

- Calcium has a calming effect on the central nervous system and can aid sleep if taken before bed.

- Magnesium is a natural sedative.

- Potassium deficiency can cause insomnia that is characterized by tossing and turning with your thoughts racing

- Zinc deficiency can also be a factor in insomnia.

- Deficiency of iron or copper has a profound effect on sleep patterns.

The amino acid tryptophan, taken at night, converts to melatonin and can help you get to sleep. Tryptophan is no longer available as a supplement but is found in milk and poultry. The amino acid tyrosine, taken in the morning, can help you stay asleep if this is your problem. These two amino acids can be antagonistic, so if taking one worsens your symptoms try the other.

Vitamins can also be useful:

- B vitamins, especially vitamin B6, regulate the body's use of many amino acids, including tryptophan, which converts to the calming neurotransmitter serotonin. Vitamin B6 can improve dream recall.

- Vitamin B3 (niacin) increases the effect of tryptophan and prolongs REM sleep.

- Folic acid deficiency was found to be linked to sleep problems.

- Vitamin B12 and inositol were found to relieve insomnia [21].

What else can relieve insomnia?

Regular exercise helps one sleep better, perhaps by more clearly delineating the periods when one is active and when one is resting. In a study done at Duke University, older men who exercised regularly slept more deeply and were awake less often during the night than sedentary controls [22]. Exercise should be done in the morning or early afternoon; exercising too close to bedtime can keep you awake by raising the body temperature and cortisol levels at a time when they need to drop to prepare for sleep.

Stress can cause insomnia, and stress reduction can reduce the amount of time spent tossing and turning. Toxic emotions such as anger, guilt, fear, and worry can keep one awake for hours.

Reducing noise and light levels can bring about sleep. Too much noise can be distracting, and too much light can fool the body into thinking it's time to be awake. Cooler temperatures are more conducive to sleep than warmer ones. A comfortable bed also helps.

Sleep restriction may seem like a strange way to go about getting more sleep, but it may be an effective way to reset your body clock. Wake up early, using an alarm clock if necessary, do not take naps, and go to bed when you are tired. After a few days of sleeping six or so hours, you may be tired enough to sleep properly.

There are about 200 sleep disorders clinics in the United States [23]. Although there are other sleep disorders, insomnia heads the list in prevalence. These clinics can be useful if all else fails. Looking at the things in this chapter should solve over 90% of sleep problems.

Herbs that are especially useful in treating insomnia include chamomile, valerian [24], linden flowers, Siberian ginseng and licorice. Chamomile and valerian should be taken about 45 minutes before bedtime [25].

What is the connection between sleep and light?

When daylight enters the eyes, the pineal gland in the brain is stimulated to make melatonin, which is a hormone-like substance that is associated with sleep and circadian rhythms. It synchronizes your sleep and energy cycles with the cycles of sunlight and darkness. Melatonin is manufactured in the brain during the day and released at night to aid in sleep. A deficiency of melatonin can lead to sleeplessness.

Melatonin is both a natural sleep regulator [26] and a powerful free radical neutralizer which has promise as a cancer preventive and treatment adjunct. One major purpose of sleep, therefore, may be the processing of free radicals, to which one is most exposed during the day [27].

Melatonin is not the same thing as melanin, the brown pigment in skin that darkens with sunlight.

How can you increase melatonin levels?
Sunglasses or colored contact lenses can interfere with melatonin synthesis by not allowing the full spectrum of sunlight in through the eyes to the pineal gland. Letting natural sunlight into your eyes without these colored barriers can increase the amount of melatonin produced. Full spectrum fluorescent lighting approximates the beneficial full spectrum light of the sun.

It is best to wake up with the sun, allowing early morning light into your house and your eyes. The antidepressant response to morning light is often accompanied by a shift of nighttime melatonin release to an earlier time [28]. There is wisdom in the saying, "Early to bed, early to rise..."

In addition, waking with the sun stimulates the adrenaline levels to provide energy for the coming day. Going back to sleep after waking in the morning keeps this mechanism from working properly, leading to grogginess that can last all day.

Night shift work, which leads to sleeping during the day, can contribute to sleeplessness because not enough sunlight enters the eyes when the person is awake. Switching to the day shift if possible can reverse the melatonin deficiency.

Melatonin is available in supplement form. It should be taken about fifteen minutes to an hour before the desired bedtime; after a few days of the supplement, your body clocks should be reset and sleep should come easier. However, if you wait until two in the morning to take it, after hours of tossing and turning, your internal clock will be reset incorrectly.

What can we learn from flowers?
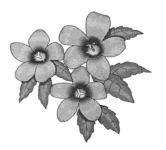
Although most flowers bloom during the day in response to sunlight, some varieties bloom at night. Such flowers will bloom at night even if they are kept in a dark closet during the day. This suggests that there may be some sort of nighttime radiation that the flowers are responding to. The same nighttime radiation may be tied to yet another reason we should sleep at night rather than during the daytime.

What are some other sleep problems?
There are sleep disorders other than insomnia. These include:

- *Sleep apnea*

- *Narcolepsy*
- *Sleepwalking*
- *Nightmares and night terrors*
- *Nocturnal myoclonus*
- *Bruxism*

Sleep apnea is a condition in which breathing stops for up to a half minute when the throat muscles become too relaxed and collapse, blocking breathing. The person, usually an overweight male, wakens in order to breathe. Although sleep apnea interferes with sleep, it is rarely fatal.

Narcolepsy is a condition causing one to fall asleep abruptly during the day, sometimes many times a day. This is different from a growing feeling of sleepiness during a dull lecture. Those with narcolepsy should not drive motor vehicles. Smoking cigarettes in bed, never a good idea, is particularly dangerous for a person with narcolepsy who could nod off suddenly and set the bedding on fire. A detoxification diet, exercise, and resetting of sleep patterns can help narcolepsy.

In **sleepwalking**, the person walks around and does things without waking up or remembering the episode on awakening.

Nightmares are frightening dreams which may or may not awaken the dreamer, while night terrors involve awakening in terror with no memory of associated dreams or images. Both of these can be tied to sugar, alcohol, fungal problems, or electrical charges given off by metals in the mouth. Past traumatic events such as war or rape can lead to nightmares as the mind attempts to use dreams to come to terms with these experiences.

Nocturnal myoclonus is a sudden jerking of the limbs during sleep which awakens the person suddenly.

Bruxism is the grinding of teeth during sleep. Bruxism can keep one from reaching REM sleep, and can lead to TMJ syndrome, a structural disorder that can cause many symptoms. It is sometimes caused by metals in the mouth that produce an electric current.

Two things that can affect sleep patterns are the effects of toxins and amino acids on neurotransmitters. Toxins can adversely affect neurotransmitter function, and one often-reported effect of detoxification procedures is improved sleep. Sleep, as well as mood, appetite and other functions, have long been known to be under the control of neurotransmitters that themselves are influenced by their precursor amino acids. The availability of certain types of hormone building blocks from protein, i.e. the avoidance of deficiencies, can thus influence sleep [29].

> **The ability to sleep well can be dramatically improved after detoxification procedures.**

Light

Light, natural sunlight in particular, enters the eyes and stimulates the pineal gland in the brain. This in turn stimulates the adrenal glands to produce adrenaline, which is why you are, or should be, energetic during the day. Without light, you would not know day from night.

Staying indoors all day or wearing sunglasses or colored contact lenses keeps all frequencies of the sun's full-spectrum light from entering the body. The result can be fatigue and sleep disturbances. So-called full-spectrum lighting used indoors can help. Ideally, you should get the sun's beneficial light by walking around outside without sunglasses. Your skin as well as your eyes will absorb the light energy and your whole body will benefit.

If the body doesn't get certain light wavelengths, it may not be able to fully absorb certain nutrients [30]. Poor illumination can contribute to fatigue, depression, hostility, suppressed immune function, strokes, hair loss, skin damage alcoholism and drug abuse, Alzheimer's disease, and cancer [31]. Poor lighting has also been linked to a loss of muscle tone and strength [32].

Exposure to full spectrum light has eased high blood pressure, depression, insomnia, PMS, migraines, and carbohydrate cravings [33]. Full-spectrum light has been positively correlated to the prevention of breast, colon and rectal cancers [34].

Sunlight, especially the ultraviolet frequencies, can have many beneficial effects from absorption through the skin and eyes [35], as shown in this graphic.

It is well known that excessive sunlight exposure can

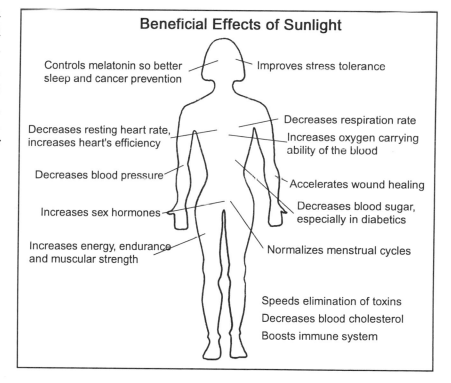

initiate skin cell changes that can lead to skin cancer, especially with repeated deep tanning or severe sunburn. These changes are particularly likely in those with light skin. However, sunlight in moderation can actually inhibit cancer formation and growth by increasing the tissue oxygen level and boosting the immune system [35].

The use of sunscreen is a mixed blessing. It can block out both the harmful burning rays and some of the beneficial effects of sun. In addition, sunscreen may also contain toxic chemicals itself. It may be better to forgo the sunscreen but instead limit your sun exposure and increase it gradually.

Sunlight has been shown to be more useful than heat from other sources in easing arthritic pain and stiffness. It can take several weeks before beneficial results are observed.

In the 1800s tuberculosis patients were exposed to sunlight and fresh air, a sign that sunlight may help kill bacteria as well as boosting the immune system.

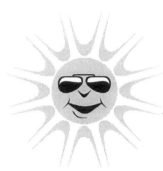

Sunlight also benefits wound healing, sores, ulcers, jaundice, gout, psoriasis and acne.

Vitamin D, long known as the Sunshine Vitamin because its effects depend on the action of sunlight, is more like a hormone than a vitamin. It is likely that sunlight has activating effects on other hormones as well. Sex hormones, especially testosterone in the male, have been shown to increase with sunlight exposure.

The importance of light and color, and the effects of different types of light and different colors, are discussed in the chapter on Electromagnetic Radiation - Other Frequencies in *Surviving The Toxic Crisis*.

References and Resources

- The Burton Goldberg Group, *Alternative Medicine: The Definitive Guide*, Future Medicine Publishing, Puyallup WA, 1994. *Chapters of interest:* "Light Therapy", pp. 319-329; "Sleep Disorders", pp. 838-848.

Water

- Batmanghelidj, Fereydoon, *Your Body's Many Cries For Water*, Global Health Solutions, Falls Church VA, 2nd ed.

- Ingram, Colin, *The Drinking Water Book: A Complete Guide to Safe Drinking Water*, Ten Speed Press, Berkeley CA, 1991.

Air

- Baker, E., *The Unmedical Miracle - Oxygen*, Drelwood Communications, Indianola WA, 1991.

Exercise

- Cooper, Mildred and Kenneth, *Aerobics For Women*, Bantam Books, New York, 1972.

- Diamond, Harvey and Marilyn, *Fit For Life II*, Warner Books, NY, 1987.

- Fixx, James F., *The Complete Book of Running*, Random House, New York, 1977.

- Kostrubala, Thaddeus, *The Joy of Running*, J.B. Lippincott Co., Philadelphia PA, 1976.

- Tulloh, Bruce, *Natural Fitness*, Simon and Schuster, New York, 1977

- Turock, Art, *Getting Physical: How to Stick With Your Exercise Program*, Doubleday, NY, 1988.

Sleep

- Dotto, Lydia, *Losing Sleep*, Quill, NY, 1990.

- Ferber, Richard, *Solve Your Child's Sleep Problems*, Simon and Schuster, NY, 1985.

- Hauri, P. and Shirley Linde, *No More Sleepless Nights*, Wiley Press, NY

- Kaufman, Daniel, and Philip Goldberg, *Everybody's Guide To Natural Sleep*, Jeremy P. Tarcher, Los Angeles CA, 1990.

Light

- Amber, Reuben, *Color Therapy*, Aurora Press, Santa Fe NM, 1983.

- Dinshaw, Darius, *Let There Be Light*, Dinshaw Health Society, Malaga NJ, 1985.

- Hyman, JW, *The Light Book*, Ballantine Books, NY, 1991.

- Kime, Zane R., *Sunlight*, World Health Publications, Penryn CA, 1980.

- Kime, Zane R., *Sunlight Could Save Your Life*, World Health Publications, Penryn CA, 1980.

- Liberman, Jacob, *Light: Medicine of the Future*, Bear & Co. Publishing, Santa Fe NM, 1993.

- Ott, John Nash, *Health and Light*, The Devin-Adair Co., Old Greenwich CT, 1988.

- Ott, John Nash, *Light, Radiation, and You*, The Devin-Adair Co., Old Greenwich CT, 1982.

- Walker, Morton, *The Power of Color*, Avery Publishing Group, Garden City Park NY, 1991.

- **Environmental Health & Light Research Institute**, 16057 Tampa Palms Blvd., Suite 227, Tampa FL, 33647. Phone 800-544-4878. *This institute continues the pioneering work of John Ott.*

- **Society for Light Treatment and Biological Rhythms**, P.O. Box 478, Wilsonville, OR 97070. Phone 503-694-2404. *Provides information on Seasonal Affective Disorder.*

Emotions Plus

-

The Psychological Connection

EMOTIONS PLUS

Your Life View - Toxic Or Terrific

What is the importance of this chapter?

Most of this book focuses on the physical, but a book on comprehensive health would be incomplete without a chapter on the connection between the body, mind, and spirit. What we feel, think and believe - our outlook in these areas - affects and is affected by the state of our physical bodies.

> **"What is true is true whether you acknowledge the author or not"**
> -Sherman Brees

An understanding of how the emotional and spiritual can influence the physical aspects of illness, including the reasons and ways you may be holding onto your illness, can lead to change. Emotional and spiritual change in turn, can be the key to your physical healing which opens the door to greater overall health.

Certain non-physical components of your make-up can either perpetuate your disease or help you overcome it. This chapter shows you how to recognize unhealthy patterns and replace them with healthy ones.

How is emotional overload related to physical overload?

Have you ever felt you were in emotional overload? One crisis after another piles up until you reach a point where you feel like, "I just can't handle another thing!" This can show itself as depression, or losing control and yelling and throwing things, accompanied by feelings of loneliness, resentment, guilt, and other unhealthy and debilitating emotions.

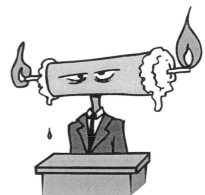

When the body is in toxic overload from chemicals, metals, and microorganisms, it, too, can reach a crisis - that "I can't handle any more" stage, with many of the symptoms described throughout this book. The body and the mind can therefore react similarly. In addition, the cumulative effect of stressors - both physical and emotional - contributes to the state of total physical and emotional overload.

What, besides the emotional, defines the non-physical side of a person?

There is more to us than the sum total of our physical being. The non-physical side encompasses both experiential and intangible attributes, such as:

- Spirituality - relationship with a higher power, or God, and a feeling that all things happen for a greater purpose, rather than by blind luck or chance.

- A sense of purpose or purposelessness; goals to strive for in achieving your life's vision; a sense of direction.

- Service to others vs. self-serving.

- Intellect - knowledge and curiosity motivating choices leading to achievement vs. fear of failing and looking stupid, causing an inability to make choices, often manifested in procrastination.

- Creativity - producing and appreciating beauty, vs. becoming closed off, stagnant and self-protected. In another and broader sense, creativity means opening up new possibilities and options, and seeing new ways of doing things.

- Social - warm caring relationships with friends and family, or hostility and a begrudging attitude leading to isolation.

- Pressure of stress, which can move us towards accomplishment or be a source of worry and debilitation.

- Habits and lifestyle - life supportive habits vs. destructive addictions

Consider the human make-up in its three components -- (1) the physical body; (2) the soul (comprised of mind, will and emotions) which through intellect and reason we receive and interpret input, and through out emotional make-up and the components of personality, gifts and creativity we make volitional choices through an act of our will tempered by conscience.

A third component is spirit - not God's but our own personal spiritual capacity to commune with the unseen, through which we can have access to a Higher Power/God.

The self can be defined as a combination of all these things -- the inner expression encompassing heart, soul, intellect, reason, emotion, personality, gifts, creativity and will, while the outer expression is manifested in how one acts out, their image and fashion and reputation.

How are body, mind, and spirit interlinked?
Much evidence has accumulated to demonstrate that what goes on in the mind and spirit can have a direct physical affect on our health.

- Prayer was found to have positive effects on people with high blood pressure, heart attacks, wounds, and headaches [1].

- Thinking positively and believing in your healing has caused remission and healing of cancer and other diseases, as shown by the work of Dr. Bernie Siegel [2].

- Willpower, a product of the mind, is responsible for many positive physical health changes as a result of being able to quit smoking, drinking alcohol, and overeating.

- Norman Cousins, in his book *Anatomy of an Illness*, described how laughter and humor worked for him and others in relieving debilitating disease.

- Service to others can take your focus off your own problems and redirect it towards a higher purpose, and in the process bring about healing and peace of mind. "If you seek to save your own life you will lose it." In other words, by focusing outward you realize an expansion of life that is continually growing and open to new experiences versus an inner focus that produces an ingrown and stifled life. You lose the full experience of life in its fullest aspects because you are bound in a small cosmos of the self, and fail to realize the fullness of potential to which the human spirit can ascribe, and for which you were created.. Could this create disharmony and an inner "dis-ease" at odds with experiencing that full potential which might eventually be manifested in a state of physical disease? - This is something to think about.

Optimism is important. It holds open the door of hope. One's own self-evaluation of health is a good predictor of well-being and future health. In other words, the healthier you think you are, the healthier you will probably be in the future [3].

Studies in England and the U.S. have shown that 50-75% of all health problems presented to a primary care facility have an emotional base or are social in origin, although they are being expressed in physical symptoms such as pain or illness [4,5].

In the overall scheme of things, our outlook has more to do with the outcome of our lives than most of us are aware of or willing to admit. There is also a lot going on behind the scenes that has a direct effect on body and mind, and is often manifested in the physical.

Hormones and prostaglandins connect the mind and body. Unresolved stress, such as worry, overworks the adrenal glands, which affects cortisol levels, and which, in turn, affects immune system function. And immune system function affects your entire body.

Adrenaline is a neurotransmitter which works in both the mind and body as a sort of "junction box" between the two. In a kind of physical/mental domino effect, if you worry cortisol is released, which can take away from the raw material, pregnenolone, which makes both cortisol and DHEA. Cortisol is an anti-inflammatory hormone which, like cortisone, suppresses the immune system. DHEA, on the other hand, can increase productive energy. A measurable physical change which can be picked up on hormone panel tests as well as affect your energy level and immune system can thus be determined by something as basic as your outlook.

How do the emotional steps to healing mirror the physical steps to healing?
Let's review the seven steps to healing which are discussed in greater detail in the closing chapters of ***Surviving The Toxic Crisis***:

1. *Eliminate toxins and allergens from your environment and your life.*
2. *Clear toxins from your body.*
3. *Unblock pathways, clear allergies.*
4. *Nutritional / biochemical support.*
5. *Align and balance body structures.*
6. *Kill / control opportunistic pathogenic microorganisms.*
7. *Optimize and fine-tune, rebuild and reinoculate the system, for example by adding protective bacteria such as acidophilus and bifidus.*

There are similar steps to psychological healing.

1. *Control toxic environmental influences where possible.*

2. *Identify toxic attitudes, such as judgment, anger, fear, guilt, greed, or control, and eliminate them from your life. Replace them with positive attitudes.*

3. *Make choices that are within your control, but accept, forgive and make peace with that which isn't within your control.*

4. *Serve and support others and thus yourself through outward service and life purpose goal setting.*

Genetics

What are some of the factors beyond your control?
You are dealt a certain hand at birth. Most parents of more than one child can notice temperament differences between their children almost from birth, such as calm, fussy, shy, outgoing, easily frustrated, etc. It becomes clear that there are factors in who we are that have nothing to do with environment.

Some of the factors that influence who we are include:

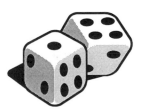

- *Gender - male, female*
- *Birth order*
- *Race and/or ethnic heritage*
- *Basic temperament*
- *Physical attributes - attractiveness, athletic ability, physical or mental handicaps*

All of these things can have a bearing on how we live our lives and how we handle illness. In these areas we can learn to play the hand we're given with the cards we're dealt. Three out of four great Americans achieved their greatest success in compensation for, and/or in spite of, the givens.

Let's look at some of the differences between males and females

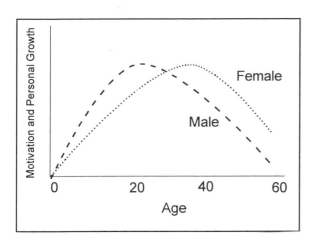

Men typically hit their peak - physically and sexually, and in drive and motivation - at around age nineteen. They get much of their identity from school, job, and sports. A woman of that age often derives a good part of her identity from the male and may look forward to starting a family. Hormonal shifts can cause a change in the scenario twenty years later, however. The woman at forty is now coming into her own. Her children are raised and married or off at school. She is going back to school or getting a job, and standing on the threshold of new challenges and opportunities. The man at forty is now losing a good bit of the sex drive, motivation, and attractiveness of his youth. He either has achieved his dreams and realized his victories, or begins to see that he won't achieve his dreams. While his dreams, motivation and sexual prowess seem to be waning, the woman at this age sees hers accelerating. This realization can precipitate a mid-life crisis and a re-evaluation of the future.

Although of course there are individual differences, the stereotypical male may tend to attack, get defensive, or cut off communication, while the female may withdraw or attack directly or indirectly. The man may hide behind his newspaper or the television while the woman may attack out of hurt - nagging and belittling him. The woman, especially, may revert to passive-aggressive behavior ("Not tonight, dear, I have a headache").

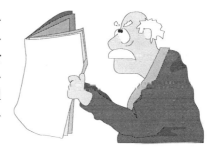

In dealing with disease, the man is more likely to seek refuge in denial of the existence of problems or illness, and the woman is more likely to feel victimized. The stereotype is of a hard-driving type-A man with high blood pressure who keeps going until he drops (11 out of 12 men die before their wives). Often the early warning sign of a heart attack is sudden death. On the other hand, the stereotypical woman experiences many small nagging symptoms, among which may be low blood pressure, which motivate her to seek help. Approximately 80% of doctor visits are by women.

In the past, both genders at an early age tended to follow the plan that was given to them by society and by their parents. Men worked, women raised the family. Today's culture, with increasing divorce rates and single parent households is sending out a whole different set of signals, so both male and female can be driven both by innate hormonal differences and by social/cultural influences. They may take their life's purpose or vision and try to pass it through their parents' belief system and then complain about undesired results. At a later age they may develop their own self-concept and set their own goals. But these two value systems can be in conflict for the rest of the person's life because they are trying to balance "because of my parents" with "in spite of my parents". And in the process, they often end up a lot like their parents.

Men and women typically go through these stages whether or not they are in a relationship. Recall the graph of men's motivation going down and women's going up with age. If one is in a relationship with the opposite sex at or near the intersection point, sparks may fly. This is around age forty, an age at which the divorce rate peaks and personal crises abound. This period is often referred to as the mid-life crisis, and interestingly enough, many women develop chronic illness at around this age (about 35-45).

By age 70 one often sees the woman leading the now compliant man - he goes along to get along, but he is just longing for a place to relax and find peace.

How does birth order influence who we are?

Each child in a family, in a sense, doesn't get born into the same family. For example, if you are a woman with an older brother, you have an older brother but he doesn't. He has a younger sister but you don't. The makeup of the family he lives among is different than the make-up of the family you live among, and this is likely to make a difference in who the person you or he grows up to be.

Birth order has a lot of influence on temperament, and a lot of this influence has to do with expectations. Although there are, of course, individual differences, the first or only child tends to grow up with a lot of high expectations and discipline, and the parents are usually more insecure in their child-rearing than they are with subsequent children. The first-born, therefore, is often a high achiever due to high childhood expectations. The first-born is also often a leader or director, since they are used to being the oldest, the one who is caretaker of the younger ones and the one they look up to. They may pick up on the nervousness of their first-time parents and develop a tendency toward perfectionism.

The last-born is typically the baby of the family. Born into a ready-made group of siblings and taken care of by relaxed parents who have benefited by the child-rearing experience, the last-born is more likely to be relaxed, independent and sociable, and less career-driven than his/her older siblings.

Middle children tend to combine the traits of both first-born and last-born children, and to be peace-makers and communicators.

What are the different temperament types?

A common model divides the different temperament types into four categories. Contemporary authors Gary Smalley and John Trent [6] have assigned animal names - lion, beaver, otter, and golden retriever - corresponding to characteristics of temperament associated with these animals. Hippocrates broke up the categories into phleg-

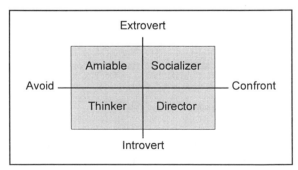

matic, melancholy (not related to sadness as the word is used today), choleric, and sanguine. Dr. Tony Alessandra [7] named the groups by function: director, thinker, socializer, and amiable. Whatever the name used, these various designations have been in use for a long time, and have certain things in common.

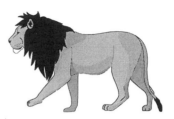

The **Director**, also called Lion (king of the jungle) or Choleric, is not afraid of confrontation, is decisive, is a leader, tells rather than sells, and wants immediate results. This is the stereotype of the New York City attitude. Such a person is more goal oriented than people oriented.

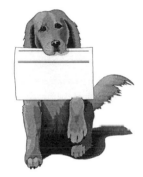

The **Thinker**, also called Beaver (industrious worker) or Melancholy, is a perfectionist, makes careful decisions, and tends to turn anger inward. Ideas and thoughts are more important than relationships. School degrees and recognition are important.

The **Socializer**, also called Otter (playful) or Sanguine, is fun-loving and a kidder, sells via confrontation and humor, is a good motivator, has many superficial friendships, and is affected by peer pressure.

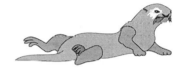

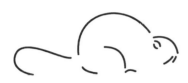

The **Amiable** personality, also called Golden Retriever (loyal) or Phlegmatic, has a strong need for close relationships, wants to make people happy, and is compassionate. Relationships are more important than accomplishments. Such a person tends to "keep score".

One's backup position (your second most likely pattern) is generally the one opposite the primary one on the chart. For example, the Thinker who is a perfectionist at work is likely to be a socializer at parties in a relaxed change of pace, especially if drinking alcohol. Amiables when forced to confront can become Directors, resenting the person who forced them to do the confronting, while Directors relax at home as Amiables, stereotypically with a poodle named Fifi which is in stark contrast with their macho hard-driving work personality. Rosie Greer, defensive lineman for the L.A. Rams, took up needlepoint in his leisure time, and nobody called him a sissy. Socializers can spend some of their backup time thinking and planning (like a Thinker) their next social performance.

Are Directors the only leaders?
U.S. presidents of the past 50 years are of all four types:

Amiable	*Jimmy Carter*
Socializer	*Ronald Reagan, Bill Clinton, Franklin Roosevelt, John Kennedy*
Director	*Harry Truman, Lyndon Johnson, Theodore Roosevelt, Dwight Eisenhower*

> *Thinker*   *Woodrow Wilson, Richard Nixon*

Playing to your strengths

One can find people of all four types in other professions as well. However, certain temperaments are found more in some choices of profession than in others:

> *Thinkers*   *Technicians - doctors, engineers, CPAs, inventors*
>
> *Directors*   *Leaders - CEOs, armed service officers, police*
>
> *Socializers*   *Sales, marketing, public relations, art, performers, motivational speakers*
>
> *Amiables*   *Service occupations, secretaries, nurses, support staff*

Each personality type contributes significantly to our society and plays a necessary role. Each character attribute has both strengths and weaknesses. Our weaknesses can keep us sick and immobile or our strengths can pull us out.

How do different temperament types react to disease?

Your predominant temperament type may have a lot to do with how you handle your personal conflicts, disease, or stress. For example, an Amiable who hates conflict may take on a victim role. The Director may either deny that there is anything that will slow him down or he can take charge and actively work to get well. Directors typically get "blowout" diseases such as high blood pressure and heart attacks, while the conflict-avoiding Amiable is more likely to develop a chronic illness such as chronic fatigue or low blood pressure.

How does the way a person handles problems affect their health?

How you handle conflict is often the way you handle disease: avoid conflict, feel unworthy and helpless and/or become a victim, keep score, hold in anger and grudges, and become depressed. Others will take action, or lay blame, deny, feel guilty, or accept the disease or problem passively.

A person who is told that s/he has a few months to live might either:

> 1. *pretend that it isn't so*
> 2. *write their will and prepare to die, or*
> 3. *research ways to fight the illness.*

> **You have a choice - fold or fight.**

You have a choice - fold or fight.

Age, gender, and personality type all enter into the way a person handles disease and the stresses of life:

> *Thinker*   *Will read articles and do research on survival methods*
>
> *Amiable*   *May feel victimized and enroll people in their story, rather than actively working to get well*
>
> *Director*   *Either denial until it's too late or an all-out frontal attack on the disease*

Socializer   *Talk to many professionals for information, use the power of positive thinking. Their backup position is to give up and enroll people in their victimization.*

Are these innate differences beyond your control?

There is very little that is beyond your control - to some degree. **Change is inevitable, growth is not**. But if you are strongly motivated to change and do what is necessary - and this applies to healing physical illness as well as personality traits - then there is a better chance that you will be successful. These differences are only as im-

> **"We are what we choose to be or we'd change."**
> John Boyle

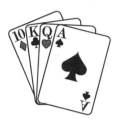

portant as you make them. Your choice - Are you willing to do whatever it takes to get well, or do you just want to not feel ill?

Life is like a card game - you are dealt a certain hand, but what you do with it is up to you. We are who we are in spite of, or because of, the cards we were dealt.

Deterministic Psychology

What variables do you have control over?

While gender, physical type, and personality type seem to be more or less "cast in stone", there are certain aspects that influence you which you may have some degree of control over, and which are environmental rather than genetic factors:

- *Where you were raised.*
- *When you were raised.*
- *How you were treated.*

How does where you were raised influence your life?

The geographical area in which you were raised also has an influence on your personality. As with any stereotype, there are many individual variations, but there is more than a grain of truth in the stereotype.

Farm country   *Hard worker, responsible, sees cause and effect, work before play*

Big city   *Less belief in cause and effect, live for the moment, getting ahead, accomplishment-oriented*

East coast city   *Confrontive, direct, hard driver, pragmatic, open to new ideas but only if they work*

Midwest   *Hard worker, traditional family values, closed to new ideas, "show-me" attitude*

West coast   *Mixed values, confrontation avoidance, passive resistance, creativity, less upfront, appearance important, peer values, open to new ideas*

Southeast   *Nonconfrontive, compliant, hospitable, traditional family values, slow to change*

These seeming stereotypes may have a greater or lesser effect on the individual. Being born or raised in a country other than the United States will also have an effect on temperament. Each country's heritage has an impact. There is some truth to ethnic generalizations: Scottish and Germans are seen to be frugal, Italians demonstrative, etc. However, **you can choose to play on stereotypes or reject them.**

How does your age play into the picture?

An important question is "What shape was the world in during your high school years?" The era in which you came of age, even more than your earliest years, has a great bearing on how you view the world and react to life's events. The eras and their effect are:

Years	Era	Values	Popular Magazine
1920-30	Prohibition	Strong moral values	Life, Look
1930-40	Depression	Security oriented, frugal	Life, Look
1940-50	World War II	Uncertainty, national pride	Life, Look
1950-60	Postwar	Carefree years, financial success, materialism	Time, Newsweek
1960-70	Rebellion	Rejection of parents' values, materialism, and hypocrisy	Rolling Stone
1970-80	"Me Generation"	Drugs, sex, self-centeredness	People
1980-90	Still the "Me Generation"	Self-centeredness	Us, then Self
1990s	Backlash	Back to traditional "family values"	Focus on the Family

If you are either a frugal, plan-ahead person or a "live-for-today" person, this may be a reflection of the time in which you grew up. As with gender and other generalizations, there are variations, and these of course do not apply to everyone. However, they were a hallmark of the times.

It is interesting to note how these things come full cycle. True values such as integrity were a part of the depression era. Then came the image of truth which spawned the hypocrisy of the

50's, a world where anything that interfered with the image - spousal or child abuse, teenage pregnancy, wrongdoing on the part of authority figures, homosexuality - was carefully hidden and denied.

The 60s were a decade of rebellion against the phoniness that characterized the 1950s. The 1970s seemed to be a decade of rootlessness, as those who knew what they didn't want didn't know what to replace it with as they had few role models. The backlash against the freedom and rebellion of the 1960s characterized the 1980s and 1990s, as the children of the 1960s did not want that irresponsibility, rebellion and contempt for authority to be characteristics of their own children. The current Family Values emphasis and the longing for community expressed by many may be a reaction to the "do your own thing" focus of the 60s.

How do the expectations of others influence your life?

Values are caught more than taught

The expectations of others can greatly influence how you perceive the world, although as an adult you have control over how much of an influence you will let this have on the rest of your life. For example, if a child is raised with love, trust, violence, discipline etc., this will have a lot of bearing on whether the adult s/he grows into will be trusting and self-disciplined or suspicious and self-indulgent.

Typecasting within a family often occurs, based initially on a slight difference which is magnified over the years until it becomes part of the person's self-definition. A child may be typecast as the smart one in the family, or the pretty one, the clumsy one, or the lazy one. People tend to live up - or down - to the expectations of others.

A word from a respected person in the child's life such as a teacher, relative or significant other can have a huge influence. How many people can remember a significant event or person from their childhood that affected the whole course of their life - for the good or the bad? Many people have given up art or music, or changed their college major, based on a single conversation with or remark from a teacher.

Childhood years are very influential for another reason also. Time seems to speed up as a percentage of our lives as we get older. For example, a year is 100% of the life of a one-year-old, 10% of the life of a ten-year-old, and only 1/60th of the life of a 60-year-old. This could explain why time seems to fly faster as one ages. Each year, therefore, has a diminishing influence on the whole as we get older. However, a slight change in the early years can alter the later years to an increasingly greater extent, just as a very slight change of trajectory angle on earth can cause a rocket to hit Jupiter or miss it by a million miles.

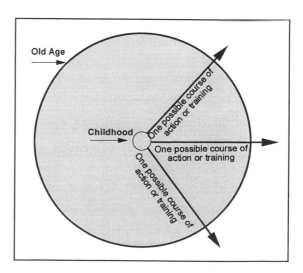

What part does race play?
There is little or no definitive evidence that race or ethnic group, by itself, has a bearing on temperament. However, the way society views our particular racial or ethnic group can have a large effect on behavior and self-concept. Certain racial and ethnic groups have been cast in the mold of being lazy, studious, hard working, dishonest, or frugal. And if one allows this to affect their life, they may become these things in part because they have internalized the projections and prejudices of others. As Carl Rogers so eloquently expresses:

> "We are not what we want to be.
> We are not what others want us to be.
> We are what we think others want us to be."
> - Carl Rogers

Jesus expressed it in another way, "As a man thinketh in his heart, so is he."

A sad aspect of human nature is the need of those who feel inferior to try to make others look bad so they can feel good about themselves. Labeling others as inferior takes away from their personhood and makes them objects of hate and less than human. This makes it easier to treat them as less than human. This technique was used to bring about the Holocaust that destroyed millions of lives.

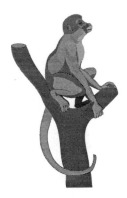

An unknown sage wisely concluded, "Throwing dirt just loses ground". Indeed the human race loses ground when any part is demeaned by the other.

The way different races are treated may be related to the universal fear of that which is different. Consider the way monkeys are driven off in Ethiopia. Villagers who want to drive off monkeys because they are stealing food and getting into mischief simply capture one monkey, paint it a different color, and release it unharmed to join its group of monkeys. The other monkeys run in fear from this now-different-looking monkey, and leave the village. In much the same way we may run in fear from that which is unfamiliar.

So what?
There are obviously many genetic and environmental influences that have an impact on who we are. These can be:

- *maximized to justify your life*
- *minimized and dismissed as "so what?"*
- *realistically viewed as a starting point for a self-examined life where you strengthen weakness and develop strength, thus exerting an influence without being*

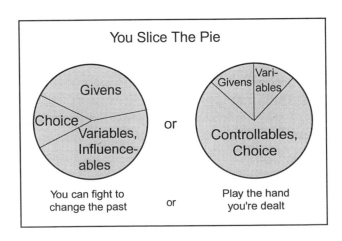

You Slice The Pie

You can fight to change the past   or   Play the hand you're dealt

controlled.

"The unexamined life isn't
worth living."
Socrates

The choice is yours.

It is important be aware of and to understand these many influences so you can make a conscious decision about whether you want to embrace a particular value or behavior in your life. This is why so much time has been devoted to understanding these influences. To get where you want to go, it is important to know where you are.

> To get where you want
> to go, it is important to
> know where you are.

What are some definitions, distinctions and concepts that are useful in the discussions in this chapter?

There are some key definitions, distinctions and concepts that are useful in following the discussions in this chapter, and which will prove to be useful in everyday life. Definitions are important in terms of semantics because some terms have different meanings to different people, which can create misunderstandings. In the following discussions, some terms may be used in ways that are not standard English usage, but they get the point across.

Distinctions, such as those between envy and jealousy, or between kind and nice, are discussed a bit later in this chapter. These distinctions are crucial so that the image of growth is not mistaken for true growth.

Three In One -- The Worlds We Live In

We exist in three worlds - the world of truth (World I), the world of image and rules (World II, and the world of rebellion (World III) against the rules of World II. As a physical example, the sunlight is truth or real light (World I), the moonlight is the image of light without being true light (World II), and darkness is the opposite of light (World III).

These concepts are amplified and examined throughout the rest of this chapter. They are, in fact, so important that they are the central theme of much of the rest of the chapter. You will be able to see which world you and others are in, in different circumstances, and see more clearly where you need to be to live in the world you choose. We all exist in, or visit, all three worlds at one time or another. But the question is - in which one are you going to build your house and live?

Clutch words - Suppose you have a car. The engine is running, but the clutch is in. The rear wheels will then not move and you can't go forward. The engine is your life's vision, and the purpose and the goals, which are steps toward achieving your life's vision. The transmission is your belief system. The rear wheels are the results. Are you moving forward in gear, or going nowhere with the clutch in?

Accomplishment knows no such thing as trying or working at - just doing

Some clutch words are: **trying, want to, working on it, going to,** or as they say in Texas, **"I'm fixin' to do."** These words give a false sense that something is really happening when in reality nothing is being accomplished. For example, *try* to pick up a book from your desk. This is impossible to do. You are either picking up the book or you're not. *Trying* to stay on your health program, for example, is just as meaningless in terms of actual results. Using clutch words gives you the illusion of accomplishment in the counterfeit world of content-free image, or hypocrisy, of World II.

Prostitute can have a wider meaning than it has in its usual sexual context. A prostitute can be said to be anyone who becomes what people want them to be for a payoff, such as acceptance, money or power.

Love - True or sacrificial love means "I want what is best for you, what best serves *your* needs". For many people, what love means instead is "I want or expect you to do or be what *I* want, and if you do as I say then I'll give you acceptance". In terms of the above definition of prostitute, this is what such a person who professes to love is asking their loved one to be.

Choices

What choices can you control? What choices control you?
There is much that is within your control. One can choose one's attitude even in the face of extremely difficult circumstances. Dr. Victor Frankl, a German Jew who spent years in a concentration camp during World War II, found that attitude and a sense of purpose often made a difference in who did and who did not survive the experience. How you view the circumstances of your life is the only part you can completely control, and can be the catalyst for change.

How important is integrity (World 1)?
Integrity means keeping your word, doing or being exactly what you say. Violation of your own integrity can contribute to illness by causing stress and conflict within yourself and with others.

What are some different ways of being?
The concept of three worlds is seen here. You can:

> 1. Live the truth (World I) . . . . *Truth seekers*
>
> 2. Live the image of truth, i.e. a lie (World II) . . . . *Self image Presenters & Rule Makers*
>
> 3. Rebel and refuse to live the lie of World II (World III) . . *Rebels Against Rule Makers*

In the chart that follows, many examples that compare and contrast the three worlds are used to convey the differences between truth, image and lie. The examples are clearer than an attempt to explain the differences. Some of the distinctions between terms are discussed following this list.

Column One, on the left, represents World I choices, i.e. living in truth. Column one choices describe that which is true and genuine, and it involves acting with integrity, having nothing to hide, and serving others with no ulterior motives.

Column Two, in the middle, represents World II choices of the rule makers or the image of truth, i.e. hypocrisy. World II choices allow one to be comfortable with a lie that has the image of truth. Here are people who can be very powerful and rich in a political organization. They tend to grow huge organizations they can control, and will eliminate anyone or anything that stands in their way.

Being self-deceived, these individuals may believe they have the truth because they look like they do, rather than being open to it and searching for it. On the surface, the image of truth (World II) only looks bad when it's compared to truth (World I); but it looks good when compared to the rebel (World III), who refuses to live a lie. On the surface, the actions of a World II person may look like World I, but the difference is they are motivated by self-serving and self-protective intentions.

According to Dr. Tim LaHay, **"In tough situations, who you are under pressure is who you really are."**

Column Three represents World III, the refusal to live a lie. World III choices are made by those who know they don't want to live a lie; they know what they don't want but have not yet found what best serves them and others. On the surface, World III choices look like the least desirable of the three alternatives. But these choices are actually more honest than those in World II, because those who choose them refuse to live the lie of the hypocrite in World II, who in turn condemn them because it makes them in look better by comparison.

In the long run, people living in World III are more likely to make a turnaround and move into the World I life of truth than are those who are living the lie of World II. When they see real truth of Grace vs. Rules, they are more likely to want more and start searching for truth, whereas the people living in World II who are content with image, believing they are the truth.

We're really talking about the choice of being a "giver" or a "taker" in life - serving or being served.

A good illustration of serving and giving vs. taking can be seen by comparing the Sea of Galilee and the Dead Sea. The Sea of Galilee has water flowing through it from the Jordan River, with lush green growth on its banks. By contrast, the Dead Sea, which is also fed by the Jordan River, is stagnant and there is nothing growing around it - it is like a barren wasteland. It is stagnant because it has no outlet. It takes, but gives nothing back.

Only by elevating our perspective are we free to change our point of view. It's the difference between being able to see the whole forest versus being surrounded by all the trees. Or like being lifted out of hostile fire by a helicopter rather than defending our foxhole.

Areas of life such as finances, outlook, physical health, and lifestyle, categorically will fall into one of these three worlds. Where we end up living by the choices we make will determine whether we dwell in the sunlight, the shadows or darkness:

- *The truth = sunlight*

- *The lie, or more accurately the shadowy image of the truth, or sunlight) = moonlight. (Without the reflection of the sunlight, there is no moonlight).*

- *Refusing to live the image of truth and having neither sunlight nor moonlight = darkness*

Here's a suggestion - circle the one description of the three on each line that best describes you, and then take a look at the overall pattern of your life and see if this is really where you want to be, realizing we exist in all three worlds. But which one do we build and set up our homes in?

Be aware that these are given as examples, for reference purposes, not as 100% definitive of the whole. It allows you the opportunity to reflect and to identify aspects of feeling, and how we see and feel about each group. Much like the trunk of the elephant being only one of many facets of the overall picture, if you discard what you don't understand you may miss out on understanding the overall picture.

WORLD I	WORLD II	WORLD III
Living the Truth (Authentic)	**Living a Lie (Counterfeit)**	**Refusing to Live a Lie**
Seeker of Truth	**Preserver of Self Image**	**Resister of Rules**
	Rule Makers	
Physical health		
Well	Not ill, feeling okay	Sick
Fix the root cause	Suppress symptoms	Feel symptoms
Feel great	Suppress pain	Pain
Natural energy	Energy using stimulants	Fatigue
Personal growth and outlook		
Integrity	Hypocrisy	Unacceptable behavior
Live in integrity	Make rules	Rebel against rules
Forgive	Excuse	Hold a grudge
Peace	Rest	Restlessness
Confidence	Arrogance	Cockiness
Joy	Happiness	Unhappiness
Actual character	Image of character	No values
Discerned reasoning	Positive thinking	Negative thinking
Unconditional love	Conditional love	Apathy or hate
Self worth	Self image	Feeling of worthlessness
Kind	Nice	Mean

406

Opportunity (get to)	Obligation (have to)	No opportunity (don't get to)
Power	Strength	Weakness
Seeker of truth	Seeker of success	Seeker for self
Request what you want	Manipulate to get	Take what you want
Authentic	Hypocritical	Don't care what others think
Do	Try	Don't try or do
Results	Effort	Give up
Free to choose	Controlled by society	Victim of society
Humble	Shy, bashful	Arrogant, proud
Secure	Self protected	Insecure
Right thing for right reasons	Right thing/ wrong reasons	Wrong thing/ wrong reasons
Play the game	Watch the game	Miss the game
Success	Achievement	Failure
Self-disciplined	Society disciplines	Not disciplined
Clear communication	Garbled communication	No communication
Hot	Lukewarm / Cool	Cold

Service, giving

Share, give	Barter	Hoard, take
Live justified life of service	Justifying your life	Self serving
"I'm here for you"	"What's in it for me"	Stealing what you want
Serve others to help them	Caretaker for own needs	Serve self
Welcome	Put up with	Unwelcome

Spiritual, Religious

Spirituality	Religious	Anti-religion
Spirituality/Freedom	Cult/Control	No Religious belief
Holy	Self-righteous	Unrighteous
Justice	Legalistic	Hedonistic
True	Good	Evil
Reward in heaven/paradise	Reward on Earth	No reward
Devotion to scriptural growth	Scripture not lived	No scripture
Praise of God	Praise from people	Condemnation
Given	Earned	Unearned, stolen
Atoned	Earned/Works	Unearned
Fear Offending God/Awe	Fear God's Judgment	Fear of conforming, being uncool

What you stand for

Committed	Involved	Apathetic
Justice	Legality	Illegality
Master = Truth	Master = Rules	Master = Self
Person of conviction	Manipulation of people	Refusal, rebellion
Life of truth	Image of right	Wrong
Absolute values	Situational ethics	No ethics

Financial, abundance

Deferred gratification	Immediate gratification	Conspicuous consumption
Investors	Savers	Spenders
Abundance	Limited resources	Deficiency
Ownership, clear title	Credit / Consumption	No money or credit
Stewardship	Ownership	Borrowing

Other, Attitude

Yes	Not now	No
Win	Beat others	Lose
Build people up	Put others down	Quit trying
Embrace	Approve	Disapprove
Friend	Acquaintance	Enemy
Praise	Flattery	Slander
Love	Infatuation, Lust	Obsession
Happy for others' success / thankful	Jealous	Envious
Discern truth for self	Judge others	Judge those who judge
Secure	Comfortable	Restless
Childlike innocence	Mature	Childish
Fairness	Equality or parity	Unfairness
Science	Political science	Science fiction
Privileges	Rights	No rights
Discernment	Judgment	No discernment
Adult	Child	Teenager
Statesman	Politician	Anti-government

Creating an image may make you appear "cool". But are you really cool?

- *It's cool to be normal but uncool to be average.*
- *It's cool to understand but uncool to ask questions.*
- *It's cool to achieve and have things but uncool to work.*
- *It's cool to be negative but uncool to be positive.*
- *It's cool to be mysterious but uncool to be open and upfront.*

Cool can't win. Accomplishment is achieved by the uncool innovators.

You reap what you sow. For example you must ask questions (uncool) before you can understand (cool).

You can choose to live in the world of light and truth (I), the shadowy world of maintaining an image (II), or the darkness of the lie (III) - it's your choice.

What are some of the finer distinctions?

Simple vs. **Easy** (World I vs. World II) - Just because something is simple doesn't mean it's easy, although the two words are sometimes used interchangeably. For example, the way to quit smoking is simple: just do it. However, as many people can attest, it is far from easy. As with changing any negative habit or pattern, it takes about 14-21 days to establish a new one.

> **Just because something is simple doesn't mean it's easy**

Shame vs. **Guilt**- Shame is for who you are. Guilt is for what you do.

Praise vs. **Flattery** (World I vs. World II) - Praise is genuine and given for the benefit of the person being praised. Flattery seems like praise on the surface, but there is often an ulterior motive - gaining the favor of an influential person, for example.

Childlike vs. **Childish** (World I vs. World III) - Childlike embodies qualities like innocence, a sense of wonder and an eagerness to learn. Childish means self-centered, victim, pouting, throwing tantrums.

Spirituality vs. **Being Religious** (World I vs. World II) - Spirituality versus being religious is the difference between a personal relationship with God versus a set of rules and judgments that produce an attitude of self-righteous superiority over others and condemnation. For as we judge, we will be judged.

Jealousy vs. **Envy** - Jealousy, for the purposes of this discussion, is wanting to have what someone else has. Envy is not wanting *them* to have it. Jealousy can be a positive motivating force for personal change so you can learn to earn what the other person has, while envy is generally destructive to anyone who has what you want.

Some people reverse these two definitions, while others feel that envy is for things (wanting a new car like the neighbor's) and jealousy is for people (the feeling some people get when their boyfriend/ girlfriend dates someone else). This is not about the right vs. the wrong word usage, but rather a means to have definitions in common so that an idea is communicated effectively. The important point here is that there is a difference between envy (beating the other person) and jealousy (wanting to win the race and have the victory).

Jealousy vs. envy is illustrated in the law of gravity of relationships. If a person is higher than you on the ladder of success, knowledge, etc., they are often willing to help you up the ladder. As you get closer to them on the ladder, they are often less willing to help you. As you are even with them, envy starts entering the picture, and as you pull ahead of them, envy may make them try to pull you down. This kind of behavior belongs in Worlds II and III.

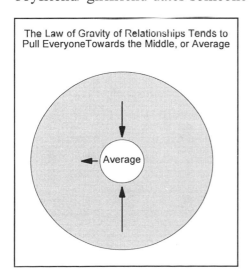

The Law of Gravity of Relationships Tends to Pull Everyone Towards the Middle, or Average

Average

Kind vs. **Nice** (World I vs. World II) - Kind is a way of being that has the other person's best interests at heart. Nice considers the person's feelings in the short run. For example, kindness is telling a friend that she has spinach between her teeth before she goes in for a job interview. Nice is refraining from mentioning it to save her momentary embarrassment, or more accurately saving yourself from the discomfort of saying anything.

Discernment vs. **Judgment** (World I vs. World II) - Discernment is making reasoned choices for oneself, while judgment is deciding what others should be doing and feeling superior when they fall short. Those in World I have given up the right to judge others.

> You can accept the way things and people are without having to approve of them

"You can disagree without being disagreeable".

-Dr. David Hawkings

Adult vs. **Child** vs. **Teen** (All 3 Worlds) - A child blindly obeys, while a stereotypical teenager rebels, i.e. deliberately does the opposite of what is expected. An adult makes her/his own decisions from a standpoint of maturity. All of these are a matter of outlook, not age.

Spirituality vs. **Cult** (World I vs. World II) - For someone involved in a particular religious belief, it may be hard to tell the difference from the inside. Very few people in a cult believe they are in one, even if it is obvious to observers. How can you tell the difference? The hallmark of true spirituality is the freedom to choose, not an attempt to control, as in a cult. Proponents of a spiritual belief system encourage you to be all you can be, rather than what they want you to be.

As discussed in the chapter on Testing Methods and Bias, any belief system with most or all of these characteristics can be said to be a cult:

- There is a central living person - a charismatic leader, guru, or priest - whom followers worship and try to emulate. This person makes the rules that you are expected to obey. Without this person's leadership the organization may well fall apart.

- Considerable amounts of your money or the value of your work ends up in the pockets of the leader or organization.

- You are told what to believe, and to the greatest extent possible, kept from reading or having other points of view.

- Information that conflicts with that which the cult wants to promote is denounced as being wrong and evil. You are strongly discouraged from making up your own mind.

- People are kept from nonbelieving family members as much as possible. Isolation from the outside world in general is typical of a cult.

- Many cults use sleep deprivation and poor nutrition to keep their adherents' minds too clouded to think or question.

Power vs. **Strength** (World I vs. World II) - Power comes from inner strength. Outward strength is situational and can go as fast as it came. For example, strength may depend on greater physical strength, having a gun or means of coercion, or being promoted to a management position.

Committed vs. **Involved** (World I vs. World II) - Commitment has a greater depth than involvement. For example, in a ham and egg breakfast, the hen is involved, but the pig is committed. In life, are you willing to commit to something even if the going gets tough - in it for the long haul - or are you involved in a cause only as long as it's comfortable? It is said that Napoleon burned his own ships so the only way his men could get home was to conquer the enemy and take their ships. His action changed the motivation of his men from being involved to being committed.

There is a parallel here in the way one can triumph over addictions - removing the metaphorical ships can lead to increased commitment. In practical terms, this means:

- *The alcoholic removes the alcohol and bars from his life*
- *The sex offender removes pornography from his environment*
- *The gambler removes himself from casinos and racetracks*
- *The overeater removes junk food from the refrigerator and cabinets*
- *The compulsive spender stays away from the mall and cuts up the credit cards*

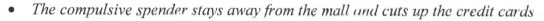

It's hard to be addicted to what you're not exposed to!

The individual then stays away from these things, acknowledging his/her weakness. As Jesus said, "Go and [do these things] no more, or a worse thing will come upon you." This is like a person who goes on a diet to lose weight, but then reverts to their old ways and not only gains back the lost weight, but more besides; now their problem is more critical and harder to overcome. They needed a commitment to a changed lifestyle, not just a temporary involvement in dieting.

Addictions are also discussed later in this chapter.

Justice vs. **Legalism** (World I vs. World II) - True justice is not situational, while the law can change or be interpreted arbitrarily. Justice, for example, is driving safely, while legality refers to the posted speed limit, which can change. Many people confuse these two. For example, if an "alternative" doctor cures someone's cancer using a method other than surgery, radiation or chemotherapy, is this legal? Strange as it may seem, no. Is it just? Absolutely. Look at the intent, not the written law.

Science vs. **Political Science** vs. **Science Fiction** (All 3 Worlds) - Science is what works reproducibly. Political science is the name sometimes given to the image of science for the sake of personal or political gain. An example of this is the governmental regulation of herbs and supplements for the stated purpose of saving people from their own gullibility, while the real reason could be to keep profits in the pockets of the pharmaceutical companies. Science fiction is not science either, but at least it doesn't pretend to be. Truth is truth, whether or not it's "politically correct".

Joy vs. **Happiness** (World I vs. World II) - True joy is long lasting and comes from deep within oneself, while happiness is usually temporary and depends on circumstances or happenstance.

Win vs. **Beat** (World I vs. World II) - To beat someone means that someone else has to lose. To win in its optimal form means that everyone wins. Our only true competition is with ourselves.

Growth vs. **Change** (World I vs. World II) - Growth is improvement, getting closer to a goal, evolving with a plan. Not all change is growth. Atrophy is change.

"Change is inevitable, growth is not" - John Boyle.

True Fairness vs. **Parity** or **Equity** - Everyone has a different view of fairness. It tends to be situational and self-serving. Reason is no preagreed absolutes. Parity is same as others in like circumstances. A good guideline is to treat others as you would want to be treated if you were them - Equity. True Fairness is Parity and Equity.

Privileges vs. **Rights** (World I vs. World II) - Rights are defined here as those things which nobody can take away. Thus the only true rights are the right to die (although not necessarily the choice of time or place) and the right to the choice of our beliefs. All else, by this definition, is privilege, including such things as: free health care, gun ownership, enough food for all children, nondiscrimination on the basis of race, sex or creed, or driving a car. Since these are privileges, not rights, they will have to be defended from time to time, or be lost by default, apathetically given away.

This discussion is about which attitude would best serve you - many things are rights, or all things are privileges. Seeing a long list of things as rights, many of which we are not in fact granted by government or circumstances, breeds resentment. Seeing as many things as possible as being privileges rather than rights breeds gratitude. Which would you rather feel, resentment or gratitude? The choice to a great extent is yours.

What are toxic attitudes?
Toxic attitudes can be as toxic to the body as are physical toxins such as chemicals and metals. Many of the choices in Columns II and III can be toxic, although for different reasons. Toxic attitudes include things like negativity, legalism, prejudice, and labeling. Legalism is focusing on the rules rather than on what is just, true and fair. If you

tend to use words like right, wrong, good and bad, this is a key that you are living in the world of rules (Columns/Worlds II and III). If you define yourself by what you are against, rather than what you are for, this is a sign of a toxic life view in general because it can bring on anger, resentment and finally depression (also known as frozen anger).

Are labels, or image, running your life (World II)? Or is content more important (World I)?

Many people let labels that they apply to other people get in their way. Do you? Imagine that you are in a conversation with someone about anything of importance - truth, philosophy, health care, politics, etc. You are seriously considering what they are saying. Then imagine that you find out that the person is a Republican, Democrat, Christian, non-Christian, a high-school dropout, a smoker, or any other label that you find distasteful, or that clashes with your values.

> **Are labels running your life?**

Would this change your opinion of the other person or his/her acceptability to you? Would you dismiss the messenger along with message? If so, you may be allowing labels to run your life, dismissing truth and value for trivial reasons and living in the world of image. Look for the truth in people rather than focusing on isolating any often trivial differences. Truth is truth regardless of who the author is.

Ask yourself: Why should others be different than what they are just because you would like them to be? You can choose not to be irritated by their differences. True love embraces even the differences, as compared with justifying one's position by only accepting people who agree with you.

Love means replacing a toxic life view with the question: how can you best serve the people you are against - for *their* best good, not your own good or beliefs?

Beliefs - spiritual and otherwise - that lead to a greater purpose outside ourselves, goals and visions, and service to others can be as healing as proper nutrition or healthful treatments.

* * * * * * * * * * * * * * * * *

Do you justify continuing your position rather than changing?

> **Do you justify continuing your position rather than changing?**

Many relationships run into problems because one or both of the participants would rather be right than build bridges to the other. Although being close is presumably their reason for being together, they seem to prefer justifying where they are and proving the other person wrong. Many people marry to make the other person happy, then they try to change the other to be more like themselves. The result: both partners are unhappy and resentful. If two people agree on everything, one of them is unnecessary. It doesn't really matter who is right or wrong; either can shift their polarized position or eliminate polarized conflict. Forgive and be free to ask forgiveness.

"Seek to understand before being understood."
- Sherman Brees

Relationships are like ligaments - when ligaments are torn, repair may take surgery and rehabilitation, rather than just rest. When relationships are torn, it may take work rather than just time.

In the area of health, many people justify staying sick by getting angry at the clinic/doctor or other health care professional or facility for reasons that are trivial compared to enduring whatever inconvenience it takes to get their health and life back - the doctor doesn't return calls, the clinic is disorganized, the health care is too expensive, the staff doesn't care. That way they can stay sick, which may have become a familiar comfort zone. They can justify being sick - "It's not my fault, it's the doctor's". They get to play the victim. Do you want involved vs. committed ownership of your life? Seekers of honest truth have a world worth living for.

How does all of this relate to disease? What is the purpose of your illness?

It may seem hard to believe, but there is probably a payoff to your disease, although not a psychologically healthy one. What does your disease buy you? What is done for you that wouldn't happen if you were not ill? These things are payoffs. Some payoffs may be:

- Do you get others to work for you - shop, prepare your food, etc.? They make sacrifices in your behalf out of obligation because you're sick. Do you ever feel in charge or control since the household now revolves around you and your disease's special needs?

- Do you ever appear to have control over the world around you, an illusion of control that you might lose if you were well?

- Does the feeling of "I can't because I'm sick" vs. "I won't" ever relieve you of responsibility and accountability? You could have a built-in excuse to avoid anything you choose not to have the energy for.

- Does your illness ever keep others from getting close to you, which can be your position of safety?

- Do you ever get a lot of sympathy and attention from your illness?

- Do you get special rights, like a handicapped parking spot or other people getting things for you?

- Do others not dare to criticize you, since you can't help being sick?

- Do you play the victim? You get to tell your story to anyone who will listen, over and over again.

- Do you get financial benefits, such as disability payments, worker's compensation, or financial help from your family since you can't work? Why work if you can get paid for being sick?

- Do both you and others expect less of you?

- Do you ever take without giving, feeling entitled because you're sick?

- I would if I could, but I can't so I won't, vs. I choose not to. Take ownership. Don't be a victim of your circumstances.

Do any of these sound familiar? Honesty is very important here. Any or all of these payoffs can be a reason, albeit an unconscious one, to stay sick. If this shoe doesn't fit you, maybe you know someone in your life that it fits very well.

Does this mean that you caused your own disease?

Assigning blame is useless if not harmful. <u>Don't fix the blame, fix the problem</u>. It is important to deal with the situation as it is now and make the changes that you can, starting today, to have the best outcome tomorrow.

If blame of yourself or others is in your way, there are seven steps to deal with this:

1. Acknowledge the problem. Tell the truth in detail and stop lying.

2. Repent - commit to and stop doing the behavior, if self-blame is the issue. Stop justifying.

3. Forgive yourself. If done right your private world of shame and the fear of discovery will lose its power over you.

4. Forgive the other person. Forgiving is giving up the right to be angry and the power of holding others accountable, thus releasing yourself from being a victim of the shame or anger that tyrannizes and controls you. Anger is like acid - it eats away at your life.

5. Ask the other(s) to forgive you. This is both a practical step and an honesty check. If you feel you can't ask others to forgive you because of your assumption that you are right and they are wrong, then you haven't truly forgiven them, only excused them. Return to step 4. You know you've conquered this when you can ask the other to forgive you for being angry, etc.

6. You are now free to change your feelings, and a change in behavior follows, along with a healing of relationships.

7. Inasmuch as it is in your power, be at peace with all people.

Forgiveness, defined as the releasing of the energy that gets trapped in an endless replay of the hurt wrapped up in resentment, is a key to healing [8].

Can you make yourself sicker? - Justifying your sickness vs. getting well to live a justified life

People sometimes get sicker to prove they are sick and reap some of the payoffs listed above. They do their best to prove to parents, spouse, children, their insurance company, the disability board, the courts, and their doctors that they are really as sick as they claim.

For example, a woman who feels generally sick and tired and achy - and she isn't imagining this - wants to see a doctor to be diagnosed. Her husband scoffs at her fears and doesn't want to use their money for this purpose. His actions lead her to believe that money is more important to him than she is. The woman then has a reason to get sicker, although this operates at an unconscious level. In her logic, if she gets sick enough, her husband will hopefully show the caring, attention, and concern she so desperately needs from him. She sees herself as a victim of the tyranny of illness, and possibly also of her husband.

Most malpractice cases don't get well because they are trying to prove in court that they are sick. They expend a good deal of effort on justifying their illness and their lawsuit, and in many cases trying (consciously or otherwise) to *not* get well until the case is over. Their body says, in effect: Fine - you want this illness/ injury that badly. Okay, it's yours.

Author Anthony Robbins has defined insanity as doing the same thing over and over and expecting different results. It's self-deceiving and it doesn't work.

Is This Really Your Goal?

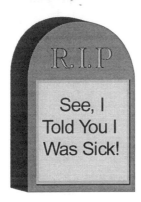

The logical outcome of this attempt to persuade others of the reality or severity of the illness, carried to its extreme, is a tombstone that reads "See, I told you I was sick!" Is this what you want - to be dead right? Stated another way, is your goal to prove you're sick or to get well? The answer seems obvious, but a surprising number of people expend more energy in telling their story and justifying their limitations than in letting go of their story and focusing on getting well. They say they want to get well, but make every excuse, rather than refusing to stay sick and doing whatever it takes to get well. With chronic illness, just wanting to get well is not always enough. You must refuse to stay sick and do whatever it takes to get well.

How can you grow from a disease or illness?
It is possible to let disease make you angry, bitter, and self-centered. On the other hand, it can be an opportunity for growth. You can:

- Develop more patience and acceptance with yourself and others.

- Develop more empathy with those who are sick.

- Change your focus from why you should grow to how you can grow. This can increase your intestinal fortitude as you will yourself to get something done in spite of illness.

- Use the understanding you gained from your disease to help others.

- Rearrange your priorities

- See your weaknesses and turn them into strengths

- Establish new healthy boundaries

True healers

This book and **Surviving The Toxic Crisis** are themselves an outgrowth of helping others by giving back the understanding learned by personally dealing with chronic disease. Many of the most effective health care practitioners have chosen their fields because they have personally dealt successfully with chronic illness. Schools and books may give knowledge which inflates the ego, but experience gives true understanding and humility. Not all healers are doctors, and not all doctors are healers. It is a blessing when you find a true healer.

> **Not all healers are doctors, and not all doctors are healers**

The house on the side of the mountain

If you are trying to get to the top of a metaphorical mountain - the top representing truth, wellness, etc. - you need a reason to get to the top. Otherwise you may camp out on the side of the mountain where it is comfortable rather than continue climbing. You become comfortable with the view, and you will justify staying where you are.

If a doctor's purpose is to build an income, s/he may stop short of being a healer, i.e. reach the top of the mountain of true healing. This can occur when he reaches an income or status level where he's unwilling to sacrifice any more comfort or status to go higher. However, if the doctor's purpose is to help heal a beloved family member, s/he is motivated to reach the top of the mountain and be a true healer. True healing - the kind that sets you and others free.

It may be hard to reach the top of the mountain. Recall the Law of Gravity of Relationships discussed previously in this chapter. For instance, you may find that you are very supported, professionally, as you climb the mountain, studying and training to become a medical doctor. As you settle comfortably into the mainstream, status quo approach to healthcare, you may be encouraged and have received much "hands-up" assistance along the way. But should you focus on a new and higher level, you may encounter a lot of resistance. You may find that the very hands that were pulling you up to their level in the beginning are now trying to pull you back down to their comfort zone. Some people are trapped in the mode of being people pleasers and respond only to the standards set by the group. They will only be pulled up to the normal, average or even a lower level mediocrity, that keeps them safely within the group mentality that affords them group approval and all the perks, including the metaphorical key to the executive washroom. Your purpose dictates your achievement level. To leave the safe status quo requires a higher level.

What is the difference between a doctor and a true healer? Think of it this way: A doctor is an achiever of knowledge which s/he applies in a prescribed manner. **A true healer strives to understand the secrets of true healing, which will never be found in the people-pleasing group mentality**.

You have to be very determined and focused on truth; what is the best and highest good for the patient, not just the doctor's income and status, in order to reach the top of the mountain. But you will find that the view from the top will more than compensate you for the struggle to get there. You will be able to look out over the vista of medical care in the 21st Century and see ever so clearly how important getting to the root cause will be in keeping people healthy and providing a key to unlock the door to more optimum health and productive longevity - a goal worthy of the true healer. Then the old maxim may have new meaning - "Adding more years to your life and more life to your years!"

So who or what are you getting well for anyway?
It is better to be motivated to get well for your own reasons than for someone else's. If you are getting well for some purpose you wish to accomplish then you can do whatever it takes to get well. You may want to ask yourself: "What would you do with your life if you were well?"

What is your motivation?
Motivation to get well often mirrors motivation in life.

A person can be motivated by feelings that are generally considered constructive, such as love and acceptance, or they may be motivated by self-protective feelings such as greed or hate. These feelings can be ranked according to service to self or to others and their resultant effect on your total health.

As you will note, indifference is at the bottom of the chart because it is an absence of feeling. The indifferent person no longer cares, even to the point of apathy. Such a person is disconnected from life and is totally self-protective.

Those above the middle line on the chart tend to be mostly other-serving givers, while those below the line tend more to be negotiators then self-serving takers. Those above the line also feel that possessions are meant to serve people, and those below the line feel that people are to be used to get possessions. Those below the line also tend to be in security and survival mode and are therefore possessed by their possessions.

What does motivation have to do with disease? or, Building a World worth living for
People who are motivated by service to others (World 1, the World of Truth) see when and how self-centeredness cripples and keeps them from reaching out and serving others. Serving others as a goal is likely to be used as an unselfish tool for healing. However, a person's self-serving motivations can cause or keep them in a disease state. Those who are motivated by greed, anger, or jealousy are likely to have a sympathetic nervous system fight-or-flight response, high blood pressure, heart disease, or cancer. Those who are fearful (fight-or-flight), worried or apathetic are more likely to override the parasympathetic systems (repair, restore, digest). Such people can develop environmental illness (EI), a disease of fear and avoidance that is characterized by a feeling that toxins like

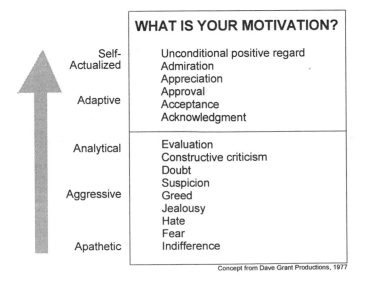

WHAT IS YOUR MOTIVATION?

Self-Actualized	Unconditional positive regard
	Admiration
	Appreciation
	Approval
Adaptive	Acceptance
	Acknowledgment
Analytical	Evaluation
	Constructive criticism
	Doubt
	Suspicion
Aggressive	Greed
	Jealousy
	Hate
	Fear
Apathetic	Indifference

Concept from Dave Grant Productions, 1977

chemicals are out to get you. Indifference breeds depression (unresolved frozen anger) and a feeling of what's-the-use, and in its ultimate self-controlling form can lead to suicide.

Healing of the whole person can involve working your way up the chart, letting go of apathy, the selfish right to be a victim controlled by the tyranny of others, and envy and hate, and starting to care about and serve others.

You can be totally healed physically but have a hard time letting go of your image of yourself as a sick person. Emotionally accepting your physical healing is a necessary step toward total healing.

If you live in the world of right and wrong (World II), vs. truth (World I) prayer and meditation reinforced by positive thinking and affirmations is better than the negative self-talk of guilt and shame (World II).

Normally if you change your desire or try harder you can go up a maximum of two steps at a time on the motivation chart. However, if you change your purpose or vision and thus your whole belief system you can jump to the top. A profound spiritual experience such as a conversion can also propel one to the top of the chart of motivations.

How important are your beliefs?
Suppose you are overweight and self-conscious about it. A near-stranger says "You're a fat slob". You may be slightly hurt or you may be able to shrug it off. Now suppose that this comment came from someone significant in your life. It would be far more painful. And suppose you are that significant person? The most powerful statements are the ones you tell yourself.

If you are consistently saying to yourself, "I'm a fat slob", the pain may not be as apparent on the surface but is capable of doing greater damage to your feeling of self worth than any comment made by someone else. You may be giving yourself this hateful message every time you look in a mirror. This can cause you to become depressed and overeat unhealthy destructive food which feeds the problem, not you. You may even feel that you don't deserve to look and feel better.

Any message, supportive or destructive, that you give yourself can profoundly affect your self-image and actions. If you believe that you aren't worthy of health or success, you create a self-fulfilling prophecy and never receive anything more. This reinforces justifying your need to be right regardless of what it costs you.

If you tell yourself that you are getting better all the time, your body can then believe it and react accordingly. Your belief system will allow you to make profound changes in your life, or stand in your way. Your body believes every word you say. If you endlessly tell your illness story, your body may believe that your illness is an unchangeable fact. If you continuously make statements such as, "That's just the way I am" or "I'm no good at that", you are looking to the past and reinforcing it in your future. This is like driving down the road and spending most of your time looking in the rearview mirror. Sooner or later you may drive off a cliff, hit a wall, or cause a serious accident that injures others as well as yourself.

The parable of the three dogs

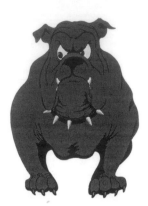

Suppose you had three dogs in the backyard - a German shepherd, a Doberman, and a Pit Bull. The German shepherd, always loyal, represents truth (World I). The Doberman, representing image (World II), appears big and strong like the shepherd, but it may turn on you unexpectedly. Then there is the Pit Bull, which, being raised to kill, without much provocation may jump to attack and destroy you (World III).

The three dogs, all fierce, strong fighters, get into a fight. Which one will win the fight? The one that you feed will have the edge over the others and will triumph. Similarly, the beliefs that you feed will have the upper hand in your life.

Health and success is 29 days of living life and one day of introspection, while poverty is one day of living with 29 days of introspection.

> **We are all what we want to be - or are comfortable being - or we would change**
> - John Boyle

We are all what we want to be - or are comfortable being - or we would change (John Boyle)

Watch what you tell yourself and others. Your ears are close to your mouth and they believe every word you say.

Why are your expectations and view of circumstances so important?

It is not the actual circumstances but your interpretation of them that affects you. Every story in your life has two components: *What happened* and *your interpretation.* "What happened" is what a video camera could have picked up if one had been present. Your interpretation may well be inaccurate and can be changed.

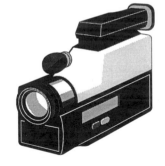

For example, suppose your father said that he would take you to the circus when you were ten years old, but he never did - this is what happened. You may be hanging onto the interpretations you formed then: He doesn't care, he doesn't love me, I was bad, I'm a victim, I'm not worthy, men can't be trusted, etc. You can look back at the event now and you are free to change your interpretations: maybe he got sick, or didn't have the money, or forgot, or was in a bad mood for some reason unrelated to you.

Accept that your interpretation of a past or present event may not be accurate, forgive those involved and move on. And maybe you need to realize that not only the interpretation but the memory may be faulty. What you heard in a conversation may not be what that person really said. Acknowledge and learn from the past but strive for a better future, either through prayer (World I) and/or reprogramming (World II). Don't let pain or anger over a possibly incorrect interpretation control the rest of your life.

What is a winning attitude?

No-lose expectations help keep you striving. Tenacity and coachability are the keys to success, not talent. Plan for the worst and work for the best - and accept whatever God gives you. If you are a praying person, **"pray as if everything depends on God, but work as if everything depends on you."** (Cardinal Spellman). ("Be thankful for whatever God gives", Kellas' addendum) You will no longer be trapped in a victim mentality. Victims win when they stop focusing on how everything affects them and put themselves in the other person's shoes.

Why is your life's vision or purpose so important?

If you had no vision or goal and nothing to work towards, life can be empty and unfulfilling. A lack of purpose is indifference or apathy, found at the bottom of the motivation chart. Children typically are excited and can hardly wait for some anticipated event, like going to camp or the amusement park. Have you lost that sense of anticipation, that childlike enthusiasm for life? Anticipation is often more important than the event itself. Getting there is more than half the fun!

Have you been disappointed so many times you don't want to get your hopes up, only to be disappointed again? Think about it - Pain and Joy both show Life.

An overriding vision or purpose, and the steps or goals that lead to fulfillment of that purpose, keep life interesting and worth living. Service to others is one of the highest goals. Whether it is for God or for other people, it gives a purpose to life greater than just serving ourselves. We can accomplish things greater than ourselves only if our vision is bigger than just serving our own selfish needs. In this respect, let your reach exceed your grasp.

> **You don't achieve results any higher than your purpose**

It is better to "shoot for the moon and miss" than never trying, living in mediocrity, with all the potential buried in anonymity, never knowing what might have been. As the saying goes, it is better to have loved and lost than never to have loved at all. The down side of the coin is "shoot for the street and hit."

How else can one develop a healthier spirit and mind?

There are an infinite number of books and courses on the subject of self-improvement. Any of these may be useful. Other suggestions:

- Identify the payoffs of your illness and eliminate them. Make your own meals. Plan ahead and set a time to give up your handicapped parking sticker and stop collecting disability payments for being sick. Replace these with steps for getting well.

- Grow in your spirituality and the belief that all things happen for a good purpose or reason.

- Look for how you can grow into the higher purpose in every situation, and then move on. Always be thinking: "What can I learn from this experience?"

- Get out of a rut. If you're in a dead-end job, try a new and creative approach to what you're currently doing and try to improve everything you can, or look for new career opportunities.

- Finish each day and be done with it. Never let the sun set on your anger. Don't hold grudges.

- Take inventory periodically (about once a month) of where you are and where you would like to be.

- Do some of the things you want to do. Invest in yourself. Your life is the sum total of the choices you make. Which metaphorical dog will you feed?

- Strive for balance in all things.

- In the morning, take some quiet time to pray or meditate. Additionally, re-program your attitude with positive affirmations to replace negative habit patterns. Stop the self-destructive limitations of clutch words and the "I can'ts" throughout the day.

- Before bed, take time to evaluate your day. Compile and prioritize a "to-do" list for the next day. This will help you to **stop wearing yourself out doing things and start getting things done**. Trade effort for results.

What are some inspirational thoughts that can help?

- Design a future that's worth living for.

- If success is 99% perspiration and 1% inspiration, that 1% is the catalyst that powers up the engine of success, but the 99% is the fuel that keeps it running.

> **Design a future that's worth looking forward to.**

- A journey of a thousand miles begins with one step. Start today.

- That which doesn't kill us only makes us stronger. (Neitzche)

- The truth will set you free. (Jesus Christ) Secrets enslave.

- We are who others expect us to be. (Carl Rogers)

- Our life's purpose defines who we are. (Erich Fromm)

- Who we are under stress is who we really are (Dr. Tim LaHay)

- The definition of insanity is doing the same thing over and over and expecting different results. (Tony Robbins)

- Once a person has deeper understanding of truth, they can never return to a lie. (Emerson)

- Just do it! (Nike) Eliminate clutch words like "try", "work" and "going to".

- You can create your own life, as opposed to accepting others' view of you.

- Everyone gets older but only some mature. Are we just big kids raising little kids to be big kids. Adults take responsibility. Not just die with the most toys, with a "Stuff Happens" sticker. Own your life!

- You can make a difference in the lives of others.

- Replace the tyranny and victimization of "It isn't fair" with the free will choice of "I'd prefer" - this can defuse a lot of anger. You can accept reality without having to approve of it.

- You expand your comfort zone with each risk you take.

- Insights must be followed by action or they are of little use. Unused potential is as useless as no potential.

- Give up looking for and focusing on what's blocking you and just do it.

- Go from "Why should I" to "How can I". Same effort - better results!

- Thoughts on fatigue: Notice how tired you get when faced with doing something unpleasant. Fatigue is a relatively guilt-free deferring device.

- Lay out the next day the night before. Finish each day and be done with it. Then attack the next day with purpose.

- When we give from a place of love rather than from a place of expectation, more usually comes back to us than we could ever have imagined.

- You must become what you want to attract. Be the kind of person you would want to surround yourself with.

- If you have a decision to make, ask which option will take you closer to your life's purpose. You can't do this if you don't have a life's purpose.

- Replace victimizing words like *can't* with volitional choice words like will or *won't*.

- Look for the best in people while being aware of the worst.

- Relationships are not good and bad, only selfish and unselfish.

- You don't achieve results any higher than your purpose.

- Let your reach exceed your grasp.

- To have a friend you must be a friend.

- Rejoice - each day is a gift of God.

"God grant me the grace to change the things I can, accept the things I can't, and the wisdom to know the difference."
                                        -- St. Francis of Assisi

What questions can help clarify things for you?

- There are some questions that you can ask yourself that can help clarify where you are now and where you would like to go.

- What would you like to accomplish in your life? Include everything from "help starving children" to "find a husband" to "paint the garage". Then set priorities. Then do it.

- What would you do if you had only two years to live? This can help put into perspective what is really important to you.

- We all get an epitaph. Design yours today, focusing on your life's mission statement - tomorrow may be too late.

- What would your life look like if you accomplished everything on your personal goals list?

- What issues or problems keep reoccurring in your life?

- Who would you be if you could become exactly the person you would most want to be. How would you describe yourself? Then put a plan in place and become.

- What would you do if you knew you could not fail?

- How would you most like people to perceive you?

- What activities would you pursue if you had unlimited time and resources to do them?

- What is your ideal physical self? Include health, appearance, physical accomplishments. What would you have to risk or change to get this?

- Most greatness comes through compensation. How do you compensate and for what?

- What do you value most about living?

Start	Stop
Loving	Hating or resenting
Life with purpose - Serve Others	Selfishness
Feeling again	Addictions - counterfeit for feeling alive

Indulgences ("What's a little going to hurt?") become habits ("Now that I've blown it I might as well indulge"), which can become addictions ("This is beyond my control now"). You can become a prisoner of pleasure at the cost of joy. In other words, the time to change anything that doesn't support you is now before it gets out of your control.

Feed the good shepherd and starve the rest - don't even allow them the crumbs from the table!

Three Steps of Choice

You can justify and excuse the life you live by blaming either your past givens or genetics, and/or environmental influences. This can make you more comfortable with who you are and content with selling everyone your "victim" story. But this can only serve to breed an attitude -- "This is just the way I am, like it or not" or "My way or the highway".

Either one of these will limit the quality of your life to the self-deception of World II, or the self-defeat of World III, when in reality you can live in the freedom of World I and the truth that sets you free.

We can use the information in this chapter to let go of our selfish, comfortable, arrogant need to be right. Repent, stop defending, and grow to be the person you were meant to be.

Again, recall the parable of the three dogs. Which are you going to feed - that which builds you up or that which can destroy you? The choice is yours. Feed the good shepherd!

--Dr. James Dobson, PhD

References and Resources

- The *Bible* (New Standard Version).

- Borysenko, Joan, *Minding the Body, Mending the Mind*, Bantam Books, NY, 1988.

- Chopra, Deepak, *Quantum Healing: Exploring the Frontiers of Mind/Body Medicine*, Bantam Books, NY, 1989.

- Cousins, Norman, *Head First: The Biology of Hope and the Healing Power of the Human Spirit*, Penguin Books, NY, 1989.

- Goleman, D. and J. Gurin, *Mind/Body Medicine: How to Use Your Mind for Better Health*, Consumer Reports Books, NY, 1993.

- Gordon, James S., *Stress Management*, Chelsea House Publishers, NY, 1990.

- Kabat-Zinn, Jon, *Full Catastrophe Living: Using The Wisdom of Your Body and Mind to Face Stress*, Pain and Illness, Delacorte Press, NY, 1990.

- Locke, Steven and Douglas Colligan, *The Healer Within: The New Medicine of Mind and Body*, EP Dutton, NY, 1986.

- Moyers, Bill, *Healing and The Mind*, Doubleday, NY, 1993.

- Selye, Hans, *The Stress of Life*, McGraw Hill, NY, 1976.

- Siegel, Bernie S., *Peace, Love, and Healing*, Harper and Row, New York, 1989.

- Smalley, Gary, and John Trent, *The Two Sides of Love*, Pocket Books, New York, 1992.

Pulling It All Together

A VISIT TO THE DOCTOR

Partners in Your Own Health Care

In this chapter you can learn:

- *How does a doctor actually do an evaluation and diagnosis?*
- *How can you assist the doctor in your mutual goal of getting you well?*
- *What exactly is blood pressure, and what do the numbers mean?*
- *How do doctors decide which diagnostic tools to use?*
- *Are imaging procedures such as MRI and CAT scan really harmless?*
- *What are your rights as a patient?*
- *Why should biopsy only be used as a last resort?*
- *What are all the strange letters and numbers on the blood test report?*
- *Is allergy testing accurate?*
- *What's the difference between diagnosis and prognosis?*

What is the purpose of a visit to the doctor?

This may seem like an obvious question with an obvious answer, but let's break down a doctor visit into its component parts. By understanding the process, you will be in a better position to work with your practitioner towards your mutual goal, a return to health.

Americans are socialized to visit their M.D. when ill, speak only when spoken to, receive instructions, and then either obey or disobey them. It's time to enter into an adult relationship with your health care provider, and become a partner in your own health care.

> **Become a partner in your own health care**

The practitioner must first arrive at a diagnosis (what is wrong). An average doctor may consider the goal of diagnosis to name the disease or condition. A good doctor feels that a diagnosis is incomplete without identifying the root causes of the condition.

The general order of events is:

1. *Questioning by doctor, medical history and symptomology*
2. *Physical examination*
3. *Testing*
4. *Diagnosis*
5. *Treatment plan*

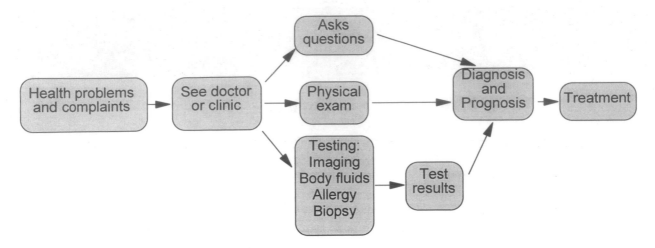

This is a simplified view of the process. An actual course of diagnosis and treatment may involve going back and forth over these five steps, or combining two or more of them. For example, a detoxification diet is both a form of diagnosis, since a person's reaction to the diet can provide information to an alert practitioner, and a form of treatment.

An overview of the first three steps, especially the various testing methods, is the focus of this chapter.

Questioning and Medical History

What is the first diagnostic step?

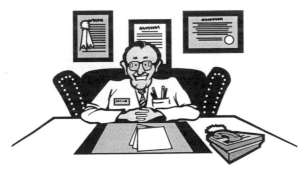

The first step in diagnosis is to listen to the patient. She, or he, is typically asked for symptoms - what is the complaint that brought the patient to the office? Both symptoms and signs are noted by the doctor. Symptoms are subjectively felt by the patient, such as headache, fatigue, or insomnia. Signs can be objectively verified by an observer, such as fever, a rash, or bleeding. The doctor will ask questions that will narrow down the range of possibilities.

What is important in evaluating a headache, for example?

Let's say a patient's main complaint is recurrent headaches. With only this information to go on, the possibilities are nearly endless - toxicity, allergies, high blood pressure, stress, TMJ, whiplash, and in rare instances, a brain tumor. Nearly all possible diagnostic procedures can be used to get to the cause of the headache, but this would be very time consuming and prohibitively expensive. The prudent doctor will first ask questions such as:

- When did the headaches **start**, and did they begin suddenly or gradually?

- Do they **correlate** with any particular activities, locations, foods, drugs? The patient may be asked to keep a diary. This information is useful for pinpointing allergies.

- **Quality and location** of the pain - sharp, dull, throbbing, all over; at the temples, frontal forehead, behind eyes, occipital (back of head at base)?

- **Other symptoms** - eye pain, vision difficulties, dizziness, nasal congestion, fatigue, insomnia?

- **When** does the headache come on or worsen? A morning headache may indicate an allergy to something in the bedroom, a headache that improves on the weekend may be due to toxins or stresses at work, and a woman's headache which has a predictable monthly pattern may have a correlation with her menstrual cycle.

- Is there anything significant going on **emotionally** - a recent loss, depression, work stress?

How can you help the doctor?
The patient can assist the doctor by mentioning anything that she or he feels may be relevant whether or not the doctor asks about it. Symptoms should be organized in a list. The patient should, however, refrain from going off into long involved stories that yield little or no useful information.

Many patients have a strong need to be listened to, understood, and taken seriously in their illness, especially if they are unable to get sympathy ("I understand") or empathy ("I know how you feel") elsewhere. This immediate need may seem to be even stronger than the longer-term goal of getting well. Be clear about what you want to communicate to the doctor and why, and stick to it. Otherwise you may find that you have taken up most of the consultation time with elaborate descriptions of exactly how your illness feels, but you have gotten little or no actual help. While a good assertive doctor can help you stay on track, it is up to you to define your goal - taking steps towards getting well - and stick to it.

Past history of the present ailment, other ailments, prior surgery, medications, and family history of disease are all important. A patient with a breast lump who has breast implants and/or a previous history of breast cancer will likely be diagnosed more aggressively, for example by biopsy, than a patient with no such history.

Don't be fooled
A statement of the symptom (such as high blood pressure), even if restated in medical language (high blood pressure = hypertension), is not a diagnosis, just a description. Don't be fooled into believing you have just obtained useful information. A true diagnosis looks at the cause, for which treatment (if not cure) can often be found.

The Physical Examination

What is involved in the physical exam, and why?

The next part of the diagnostic process is the physical examination, which can be done both with and without the use of instruments. A good doctor will observe the patient's appearance and demeanor - is the skin pale, yellowish, slack, or is there a rash; is the person draggy and listless, or agitated; does the person walk and sit straight or might there be a structural problem?

Observation of certain parts of the body can provide additional information. For example, much can be told from the color, shape and texture of the fingernails, and the inside of the eyelid, if too pale, can indicate anemia.

The beat goes on

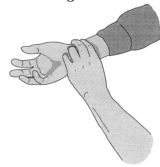

Pulse and blood pressure are taken routinely to determine the general health of the heart and circulatory system. The resting pulse should be about 80 beats per minute for a woman, 72 for a man; a weak, rapid, or irregular pulse may or may not be significant. The severity of the irregularity and the presence of other symptoms may dictate the need for further testing. Irregular pulse, i.e. irregular heartbeat, can result from excessive caffeine consumption, indicate a magnesium deficiency, be a normal individual variation, or can be a sign of a life-threatening process. A rapid pulse can indicate a potassium deficiency.

The pulse is usually taken in the wrist of either arm just below the thumb, and blood pressure is generally taken from one arm, both tests done at rest in a sitting position. If a cardiovascular abnormality is suspected, however, the pulse may be taken at different points or the blood pressure taken in both arms, or the patient may stand, lie down, or exercise during these two tests for additional information. A difference between the sitting and standing pulse may indicate adrenal problems. Male sexual impotence, in the absence of an obvious physical or psychological cause, may be due to decreased lower body circulation, which would be revealed by the taking of the groin pulse.

After the pulse is taken, the nurse may hold the pulse-taking position, but will actually be counting the breathing rate. It is done in this way because the breathing rate can change if a person's attention is drawn to it. A too-rapid breathing rate can indicate diminished lung or heart function.

What exactly is blood pressure?

Blood pressure is a measure of how hard the heart has to work to pump the blood throughout the body. Blood pressure is expressed as two numbers, one over the other. Normal (ideal) blood pressure is 120/80. The first number, always higher, is the systolic pressure and the second number is the diastolic; these numbers refer to the maximum pressure and resting pressure between heartbeats respectively. If the blood vessels are narrowed due to arteriosclerotic buildup or spasm, the blood pressure goes up, just as the pressure of water in a hose goes up when the hose is pinched. A blood pressure of 140/90 is borderline high, and 200/150 is life-threatening if prolonged. A low blood pressure, under 120/80, is rarely significant in itself unless unmistakable symptoms of shock are present, although a low blood pressure may be an indication of other conditions such as suppressed, deficient or weak adrenals. Blood pressure that varies considerably from time to time may be due to allergies, as compared with a consistent high blood pressure that may be due to toxins.

What are some other tools of the trade?

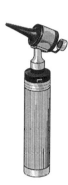

A small lighted magnifying glass may be used to look at the throat, nose, and ears for signs of infection. It can also be used to view the expansion and contraction of the pupil of the eye, and to look within the eye at the capillaries to check for cardiovascular and eye problems. A thermometer is most often used to detect fever, which is a sign of infection. Body temperature is also important in detecting thyroid problems - a lower than normal morning temperature can indicate low thyroid function, and can alert the doctor to order thyroid function tests.

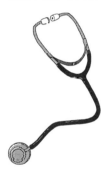

A stethoscope is used to listen to the heart and lungs. When applied over the heart, the doctor is listening for heartbeat regularity and for any clicks or murmurs that may indicate heart disease or a structural problem. When applied to the lungs, both front and back and upper and lower, the doctor is listening for rattling, wheezing, or crackling noises which can indicate pneumonia, tuberculosis, bronchitis, or other lung diseases. This finding often indicates the need for a chest x-ray or other further diagnosis.

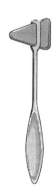

A special, small triangular rubber hammer is sometimes used to check the reflexes of the knee or elbow. This is a rough test of neurological function; a lack of these reflexes can indicate a nervous system problem.

What the well-trained hand can find

The doctor may feel the patient's neck for enlarged lymph nodes (infection or lymphoma), or an enlarged thyroid gland (goiter or tumor). The abdomen is palpated (felt) for enlargement of the liver (right side) or spleen (left side) which would be abnormal, and also for any pain or tenderness.

Testing

What is the purpose of diagnostic testing?

Before a diagnosis can be made, testing of some sort is generally done. The results of the testing confirm or disprove the preliminary educated guess as to what is wrong. Once a diagnosis is made, treatment can proceed.

There are three purposes to testing - to find out:

1. *What is wrong*
2. *Why it's wrong (cause)*
3. *How it can be fixed*

So what?

Before any kind of testing is done, the question should be asked by the doctor or patient, "So what?". If a particular test result does not alter any treatment decisions, or if the doctor doesn't know what to do with the results, then there is no purpose to doing the test. One patient, for example, was in a horseback riding accident as a teenager. The doctor suspected a fractured tailbone, which would have shown on an x-ray. However, since there is no treatment for a fractured tailbone, the doctor wisely declined to take x-rays, since the procedure carried some risk and would provide no useful information.

What types of diagnostic testing are there?

Diagnostic testing can be separated into several categories:

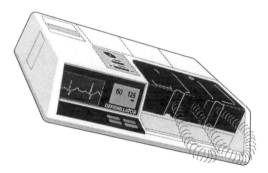

- *Imaging techniques, including x-ray diagnosis of various types, ultrasound, and MRI*

- *Electrical monitoring such as EKG and EEG*

- *Invasive procedures such as biopsy*

- *Allergy testing of various types*

- *Body fluid testing of blood, urine, saliva, stool, sputum*

- *Other techniques such as live blood cell analysis*

- *Energy medicine techniques such as kinesiology or EAV*

Are imaging procedures harmless?

Western medicine usually uses the more invasive technologies, such as biopsy and imaging. Imaging techniques such as x-ray are not often considered invasive, but they can be invasive in the sense that they can have adverse effects on the body, as discussed in the Electromagnetic Radiation chapters in *Surviving The Toxic Crisis*. Alternative/comprehensive medicine generally prefers the non-invasive procedures, as its practitioners recognize the harm that can be done to the body by biopsy and imaging techniques.

There is a place for these comparatively invasive procedures even in alternative medicine, however. It is best to look at all of the tools available and weigh the pros and cons of their use for a particular diagnostic problem.

With such a wide range of diagnostic tools at their disposal, how do doctors decide which one to use, and in which order?

After questioning and examining the patient the doctor has a pretty good idea of what to look for, such as low thyroid function, mineral deficiencies, a broken bone, a tumor, parasites, food allergies. Many times more than one problem is suspected. A person with chronic fatigue, for example, may have many or all of the following: nutrient deficiencies and/or imbalances, toxic buildup of chemicals, heavy metals in the body, parasites, a viral infection such as Epstein-Barr, or structural abnormalities. However, whether the problems are single or multiple, they must be diagnosed to be treated effectively.

Many causes = One symptom   One cause = Many symptoms

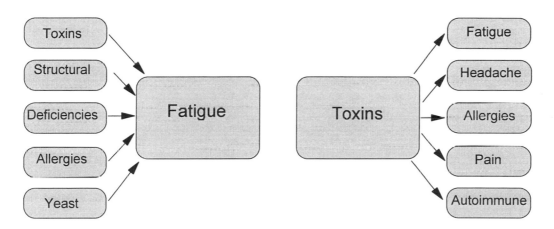

One symptom may have many causes as just discussed, but one cause may result in many different symptoms depending on a person's genetic weak link. Almost any toxin discussed in this book, such as mercury, pesticides, or giardia, can cause any of a list of symptoms that may seem to be unrelated.

The type of problem suspected dictates what type of testing is done. In many cases a screening test such as a blood panel or Live Blood Analysis (both discussed later in this chapter) is used to get an overview of what may be going on. A screening test tells a little about a lot of things, in contrast to a specific test which tells a lot about one specific thing, or more accurately, a narrow range of focus. For example, Live Blood Analysis (LBA) can see indications of parasites or metals in addition to several dozen other things, but can't give more information than that on any one thing. From the screening test results, the practitioner can order more specific tests such as stool tests for particular parasites or a mercury vapor or hair test for metals.

With a preliminary diagnosis, or diagnoses (plural of diagnosis) in mind, the doctor may recommend further testing. In almost all cases there are two or more different tests that will give almost the same information. Rarely will one test be the only possible correct choice, although many doctors act as if this were the case.

Why would one type of test be favored over another by an individual (doctor or patient) given the same set of symptoms?

- **Belief** - American physicians are trained to believe that invasive tests and expensive machinery are more accurate than simpler tests. This is because they are trained to stop acute symptoms. Also, they tend to trust the complex numerical output of an expensive modern instrument more than the judgment and interpretation that are usually part of simpler tests.

- **Cost** or insurance coverage

- **Availability** of instrumentation or trained personnel

- **Specialty** - allergists are more likely than other doctors to order allergy testing; cardiologists are more likely to order an EKG.

- Potential **health risk** to the patient

- **Complexity** of information required - is a three-digit numerical readout necessary, or would a simple yes or no be sufficient?

- **Habit** - most doctors order the tests they have ordered in the past, regardless of whether they are all necessary for this particular case.

- **Knowledge** - A doctor can only order a test if s/he is aware that it exists and what it does. For example, many if not most American doctors do not order a Live Blood Analysis because they were not taught about it in medical school in this country, although it is in comparatively wider use in Europe. Stool or saliva tests for parasites, or mercury vapor or voltage tests for dental problems, are often not ordered because most doctors don't realize how important or widespread parasite and dental problems are as root causes of health problems.

What are your rights as a patient?

Contrary to the belief fostered by some, you, the patient, have every right to question the diagnostic procedures suggested, weigh the options, refuse certain tests, request others, and in short act like a free-thinking adult who is taking part in her or his own health care. In order to ask the questions and make the decisions, however, it is necessary to know what kinds of testing are available. This includes the methods your doctor may not tell you about or denounces as quackery. This chapter will review the options, what they can and cannot do, how they work, and their pros and cons. It is not our purpose, in this chapter or anywhere in the book, to say "do this, don't do that" but rather to provide some balanced information so you can make your own decisions.

If nothing is found in the testing, does this mean that nothing has been accomplished?

As with all diagnostic tests, negative findings, or the absence of any abnormal signs, are as important as positive findings. Both negative and positive results give the doctor information which:

- *is diagnostic in itself to either confirm or rule out a problem, such as parasites*
- *is used to confirm another diagnostic procedure*
- *is an indication of which other tests should be done.*

What is the difference between diagnosis and prognosis?

Two terms which sometimes cause confusion are diagnosis and prognosis. Diagnosis refers to what the problem is, the cause of the symptoms - a cold, cancer, a sprained ankle. A prognosis is an educated guess, based on the diagnosis along with statistics and previous experience, as to the probable course of the disease or condition with or without treatment - for example, the cold will heal by itself, the cancer has a 75% fatality rate, the broken bone will heal completely but only if set. Diagnosis is about the present. Prognosis looks to the past to predict the future.

Prognosis can also be predictive or preventive, as in "If you keep smoking you may develop cancer or heart disease". It can be used to stop the train before it goes off the track.

Two terms which come up in discussions of prognosis are treatable and curable, which are also easily confused. Treatable means that, with treatment, some improvement in symptom severity is expected, or the degenerative process can be slowed down, or one's lifetime may be extended as with cancer, or a disease such as diabetes is manageable. Curable, on the other hand, means that with treatment the problem will likely disappear entirely, i.e. be cured. If your illness were an airplane heading for a crash, treatment would be stopping or slowing the plane's descent, while cure is reversing the descent - or the course of the illness.

Imaging techniques - Not just taking a picture

What are imaging techniques, and are they harmless?

Imaging procedures use x-rays, high frequency sound waves, magnetic fields, or gamma rays to differentially penetrate various tissues of the body and project an image onto sensitive film. Alternatively, the image can be analyzed by computer to construct a picture of what is inside the body. These techniques are much less invasive than biopsy and are often just as useful or more so providing microscopic analysis is not needed. Although imaging techniques are safer than biopsy, they have their risks which should be weighed against the benefits.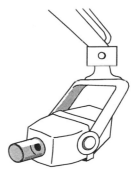

The various types of imaging tests and their risks and benefits are discussed in the Electromagnetic Radiation chapters in *Surviving The Toxic Crisis*. As with all treatment and testing techniques, it is important for you to know and weigh the risks and the benefits to decide what is best for you.

Biopsy

What is biopsy, and why should it usually be a last resort diagnostically?

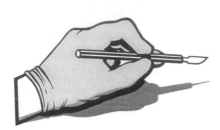

Biopsy is the most drastic diagnostic procedure. It involves taking a sample of the suspected diseased tissue by surgical means and looking at it microscopically to diagnose, for example, a malignancy. Treatment is recommended based on the results. It is less common now that sophisticated imaging techniques are available, but still has its uses. For example, a suspicious breast lump or mole can be removed in its entirety. It should be removed anyway whether or not it is malignant, so the biopsy is also part or all of the treatment. Microscopic examination of the actual tissue is sometimes the best way to get an accurate diagnosis.

Biopsy is of three types:

- *removing the entire suspicious mass for combined diagnostic and treatment purposes*

- *cutting out and removing part of a mass for diagnostic purposes*

- *taking a sample by large-gauge needle, most often used for internal organs such as the liver or for breast cysts*

Is a biopsy a safe method of diagnosing cancer?

The needle technique is less invasive than cutting, but both of these carry with them the possibility of opening a previously encapsulated tumor and spreading cancer cells into the blood stream. An event dreaded by surgeons is the accidental cutting or piercing of an encapsulated tumor, but this is what a needle or partial biopsy does by design. If cancer is suspected, removal of the entire mass as a whole is best. Any biopsy is surgery with its attendant risks, especially if general anesthesia is used. Biopsies are generally more expensive than other tests, but are ironically ordered sometimes to save the patient money, as some insurance plans will pay for biopsies but not for simpler procedures.

Biopsy Risks	Biopsy Rewards
Spread cancer	Can also be treatment
Anesthesia risk	Accurate diagnosis
Expense	Insurance coverage
Scarring	

One patient, a 45 year old female missionary, had a breast cancer biopsy done after being told that she was in remission. The cancer metastasized, spreading to her bone and brain like wildfire, eventually killing her. Cancer, like fire, must be stopped by eliminating the cause; much like arresting the arsonists before the match is lit. In her case, dental mercury levels were five times higher than OSHA's maximum limit.

Body Fluid Testing

Body fluid testing is used by both standard Western and progressive comprehensive-alternative practitioners, although their interpretation of the results may be different.

What body fluids can be tested?
Nearly any body fluid can be tested where appropriate. These fluids and typical tests include:

- *Whole blood - many tests*

- *Plasma - the liquid left after red blood cells are centrifuged (spun) out - many tests*

- *Serum - same as plasma, but with fibrin (clotting factor) removed - many tests*

- *Urine - sugar, proteins, bacteria, drugs, other tests*

- *Stool - parasites, blood, yeast*

- *Vaginal fluids - candida (yeast), sexually transmitted diseases*

- *Saliva - adrenal function, can be tested for marijuana, hormones, vitamin deficiencies, IgA (immune component), some parasites*

- *Spinal fluid - meningitis, cerebral hemorrhage*

- *Gastric juices - parasites, sufficient HCl*

- *Sputum - lung infection*

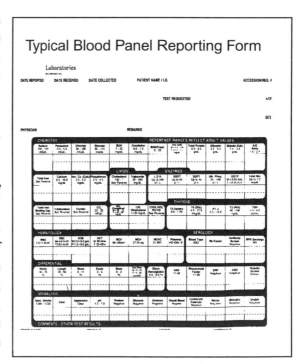

Blood tests, including serum and plasma, can measure a great many things depending on what is being tested for. The most common blood tests, which are done routinely in many medical facilities, are shown here on a typical reporting form. This form includes, for each test, a range of normal responses. Values higher or lower than these are an indication of abnormality.

What is the difference between out of range and abnormal?
Some doctors, especially these with an allopathic orientation, look only at those values that are out of range, dismissing all others as normal. Progressive practitioners, who look not only for clearly defined disease but for any departure from ideal wellness, will usually also take note of values that are on the low or high side of the normal range, or look at the

relationship between two or more values. Some values that are more than a few percent from the *average* value within the so-called normal range may be significant. Progressive practitioners have learned that out of range values may be sufficient for detecting acute problems, but chronic conditions often have more subtle patterns.

It is not uncommon for an allopathic doctor to look at a blood panel result, see nothing out of range, and say "Your blood test doesn't show anything". The fact is, this is a little misleading. In order to pick up on the more subtle patterns relating to chronic conditions, one needs to know how to interpret the finer subtleties between just average versus optimum levels.

How would this work with an actual patient?

One patient, a woman in her mid 30s, came to a comprehensive clinic with multiple symptoms. She had had a blood panel test done elsewhere, which supposedly turned out normal - no out of range values. Knowledgeable interpretation revealed patterns that showed her problems. Although all of her values were within the listed ranges, when compared to the average she had low potassium, low glucose, high chloride with normal sodium (digestive problems), allergy, low A/G ratio, and high triglycerides. Treatment based in large part on the correct interpretation the finer subtleties of a "normal" blood test restored her health.

She had mercury from her dental fillings, which caused her to be low in potassium and set up an environment for growing microorganisms by killing the protective bacteria. This allowed allergy to come in because of the undigested protein, inferred from the high chloride readings on her blood test. Her high globulin and low albumin/globulin ratio also indicated poor protein digestion, and her high triglycerides showed she was eating more simple carbohydrates than she could handle.

In addition to the indicated dietary changes, including a low-yeast rotation allergy diet, she had her mercury removed and had treatment for yeast and other microorganisms. She also took potassium, lipogen (by Metagenics) for the triglycerides and fat digestion, a women's supplement by Professional Preference, the antioxidant ACES (by Carlson), and acidophilus to control microorganisms and aid in digestion.

What are all the strange letters and numbers on the blood test report?

A look at the standard blood tests on the reporting form reveals a bewildering list of unfamiliar words and sets of initials. The following explanations, although brief, should help to resolve the confusion. Much more information than this can be obtained from a blood test when it is evaluated by a trained practitioner.

Minerals - Sodium (Na+), chlorine (Cl-), and potassium (K+) are essential minerals. Na and Cl are measures of the salt content of the blood, while K is a measure of adrenal gland and kidney function and is responsible for muscle strength. Low sodium can indicate adrenal gland failure.

Glucose is blood sugar. A high value can indicate diabetes, while a low value can mean stressed adrenal glands or hypoglycemia.

Kidneys - BUN is blood urea nitrogen, a breakdown product of protein; creatinine is a breakdown product of muscles. High levels of either or both are an indication of kidney dysfunction. Uric acid is a breakdown product of urine metabolism. High levels indicate a predisposition to gout or gouty arthritis.

Liver - The enzymes LDH (low = dry liver, high = fatty liver), SGOT (gallbladder function), SGPT (fungus), alkaline phosphatase (cell destruction), and GGTP are all measures of liver function. High levels may indicate liver damage as from alcohol and chemicals. GGTP is most sensitive to alcohol, and detects liver damage due to alcohol at an early stage. Bilirubin measures bile, and a high level can correlate with jaundice (yellowed skin) due to a blocked liver duct or immune dysfunction.

Protein - Total protein is a measure of the body's nutrition. Albumin, which is manufactured by the liver, transports minerals, and globulin is part of the immune system. Both albumin and globulin are protein fractions. A/G ratio is the ratio between albumin and globulin, and should ideally be around 1.8.

Lipids are blood fats, and the various types (cholesterol, triglycerides, LDL, HDL) are discussed in the chapter on Oils and Fats. The LDL/HDL ratio should be 3.5/1 or 4/1, and the lower the ratio, the lower the cardiovascular risk. However, if the ratio is too low, this can indicate dry liver, and low oils and oil soluble vitamins A, D, E, and K.

Thyroid function tests are T4, T3 uptake, and FTI. T4 is the amount of thyroxin released from the thyroid gland, while T3 is a measure of its uptake by the cells. Low and high values indicate hypo- and hyperthyroidism respectively. Hypothyroidism may be due to low iodine or tyrosine.

Blood / hematology - RBC are red blood cells, and HGB (hemoglobin) and HCT (hematocrit) are also RBC measures. Low values mean anemia or vitamin B12 or folic acid deficiency. MCB, MCH, and MCHC are other RBC measures. Platelets are blood clotting factors, and low values indicate a tendency to bleed excessively and high values indicate a tendency to form blood vessel clots.

Iron - Ferritin is the most sensitive measure of iron stores in the body. A value lower than about 80 indicates an iron deficiency, which can affect red blood cell (RBC) count, hematocrit, hemoglobin, and can indicate anemia.

White blood cells WBC are white blood cells. A high value indicates active infection, a very high number can mean leukemia, and a low number can mean a chronic viral infection. The differential count refers to the types of white blood cells. The neutrophil/lymphocyte ratio should be 60/40. If neutrophils are too high, a bacterial infection may be present, while a low level points to a depressed immune system. Monocytes are also a measure of immune system function. A high level of lymphocytes may mean a viral infection. A high level of eosinophils can indicate allergy or parasites. Basophils are also white blood cells.

Are test results absolute?

Blood test results are usually indicators of a possible problem. For example, elevated liver enzymes point to a potential liver problem, but don't actually prove that you have something serious like cirrhosis of the liver or hepatitis [1].

The absence of test evidence of a problem does not definitively rule out the problem.

What is the difference between a screening and a diagnostic test?
Screening tests, such as the blood panel, LBA/OSA (described later in this chapter), urine tests, and some others are for screening purposes. They look at the whole body or much of it, but don't give a lot of information about any one thing. They can indicate a potential liver problem, the possibility of parasites (but not what kind or where), the likelihood of a buildup of toxic heavy metals, etc. Their value lies in their providing an overview of what the problem areas are likely to be, and point towards which diagnostic tests would likely be of most benefit. There are so many diagnostic tests that it would be prohibitively expensive and time-consuming to run them all, so a screening test is a good place to start unless the probable source of a problem is known.

Diagnostic tests are as specific as screening tests are general. They look at a particular potential problem or body system and give more definitive information.

For example, a screening test might show indicators of heavy metals. The LBA/OSA test might show dark crystals, or the white blood cell differential part of the blood panel test might show high monocytes. A more diagnostic test, hair analysis, can show how much of particular toxic metals are eliminated in the hair.

What can urine tell about you?
Urine testing, or urinalysis, can also reveal many things depending on the tests done. When done as part of a routine analysis, the following are usually tested for:

- Specific gravity is the concentration. 1.00, the specific gravity of water, is the lowest possible value, but not the ideal, which is 1.02. The first morning urine is usually the most concentrated and highest in mineral content.

- Color is obviously yellow, but there are variations - reddish, brownish. Appearance refers to clear or cloudy; clear is normal and cloudy often means a bacterial infection is present. Certain drugs can affect the color and appearance of urine. Certain food substances can temporarily and harmlessly color the urine, such as deep yellow from vitamin B2 (riboflavin) or reddish from beets.

- pH measures the acidity of the urine, with 5.5 to 6.5 being normal.

- Protein, glucose, ketones, leukocytes, blood, nitrite, and bilirubin should not be in urine. "Negative" means normal. Ketones are breakdown products of fat, and can indicate diabetes or a fasting state. Leukocytes are WBCs, and indicate a probable urinary tract or related bacterial infection. Nitrites are also a test for bacteria.

What other fluids can be tested, and what for?
Stool, while not officially a fluid, and gastric juice can be examined for parasites or their eggs. Blood in the stool, called occult blood, can indicate a bleeding ulcer, cancer, or other gastroin-

testinal tract abnormality. Bright red visible blood in the stool is usually from anal fissures or hemorrhoids and is rarely serious in itself, but it can indicate constipation, vascular fragility, low antioxidants or bioflavonoids, the cause of which should be evaluated and treated. On the other hand, dark red or blackish blood or clots can indicate deep bleeding or other serious conditions. Stool assay is not routinely done unless these conditions (parasites or internal bleeding) are suspected.

Stool testing for parasites, described in more detail in the Microorganisms chapter in *Surviving The Toxic Crisis*, is only about 60% accurate on negatives but nearly 100% on positives. This means that if the test result is negative, there is a 60% chance that you don't have that parasite, but if it's positive, it is almost certain that you have the parasite. Repeat testing can improve the accuracy rate since parasites are more easily seen during certain parts of their life cycle.

Sputum is the mucus brought up from the lungs or bronchial tubes. It can be cultured to determine the cause of a lung or bronchial infection, such as pneumonia or tuberculosis.

Spinal fluid is obtained by doing a spinal tap, which is the insertion of a needle into the spinal column. Spinal fluid should be clear and water-white; cloudy fluid or the presence of white blood cells can indicate meningitis or other spinal infection. Red blood cells in the fluid can indicate a cerebral hemorrhage.

LBA/OSA

Are there other types of blood testing?
Two other types of blood test are Live Blood Analysis (LBA) and Oxidative Stress Analysis (OSA), also called Dried Layer Testing. These tests are very effective for screening and prediagnosis of many conditions of bodily imbalance or toxicity. Although not approved by the FDA here for direct diagnosis (they are legal for screening / research purposes), they are used more widely in Europe, where they can be legally used diagnostically.

What is a screening test?
A screening test can alert the practitioner to possible problems such as metals, parasites, or digestive difficulties so more definitive diagnostic testing can be done in these areas. A screening test is a more efficient way to decide what tests need to be run to diagnose disease, rather than groping in the dark, guessing as to a cause, and ordering expensive tests, (e.g. for metals or parasites) randomly.

What do these tests cost?
LBA and OSA together usually cost around $100. These tests can actually save the patient time and money by pinpointing other tests that need to be done.

What is the basic premise of these tests?

The blood is a mirror of all parts of the body, and conditions and disease states in nearly any part of the body can show up in a drop of blood. The idea that a tiny part can contain all of the information of the whole is the basic premise behind the re-creation of dinosaurs in the movie Jurassic Park.

If you are skeptical of the statement that the blood reflects the body, consider the widely used and accepted blood panel discussed earlier in this chapter. In the blood panel, a tube of blood is sent to a laboratory and the results are sent back to your doctor in the form of a computer print-out. Among the things that can be determined from your blood using the blood chemistry panel are:

- Liver function from levels of liver enzymes such as GGTP and LDH

- The health of your cardiovascular and digestive systems and gallbladder function from cholesterol, SGOT and triglyceride levels

- Your thyroid function (metabolic rate), determined from T4 and T3 readings which measure output from the thyroid gland in your neck

- Your blood sugar level (glucose) and triglycerides can be a measure of how well your pancreas is handling your diet.

- Your red and white blood cell count can show how well your bones are producing blood cells, and how well your liver and spleen are removing old ones.

- Blood urea nitrogen (BUN) and creatinine are indicators of kidney function.

- The types and numbers of white blood cells can indicate an infection, and even narrow it down as to type of infection - viral, bacterial, etc.

It becomes clear that your blood represents your body in microcosm or miniature. Other types of blood testing can also make use of this relationship between the blood and the body. This is the basic premise behind all blood tests.

How are these tests done?

There are slight variations in procedure depending on the practitioner, but the general procedure is this: Your finger is pricked with a sterile disposable lancet and a drop of blood is gently squeezed out and allowed to sit on your finger for a minute. A glass microscope slide is touched eight times to the drop to form the layers for the Dried Layer (OSA) test. This slide is set aside to dry. Another drop of blood is put onto another slide and looked at immediately for Live Blood Analysis.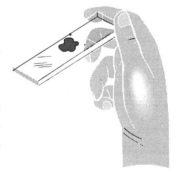

A checklist of several dozen things is used to let the practitioner know what to look for and what these things can mean.

How do you know that these tests are accurate?

Many findings can be explained based on a knowledge of body processes and what these can do to the blood. Other findings can't be explained as easily, but are still reproducible and thus valid. Science is not necessarily that which is understood, but that which is repeatable, predictable and verifiable. Gravity was a scientific fact long be-

> **Science is not necessarily that which is understood, but that which is repeatable, predictable and verifiable**

fore it was understood by scientists and is a scientific fact even for a five-year-old who has no idea what it is. LBA and OSA results have been shown to correlate with certain processes in many thousands of patients, and for this reason are considered to be as accurate, i.e. scientific, as most other tests.

What can be seen in Live Blood Analysis?

First, to clear up any possible confusion about the name of the test, Live Blood Analysis, also sometimes called Live Blood Cell Analysis or even Live Cell Analysis, is not the same thing as Live Cell Therapy. Live Cell *Therapy* is a type of treatment that is not related to Live Blood *Analysis*.

Many things can be seen in a drop of your blood. Number and types of white blood cells, shapes of red blood cells, whether the blood cells clump, and other matter in the blood all indicate certain conditions. These observations and indications include:

- Parasites of certain types, such as L-form bacteria and worms, can sometimes be seen directly.

- Spicules, or needle-like structures, can indicate liver stress. This can be from abuse or toxicity and thus would be a bad sign. However, if you are undergoing detoxification procedures of any kind, such as diet, sauna, colonics, or liver flush, the presence of spicules can be a positive indication that the liver is processing toxins for elimination.

- Infection is shown by increased numbers of white blood cells. The type of white blood cells in excess are an indication of the type of infection (viral, bacterial, etc.)

- General health can be determined by the general look of the blood.

- Digestive problems show up in the form of lemon-shaped red blood cells.

- Toxicity, as from chemicals or dietary toxins (coffee, fried foods, microwaved foods), or allergy can show up as stacked, stuck-together red blood cells.

Many other things can be determined from your one drop of blood.

What is Dried Layer Testing, and how does it work?

In Dried layer Testing (Oxidative Stress Analysis, or OSA), a drop of blood sits on your finger for about a minute to allow heavier particles to settle to the bottom of the drop or go towards the outside or it. The glass microscope slide is touched to the drop eight times in succession to make eight dots of blood on the slide. This slide is then observed through the microscope at a lower magnification than the Live Blood Analysis. While LBA looks at individual cells, OSA looks at the patterns formed by the drop.

What can be determined using OSA?

As is the case with LBA, many things can be determined using OSA. For example:

- Small white areas can indicate stress, emotional or physical, including allergy.

- Tan/grey areas can indicate yeast overgrowth. This is an *indication* of yeast, as compared with a *diagnosis* of yeast as obtained from a stool test, in which the actual yeast is seen.

- Black and white areas in a lotus-root pattern in the center of layer three, four, or five can indicate a lower colon or digestive problem, often accompanied by a dull ache in the lower back. These two things (digestive problems and backache) are often found together, as the nerves from the lower back serve the lower intestinal area and a problem in either one can affect the other.

- A dark ring or dark spots around the outside of the drop usually indicate metals. The metals, heavier than other blood components, go to the outside of the drop by centrifugal action.

- Dark areas within the drop may indicate parasites.

- A white or black line can indicate a structural or circulatory problem or injury. The location within the layer may show where in the body this is located. This may or may not correlate with the location of pain.

- Other formations can indicate thyroid problems, heart rhythm irregularities, overall degenerative conditions or systemic problems, or other conditions.

Although these indications should be verified with diagnostic tests, avoiding costly dead ends or misdiagnoses can easily recoup the cost of the test.

What are the limitations of these tests?

The limitations of these two tests are more legal than actual. These tests have been used on an international basis for a long time, but since they are not mainstream medical tests approved by the FDA, they can't be legally used for direct diagnosis. But the information they provide, along with medical testing and symptoms history can help the practitioner to arrive at a diagnosis in a more timely manner, and save the patient from doing a whole bank of testing just to cover everything. The practitioner may see clear indications of, say, a thyroid or bowel problem but cannot legally make a diagnosis based on these tests. But s/he can then order specific tests to rule out or confirm what seems to be indicated. Thus they are considered to be screening tests, useful for indicating which more specific tests might be required.

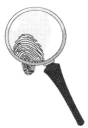

A practitioner who performs these tests can be compared to the forensic scientist who goes to a crime scene to gather fingerprints, hair samples and other evidence. Although these clues are crucial to solving the crime, the person who gathers evidence can't say who did it. Similarly, the practitioner who does these tests is gathering clues to be evaluated by the doctor who will do the actual diagnosing.

There is no test which is 100% accurate, and these tests are no exception. They are, however, valuable tools when used in conjunction with medical testing and symptoms history.

Allergy Testing

Who needs allergy testing?

Many of you reading this book have allergies, either known or suspected. It is important to know just what you are allergic to so you can either avoid the substance(s) or have desensitizing treatments. Allergy testing will, in theory at least, give you this information.

What is the basic principle behind allergy testing?

There are many types of allergy tests, but their general principle is the same. A suspected substance is introduced to the body and/or blood, and a response of some sort is looked for. A positive response, i.e. a change which is a sign that the body is reacting to the substance, means that the person is allergic to that substance. No change, no allergy.

What are some of the limitations of allergy testing?

Allergy testing can provide some valuable information, but it has its limitations. It is important to realize that allergy test results, even if they are in the form of an impressive computer printout, are not necessarily very accurate. Accuracy in this case refers to the correlation between the test results and the actual symptoms experienced or not experienced by the person exposed to the allergen. Other drawbacks to allergy testing are:

- **Daily variation** - If you have a known allergy, you have probably noticed that you don't react in exactly the same way, and to the same degree, to the same amount of allergen each time. Reactivity depends on, among other things, the total body burden that your body is coping with at that moment. Therefore it is not surprising that allergy tests would show different results on different days.

- **Variability between tests** - If two or more different types of tests are given, it often happens that the results don't match. This can be due to daily variation, or due to the fact that different people respond more strongly to some types of testing than others. If two people are allergic to a substance, one may develop a skin rash and the other may become tired; the first one is more likely to have a positive response to a skin test although both are allergic.

- **Dose** - Allergic reactions are often dose dependent. While it makes sense that a larger amount of an allergen is more likely to cause a reaction, or a more severe reaction, than a smaller one, this is oddly not always the case. If the dose tested is not the same as the dose encountered in real life, a false test result may be obtained.

- **Severity** - Most tests are most accurate with a severe allergy. In such a case, however, the allergen is usually already known so no new information is gained.

- **Qualitative** - Most test results are only qualitative (yes or no), not quantitative (how severe is the allergy). A skin test may be strongly or weakly positive, but the strength of the test reaction correlates poorly with the degree of change in how you actually feel. Suppose you test positive for animal fur and you want to know whether the potential amount of health improvement is worth giving up your beloved pet for. In other words, how allergic are you? Tests cannot reliably tell you this.

- **Skill** - Results can vary due to the skill, test application technique, and interpretation of the operator.

Even with their many drawbacks and inaccuracies, allergy tests certainly have their place. They can give you ideas as to what to eliminate in order to see whether you feel better. They can allow you to avoid substances to which you might have a life-threatening reaction. They can point to other more detailed tests that could be done.

What are the types of allergy tests?
Allergy tests can be provocative, noninvasive, or direct.

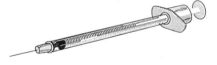

Provocative testing involves trying to provoke a response by putting the substance in the body in some way - injection, ingestion, inhalation, or on the skin. The immune system reacts to provide a recognizable response. Severe reactions or increased sensitization may result, even to homeopathic-level doses. At best the deliberately induced allergic reactions are unpleasant. However, if allergies are ruining your quality of life, then the discomfort of testing is a small and worthwhile price to pay.

Noninvasive testing does not affect the body directly. Noninvasive tests include blood tests, in which the reaction is observed in the blood sample rather than in the body. Energy medicine tests such as Interro and kinesiology (muscle testing) are also noninvasive, and measure the body's energetic response to substances.

Direct testing involves removing as many potential allergens and toxins as possible, as through an elimination diet, and then carefully observing your reactions to ordinary exposure to individual substances. This is the best method, as it measures your body's reactions in real life situations.

Not all types of allergy testing give the same information. Some types of testing are better for, say, food allergies than others, although not all doctors agree as to which is which. These types of testing are discussed here.

Skin tests - In skin tests, a drop of allergen extract is placed on the skin, after which the surface of the skin is scratched or punctured. Alternatively, the substance is injected between the layers of skin (intradermally). Skin testing is usually done on the inside of the forearm, and a number of substances can be tested at once. If the substance provokes an immune response, the mast cells release histamine which produces a reddened wheal (bump) at the spot on the skin where the allergen was introduced. This usually occurs within fifteen minutes. There will be no visible response to a substance if there is no allergic reaction. A control dose of saline solution is sometimes used to compensate for any reaction to being scratched or pricked.

The scratch test is less uncomfortable and safer than intradermal injection, as the material can be wiped off if a severe reaction is encountered. The injection test is usually more sensitive. Skin tests are generally better for diagnosing the cause of asthma or hay fever than the cause of hives or eczema. Skin tests are rarely useful for diagnosing allergy to stinging insects or to drugs other than penicillin. They are more useful for food and inhalant allergies and to determine the cause of contact dermatitis.

Skin tests are most accurate for pollens and molds, but are not very accurate for food allergies / sensitivities [2].

Don't try this at home, folks - it could be dangerous. Have it done ONLY by a qualified practitioner.

Sublingual testing - In sublingual testing, a drop of the allergen is mixed with glycerine and placed under the tongue, an area rich in blood vessels close to the surface that can carry the substance through the body. The patient watches for signs of allergic reaction such as sudden fatigue, weakness, irritability, or difficulty breathing. If necessary, the reaction is neutralized with a dilution of the same extract. Sublingual testing is best for food allergies and sometimes inhalant allergies. Allopathic and alternative doctors differ sharply on the effectiveness of the test, with alternative practitioners more likely to support it. The main drawback is that a systemic allergic reaction is necessarily induced. If the person is very allergic, the systemic reaction can be as severe as anaphylactic shock, which can be fatal. This is obviously not a trivial matter, and this risk should be assessed against the benefit.

Inhalation testing - The inhalation challenge is sometimes used to determine inhalant allergies such as molds, dust, pollen, or grasses. A small amount of the dried, sterilized substance is sniffed, and allergic symptoms should occur within five minutes. Since the substance is inhaled, the test tends to be more accurate than other types of testing for inhalants. As with skin and sublingual testing, the main drawback is the deliberate provocation of an uncomfortable and potentially dangerous reaction.

What are some of the safer testing methods?

RAST stands for radioallergosorbent test. It measures the amount of IgE (an allergy provoking antibody) in the blood after stimulation with a suspected allergen. It is safer than the invasive methods, as the allergen is applied to the blood sample rather than to the body. Precise measurement of IgE can approximate the degree to which one is allergic, and can provide information on the best dose for desensitization treatments. The sophisticated instrumentation and impressive computer printout can lull doctors and patients into believing that this test is more accurate than other tests, which is not necessarily the case. RAST is also more expensive than most other tests, but it is also simpler and quicker. You simply have some blood drawn and send the vial to the lab, along with a hefty check, rather than enduring multiple visits, needle pricks, scratches, and reactions.

For unknown reasons, IgE levels tend to be higher in smokers than in nonsmokers. For this reason it is a good idea to let your doctor know if you smoke, to avoid possible misinterpretation of the test.

Cytotoxic testing is another blood test; this one is specifically for food allergy. Cells in the blood sample are mixed with sterile water and applied to microscope slides smeared with food extracts in a base of petroleum jelly. The slides are observed microscopically at several intervals ranging from ten minutes to two hours. Certain cell changes are interpreted to be a sign of allergy with both the intensity of cell changes and the amount of time they take to occur correlating to the degree of allergy. There is controversy as to the accuracy of the test, but it is probably no less accurate than skin testing and is safer and more convenient. Many foods can be tested with one blood sample.

What allergy test can be done by the patient at no cost?

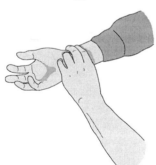

Pulse - A simple test that can be performed by the patient is the pulse test. It has been observed that a person's pulse will often increase noticeably when the person is exposed to a known allergen. In the pulse test, the person will take her/his pulse both just before and just after exposure to a suspected allergen. To take the pulse, put a finger (not the thumb, which has a pulse of its own) on the pulse point of the wrist just below the base of the thumb. Alternatively, the pulse at the temple can be used. Count the number of beats in fifteen seconds and multiply by four to get the number of beats per minute. Get a baseline pulse reading, and then take the pulse again a few minutes after eating or breathing the suspected allergen. Don't change your basic posture (sitting, standing, lying) or activity level during these few minutes.

An elevation of at least ten beats per minute, especially if confirmed by repeat testing, is considered to be evidence of allergy. The accuracy level of this method as compared with the other methods is not known, but it costs nothing, involves no needles, and can be done at any time without a doctor's assistance. Eliminating or reducing food allergens and then introducing foods back one at a time, as described later in this chapter, is a good general way to identify food allergens. Pulse testing can be utilized as foods are added back.

Weak instead of strong? It may be an allergy

<u>Kinesiology</u> - In kinesiology testing, the person being tested holds one arm out and resists the downward pressure on the arm applied by the tester. Once this baseline level of resistance is noted, the person holds some of the suspected allergen in the other hand and pressure is exerted on the arm again. If the degree of resistance is about the same, the substance is not an allergen. If the patient's arm lacks the strength to resist with certain substances, the patient is allergic to them. The amount of substance tested can be small, and it can even be in a glass vial or other container. In an alternative method of kinesiology testing, the person puts the thumb together with the first or second finger, and a second person tries to pull the thumb and finger apart. This is repeated with the test substance held in the other hand; a lack of strength indicates an allergy.

The body electric

<u>Electrodiagnosis</u> makes use of the pathways, or meridians, in the body. Electrodiagnosis is sometimes called EAV, for Electroacupuncture According to Voll, the researcher who developed it. Devices such as the Computron are used for treatment purposes as well as allergy diagnosis. When the Interro is used for allergy testing, the patient holds a metal electrode in one hand and the tester places a metal probe against the acupressure points on the sides of the fingers or toes. The baseline reading should be around fifty on a scale of zero to one hundred. The wavelength of the suspected allergen is stored in the computer, or alternatively the actual substance is placed in a test well on the machine. If the wavelength of the substance causes a galvanic skin response reading significantly different (usually lower) than the baseline reading, the substance is a probable allergen.

Electrodiagnosis is a controversial technique, ridiculed by many Western doctors (including those who are not at all familiar with it but presume to "know" that it doesn't work), yet it appears to be as accurate as, or more than, most other methods. The results depend a great deal on operator skill and consistency in applying probe pressure. The procedure is harmless and there is little or no discomfort involved.

Many types of substances can be tested - foods, inhalants (by using the lung meridian point), liver toxins, chemicals, metals, and other substances. Substances can be tested as a large or small group by combining wavelengths, and then tested individually if there is a response to the group. For example, foods may be tested as a group. A negative or weakly positive response to foods in general means that food allergy is unlikely to be your problem, and foods are not tested further. A positive response to foods requires further testing, but whole groups such as grains, meats, or fruits can be tested at once. If a person tests negative for fruits and meats but positive to grains, then individual grains can be tested - wheat, rice, rye, oats. The test is quick - about five or ten seconds per substance or group, but given the many thousands of possible allergens, the test would still be impossibly time-consuming if group testing were not possible.

Electrodiagnostic testing can also be used to determine and even produce homeopathic remedies and doses to neutralize food allergies.

When diagnosis is also treatment

Elimination or detoxification diets - Imagine listening to an entire symphony orchestra and trying to pick out one single violin by ear. It would be nearly impossible. Now mentally remove most members of the orchestra and again listen for the single violin; now it can be recognized. This is the principle behind elimination diets. If you are allergic to many foods, you probably feel pretty badly overall, and eating one of those foods will not allow you to feel enough difference to identify any one food causing you problems. If, however, you eliminated all or almost all of these foods, and then reintroduced them one at a time, a clearly defined change in the way you feel will allow you to pinpoint the allergens individually.

There are different types of elimination diets, ranging from total fasts (pure water only) to juice fasts to diets composed only of foods with low allergic potential. It takes four days to clear allergens out of the system completely, and eight days to reintroduce foods. One effective elimination diet allows nonallergenic supplements, protein powder and enzymes to digest parasites as well as non-sweet green and root vegetables and healthy oils for four days, with a different non-gluten grain added to these each day from days five to eight. Typically a person on such a diet will feel worse on days two through four, better on addition of grains, and much better by day eight. The degree of improvement as compared with the pre-diet level is a measure of the degree to which food allergies are responsible for your symptoms.

How badly you feel after beginning the diet is also a measure of allergy (or microorganism toxicity), as allergy and addiction are related - a good allergist will often ask what foods you eat daily and feel you can't do without as a starting point. The feelings of illness are actually very similar to withdrawal symptoms for this reason.

After day 4 you add in one low gluten grain per day. After day eight you are starting with a relatively clean slate, and food groups are then individually added. Carefully note any symptoms on adding these foods, which should be much more obvious now that your increased feeling of health and well-being is used as a baseline. If a food elicits no apparent allergic response, it can be eaten while other foods are tested, but no more often than once every five days to minimize chances of an allergic reaction developing.

The detoxification/elimination diet can be inconvenient and time consuming, but it is much more accurate than most other tests. It also has the advantage of being curative as well as diagnostic.

Be aware

Observation - It is more difficult to eliminate non-food potential allergens from your environment to do a type of elimination testing, but an important part of the elimination diet can be utilized - observation of symptoms. Take careful note of any change in the way you feel and try to correlate it with something you are exposed to. for example:

- Itchy earlobes when wearing cheap earrings - this can be a sign of nickel allergy.

- Foggy thinking after pumping gas can be an allergy to petrochemicals or to any of the components of gasoline.

- A flash of anger or irritability after smelling cologne on a passerby can indicate an allergy to artificially scented products, an allergy which is quite common and often unrecognized.

- Feeling poorly after a trip to the dentist - increased mercury exposure or allergy to any of a number of dental materials such as formaldehyde can cause this.

- The "allergic salute" is the upwards rubbing of an itchy nose - see if this correlates to any particular inhalant exposure.

- Sore, itchy, or red eyes - does this occur during smog alert days, pollen season, when wearing contact lenses, or when reading the newspaper?

- Fatigue can be a major allergic symptom - take a look at what you did an hour before to a day before.

- Aching

- Mucus, throat clearing, stuffy or runny nose

- Higher pulse rate, as previously discussed

Like the elimination diet, careful observation is more accurate than most tests because it measures actual responses. A written diary of exposure and symptoms may be helpful.

How can you increase the accuracy of tests?
It may be a good idea to do another test or two for verification. If results of any two or more tests agree with each other, the accuracy of the result is more likely. For example, if Live Blood Analysis, liver panel testing, and muscle testing all indicate liver stress, then chances are very high that you have liver stress. Multiple testing reduces the high inaccuracy rate of many tests. Ideally, tests will be combined with observation of your own symptoms.

Treatment

What is the next step?
Once the arsenal of tests has been utilized and a diagnosis or diagnoses (plural of diagnosis) has been reached, it is time to begin treatment. The different types of treatment for many different conditions are discussed in the book *Alternative Medicine: The Definitive Guide*, The Burton Goldberg Group, Future Medicine Publishing, Puyallup WA, 1994. The *Alternative Medicine* book can be considered to be a companion volume to this book for this purpose.

Allergy testing and treatment by NAET, developed by Dr. Devi Nambudripad [3,4] can also help to identify and eliminate allergies. This technique is described in the Toxic Immune Syndrome chapter.

References and Resources

- The Burton Goldberg Group, *Alternative Medicine: The Definitive Guide*, Future Medicine Publishing, Puyallup WA, 1994.

- Nambudripad, Devi, *Say Goodbye To Illness*, Delta Publishing Company, Buena Park CA, 1993.

- Nambudripad, Devi, *The NAET Guidebook*, Delta Publishing Company, Buena Park CA, 1994.

From The Womb To The Tomb

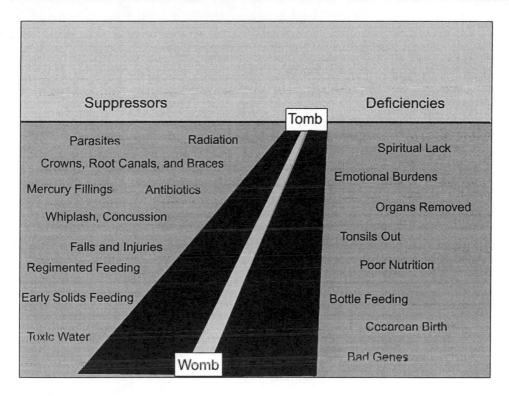

There are many things, even starting while you were still in the womb, that have added up over the years until your present state of ill health was reached.

Your body, or your immune system, can be thought of as a rain barrel. The size of your rain barrel is determined in part by genetics. The weakest link, genetically, can be likened to the weakest place in the barrel that is likely to spring a leak. Each stressor throughout our lives, whether physical or emotional as described here and throughout these books, acts like a drop, a tablespoon or a cup full of water in our rain barrel. The point at which the barrel overflows is the point where your body can't take any more, and illness develops.

The ways to deal with this are to reduce the amount of stress on the body (lower the water level in the rain barrel) and build up the immune system (patch the areas most likely to leak and thereby increase the capacity of the barrel). These books become your roadmap to find an exit off of this road to bad health you may have been stumbling down and out onto the expressway to optimum health!

And now, here are some guideposts to speed you on your way.

Why is it important to go over stuff that happened a long time ago?
The more you understand about where and how your health first went off course, the more likely it is that you will be able to make the necessary changes to get back on course.

Some of the stones on the road to bad health are:

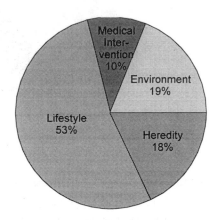

Sperm   Ovum   You!

Bad genes - As soon as you were conceived, the fertilized cell that became you contained genetic information from both of your parents. In addition to inheriting your mother's eyes and your father's nose, you may also have inherited your father's predisposition toward multiple sclerosis or your mother's tendency to arthritis. This is known as your genetic weakest link, where a problem or imbalance is most likely to be expressed.

Some things that may seem to be genetic may be from your mother's (or father's) bad health before your birth. You may have "inherited" their microbiology (parasites such as fungus) or have less than optimal health due to your mother's smoking, mercury fillings, or poor nutrition. For example, it is thought that alcoholism may have a genetic component because it seems to run in families. However, it is likely that fungi or other microorganisms shared between family members are at least partially responsible for the fact that more than one family member is alcoholic.

The baby can get its mother's microbiology (parasites) from birth. This can have a lifelong effect that is often mistaken for heredity.

Only about 18% of health problems are due to heredity. The remaining 82% are preventable.

Cesarean birth - Some babies are delivered by Cesarean section, in which the uterus is opened up surgically and the baby is lifted out, rather than vaginally as intended by design. Such babies are deprived of the protective colonizing bifidus bacteria normally picked up in the mother's vagina, provided that she has enough. They are also deprived of the uterine contractions which have beneficial effects on the circulatory system, lungs, and muscle tone.

Bottle feeding - Check out the logic here:

- *The best milk for kittens is cat's milk.*
- *The best milk for puppies is dog's milk.*
- *The best milk for calves is cow's milk.*
- *The best milk for human babies is...soybean milk? cow's milk? goat's milk? vitamin powder? corn syrup? Apparently somebody thinks so.*

Artificial (bottle) feeding has replaced most breastfeeding in this country for decades now, as scientists and formula marketers (who had a lot to gain financially) felt that they knew more about infant nutrition than God. Breastfeeding is superior to bottle feeding for several reasons besides mother-child bonding:

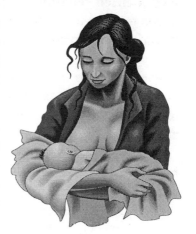

- **Good stuff** - Breast milk contains just the right mixture and types of protein and fat, as well as colostrum which contains antibodies to the bad guys the mother is fighting. These transferred antibodies work like the operating system of a computer, setting up an optimal program for the baby's immune system to follow.

- **Bad stuff** - Formulas from the 1950s contained cow's milk, corn syrup, and water. Milk, soy, and corn products contribute to later food sensitivities, ear infections, and tonsillitis, and the sugar contributes to later addictions. Milk, soy, corn, and wheat are the top four allergens in children and adults, and artificial feeding may have something to do with this. Today's formulas contain protein of a type that babies are not equipped to digest properly.

- **Tooth problems** - The sugar in formulas, and the tendency to keep the bottle in the mouth, leads to tooth decay (and mercury fillings and their attendant problems). Prolonged sucking on the bottle nipple can cause later orthodontic problems.

- **Fermentation** - A loaded diaper from a totally breastfed baby really doesn't smell too bad, while a formula-fed baby's stool is hard and foul-smelling. This rotting smell is due to putrefaction (putrefaction by bacteria is why a dead animal smells) and fungal fermentation. The baby's immature digestive system coupled with a lack of protective breastfeeding bacteria is not equipped to handle formula components. The toxic byproducts of fermentation suppress the immune system and can cause disease. This disease state may take hold so early you'd think you had been born with it.

Early solids feeding - Babies get their first tooth at about six months for a reason: they were not meant to take in solid food other than mother's milk until then. A baby should be breastfed until it is at least three times its birth weight. The baby does not have the necessary digestive enzymes until then, leading to later allergies.

Several decades ago, the prevailing wisdom was "a fat baby is a healthy baby". Your mother was misled by scientists, doctors, and baby food advertisements to give you cereals, fruits, and other types of mush as early as age two weeks. We know now that a fat baby is actually a toxic puffy allergic baby with a probable future of battling weight gain and ill health. The greater fat cell content may be to store toxins or due to allergy.

Regimented feeding - A normal baby is born equipped to know when, what, and how much it needs to eat with a minimum of instruction, since any animal that can't figure this out on its own would have starved itself into extinction long ago.

However, since the day you were born, someone else - the scientists, your doctor, baby books, and your mother - probably determined what, when, and how much you should eat. Maybe you remember the food battles from your childhood and teen years. These battles can be carried into adulthood.

By the time the average American reaches adulthood, s/he has spent twenty years or so eating when s/he is not hungry, not eating when s/he is hungry, and eating types and amounts of food that have been determined by someone else. At this point you may not be able to tune into your body's inner wisdom and know what and how much to eat.

In addition, much of the food you were force-fed or given as treats - white flour, beef, yeast, sugar, fried foods, and processed foods - is unhealthy in itself and never meant for human consumption. You may grow up with a craving for these foods because you were sensitized to them in childhood.

Other steps in the road to bad health are numbered in parentheses to correspond to the numbers and letters on the circular chart.

Falls and injuries (1) - If you ever fell down and got a concussion, there may have been some injury to sensitive parts of the brain called the limbic system. If you have ever gotten whiplash in an automobile accident, there may have been some damage to some delicate structures, such as the pituitary, or master, gland in the base of the brain, the thyroid gland in the neck, or the larynx (voice box). There can also be damage to the connection between the limbic system and the body. This is like having an army which has only garbled or limited communication with headquarters.

Childhood bone and joint injuries can contribute to bone and joint pains and swelling decades after the injury is healed and forgotten.

Antibiotics (5) - Do you remember having earaches and sore throats as a child? Chances are the doctor repeatedly prescribed antibiotics for earaches and other bacterial infections, as well as for viral infections and even allergies, and later for acne.

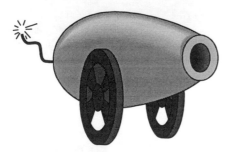 Picture a battlefield with both enemy soldiers (disease-causing bacteria) and good soldiers (protective bacteria). A bomb (antibiotics) is dropped onto the battlefield (your body) and wipes out both types indiscriminately, like using a neutron bomb to kill a terrorist. For this reason antibiotics will usually do more harm than good. The bad-guy bacteria usually come back first.

A large percentage of adults with CFS have a history of frequent and recurrent antibiotic treatment in childhood or teen years [1].

Toxic water (5) - Most water that does not come from private wells has been treated with chlorine, which is intended to kill unfriendly bacteria and other potentially harmful living organisms. In the body, chlorine (and its relatives fluoride and bromine), like antibiotics, kills some of the protective bacteria along with the bad. In sufficient quantities, it can also cause damage to your tissues and cells.

Sodium fluoride or fluoride in another form is added to some city water because it is erroneously believed to reduce tooth decay in young children due to its calcium-binding capacity. This is not a good idea because:

- *The amount each child - or adult - gets can't be controlled.*

- *Too much fluoride can be toxic, causing tooth mottling, lowered calcium leading to brittle bones, and liver cancer.*

- *Adults, who get no known benefit, are ingesting a harmful chemical.*

Chlorine, fluorine, and bromine and their adverse health effects are discussed in greater detail in the chapter on Water Pollution, Fluoride and Chlorine in *Surviving The Toxic Crisis*.

Although there is testing and treatment, other contaminants such as bacteria and leaking chemicals can get into the water supply. Lead, copper, and PVCs from metal or plastic water pipes can also be leached into the water.

Mercury fillings (5) - Almost all tooth fillings, until recently, were made of a silver-mercury amalgam composed of about 50% mercury. Contrary to previous belief, mercury in an amalgam is quite toxic. It is listed fifth on the list of most toxic substances and ranks as more poisonous than arsenic. Mercury and its toxicity is discussed in depth in the chapter on Mercury in *Surviving The Toxic Crisis*. Most of us have had mercury amalgam fillings in our mouths since childhood; even slight toxicity would have a noticeable effect after nearly a lifetime of continuous exposure.

Tropical diseases (6) - Did you ever go on a trek into the Amazon Basin? No? Then you may think that a section on tropical diseases and parasites does not pertain to you, but it does. Most of the southern United States has a subtropical climate, meaning that it doesn't freeze in the winter, which allows the proliferation of tropical diseases, anaerobic organisms, and parasites. Some of these don't even require a tropical climate.

Toxoplasmosis, dangerous to a developing fetus, can be acquired by changing an infected cat litterbox. Giardia, which causes acute diarrhea at first and then later problems, can be picked up from contaminated water, even from clear mountain streams. It is possible to acquire one of these or related diseases

> **Microorganisms can lead to degenerative disease.**

without knowing it, but they can cause years of fatigue, gastrointestinal distress, and other symptoms such as tight shoulder muscles, pain between the shoulder blades, stiff neck, headache, fatigue, and nausea upon eating fatty food.

Many doctors don't think of microorganisms and tropical diseases when presented with certain symptoms. These microorganisms can lead to many degenerative diseases.

Irradiation of the thymus (7, B) - The thymus gland is found in the upper chest cavity behind the breastbone. In the 1940s and 1950s, it was believed that the thymus had no function after early childhood, since it usually shrunk after that time. If it didn't shrink, it was sometimes irradiated, or bombarded with x-rays to cause it to shrink. The damage this caused was threefold:

- X-rays often damaged the nearby thyroid and parathyroid glands, which caused retarded growth and mental development in children, and lifelong sluggishness and overweight.

- X-rays to any part of the body can harm the rest of the body, and the effects accumulate over a lifetime, possibly ending up with mutated fermenting cells called cancer.

- Scientists again thought they knew better than God what belonged in the body. In their arrogance, they irreparably destroyed a major part of the immune system.

Removal or destruction of the thymus and other organs is discussed in greater detail in the chapter on Treatment-Caused Trauma.

Radiation (7, B) - Dental and other x-rays, used in previous decades with far less caution than today, have a cumulative and toxic effect. The primary danger is cell changes, which can cause cancer.

If you were born prior to 1955, you may remember fluoroscope machines at the shoe store, another type of x-ray. Radium-dial clocks and watches were also common in those days.

Electrical appliances emit radiation of a sort, called electromagnetic fields (EMF), discussed in its own chapter in *Surviving The Toxic Crisis*. Possible associations have been found between EMFs and reproductive problems (miscarriages, birth defects) and cancer (especially leukemia, lymphoma, and brain cancers) [2].

Tonsillectomy (8) - Perhaps you remember going into the hospital as a child to have your tonsils out. The adenoids (also called pharyngeal tonsils) were often removed along with the tonsils (also called palatine tonsils). There are also masses of lymphoid tissue, called lingual tonsils, at the root of the tongue. All three sets of two tonsils are involved in that part of the immune system called the lymph system, and play a role in the protection of the body from invading bacteria and viruses.

460

Back when you were young, it was believed that swollen tonsils were the cause of sore throats, when they were actually the lymph's escape valve and the body's means of fighting the sore throats. So out they came, and your immune system is a bit weaker as a result. Allergies and lung and bronchial problems can be caused in part by the removal of the tonsils.

Braces (5,2,3,4,7) - Tooth braces are made of nickel and tin, which are part of stainless steel, crowns and caps are made of nickel or gold, and posts for dental implants and root canals are stainless steel, which contains nickel. Nickel can contribute to the development of cancer; it is in fact what scientists inject into laboratory rats to give them cancer. Nickel 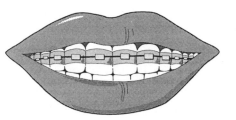 allergies are the most common metal allergy, found in about 33% of women and 12 % of men. In addition, almost any two different metals in the mouth, including those fillings, can cause what is in effect an electrical battery. This is harmful to the body as discussed in the chapter on the Battery Effect in *Surviving The Toxic Crisis*.

> **A surprising number of people with chronic illness were found to have been molested as children.**

Emotional burdens (A) - Each of us has an accumulation of small and large emotional burdens gathered throughout life. Fears, hate, disappointments, low self-esteem, rejections, abandonment, and many types of emotional stress tend to drag you down and place a burden on your immune system. A surprising number of people with chronic illness were found to have been molested as children.

Spiritual lack (C)- Although many people do not feel the need for a spiritual base, the lack of such a base can cause a person to feel responsible for everything in their life, alternating with a feeling of helplessness. Those with a spiritual base have a source of grounding and purpose which can give comfort and answers that can reduce the overall stress level of the individual. Having a life's purpose or vision can be similar in effect to having a spiritual base.

How do the stones in the road to bad health affect you?
Most of these "stones" are linked to medical intervention which was not only unnecessary, but harmful. Most of the harmful effects are related directly or indirectly to impaired immune system function or removal of the buffers and filters such as tonsils, gallbladder, and appendix.

Digestive problems (3) - Early feeding of the wrong foods can lead to later digestive problems:

- Protein digesting enzymes in the liver are lowered, leading to difficulty in digesting complex proteins like casein (milk and soy protein).

- The liver's bile production to the gallbladder is lowered, leading to difficulty in digesting fats, especially saturated fats and fried foods.

- The pancreas lowers carbohydrate digesting enzymes so that digestion of gluten-containing grains such as wheat, rye, oats, and barley is impaired. This can lead to an increase in fermenting yeast and bacteria.

- The insulin producing function of the pancreas is also impaired, so that it is less able to deal with the excess of sugar that you are taking in. A rise in triglycerides, artery-clogging fats in the bloodstream, can result.

- Poor digestion leads to slower bowel transit time, which can in turn lead to food sensitivities.

Allergies and food sensitivities (4) - Early introduction of cow's milk into the diet can cause lifelong milk and other food sensitivities. This is especially the case after a Cesarean birthas 80% of babies deprived of bifidus bacteria have milk sensitivity. Too-early introduction of fruit juices and other foods will also predispose a person to later allergies to these foods, as well as addictions. Alcoholism is sometimes an allergic addiction to corn (bourbon), grapes (wine), beer (malt) or other ingredients called congeners.

Bacteria (5) - All bacteria are germs, and germs are bad things that cause disease, right? Wrong. Most bacteria are protective (beneficial) and even necessary for digestion. The bifidus bacteria, which the baby is intended to pick up at birth from the vaginal canal and is deprived of if a Cesarean section is done, is the baby's first line of defense against disease. Bifidus is also responsible for making B vitaminsespecially biotin, which help to control yeast.

Breast feeding, unlike bottle feeding, passes along some of these good bacteria from the mother, which protect the baby and aid in digestion.

Metals (5,2) - Heavy metals such as mercury are toxic to cells and have an antibiotic effect, and a combination of metals in the mouth cause an electrical effect similar to that of a battery.

Yeast (6) - Yeast can cause a number of problems, as discussed in the chapter on Yeast Infections in *Surviving The Toxic Crisis*. Yeast buildup is caused by:

- *A shortage of beneficial bacteria to keep them under control.*

- *A poor, yeast-enhancing diet: sugar-sweetened cow's milk, followed by fruit, yeasted bread, white flour products, and vinegar.*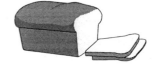

- *Antibiotics, including prescription drugs, chlorine in water*

- *Mercury fillings in the mouth.*

Radiation (7) - The immune system is damaged by radiation, which you were exposed to from a number of sources:

- *x-rays of teeth and suspected broken bones; fluoroscopy*
- *irradiation of the thymus*
- *radium-dial clocks and watches*
- *power lines over your childhood home*

- *water bed heaters and electric blankets*
- *motors such as clocks*
- *more recently, cellular and portable phones*

Radiation also causes cell changes called free radical damage which can lead to cancer.

Immune system effects (7,B) - Removal of parts of the immune system, such as the tonsils and adenoids by surgery or the thymus by irradiation, will make the immune system less effective (see chapter on Treatment-Caused Trauma), as will radiation and yeast.

Weight problems (8) - Much of the epidemic of obesity in this country is linked to diseases such as hypertension and is really caused by:

- Toxic water weight from poor foods and poor elimination.

- Excess fat cells formed early in life due to early solids feeding and overfeeding, and to protect the body by absorbing toxins.

- Regimented feeding from birth leads to difficulty in recognizing true hunger and knowing when to stop eating, and in knowing what your body needs.

- Water and fat retention from the body's attempt to dilute chemical toxins in the body.

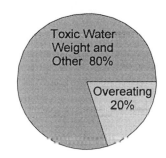

In fact, about 80% of all overweight is due to the retention of water to dilute toxins and allergens rather than to overeating.

* * * * * * * *

Now that you have had a chance to think about some of the things you may have experienced in your "travels" on this road to bad health, you can take steps towards overcoming the challenges you face. And the first step in overcoming chronic health problems is to understand what got you to where you are. Hopefully this book has given you some insights.

The second step is finding the kind of doctors and practitioners who are knowledgeable about your situation, and have been helping others achieve their goals of more optimum health. Yes, it can happen for you, too.

This book has reviewed the source of many of the toxic suppressors that must be dealt with in order to get your health back. Once you have made the decision to start on your journey to health, it's important to have the right kind of help and expertise to provide the kind of direction and guidelines that enables you to take responsibility, and take action that will put you on the Road to Good Health.

To that end, you need the type of facility that encompasses the kind of comprehensive, integrated approach needed to deal with the multi-level of problems that may be part of the root cause of your problems. You need to find the Ideal Clinic -- This aptly describes what you will find at Comprehensive Health Center - Medical, a clinic that has evolved to provide the resources under one roof to deal with a multiplicity of patient needs.

Let's take a look at how this type of ideal clinic came into being and how the guidelines and integrated approach developed and grew to be what it is today.

BUILDING THE PERFECT CLINIC

AND SUMMARY

How do people get sick?

The Centers for Disease Control (CDC) have divided the primary causes of disease into categories as shown by this pie chart. Heredity plays a role of about 18% in causing illness. Restated, the remaining 82% of disease is within our control: environment, avoiding medical intervention, and especially making lifestyle changes.

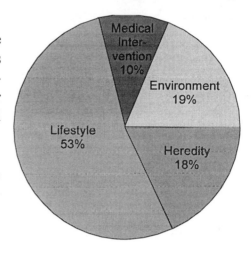

The CDC is validating what progressive practitioners have known for years. The mainstream is shifting in this direction.

What is the nature of illness, and why is it important?

The first step to setting up an effective clinic lies in understanding the nature of illness itself. A medical practice may start with a faulty premise, such as: "All parts of the body are separate from each other, and some are unnecessary." or "Most illness is hereditary or beyond our control so the doctor's role is to treat the symptoms." Once these faulty premises are set up, the clinic will not function well in its primary role of helping the patients get their health back.

To work effectively, a clinic must be based on an understanding of the nature of chronic illness:

What are the basic premises that the ideal clinic is based on?

- There are many steps in the patient's road to bad health, including metal dental work, chemical toxins, surgeries, electromagnetic radiation, structural problems, and poor nutrition. These primary toxic suppressors can then set up conditions for microorganisms - secondary toxic suppressors - to move in and do their damage. Both types of suppressors have to be eliminated and dealt with before medication or other approaches will have much permanent effect.

- These suppressors can adversely affect the immune system, the key to the optimum functioning of the body's systems. This suppression and the resulting symptoms was given the name "Toxic Immune Syndrome" seven years ago. The symptoms can vary according to the patient's genetic weakest link - chronic fatigue, headaches, fibromyalgia, irritable bowel, and others. These and many other symptoms have no single cause. The CDC now agrees with this approach.

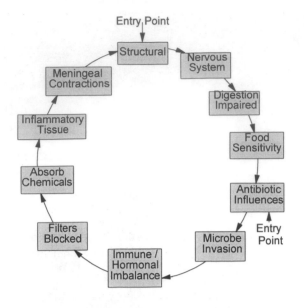

- All of the body's systems are interrelated.

- There can be a "domino effect" of poor health. As this chart shows, structural problems can leadto nervous system problems, which can lead to digestive problems and continuing on around the circle, with a problem in one system setting you up for and making you vulnerable for one in the next.

- The bad news then is that health problems can leadto a negative domino effect -- a vicious cycle. The good news is that the interrelatedness of the body's systems can also lead to a positive domino effect, where clearing up one problem can enable most or all other systems to function better, which can help clear up further problems all the way around the circle. For example, fixing a structural problem can lead to better nerve transmission, which can lead to better digestion, until finally you come full circle. And you find it's a good place to be. Because you are once more experiencing what it's like to feel good again. And you may have felt so bad for so long that you forgot what it feels like to really be healthy!

How does one gain perspective - and regain health?

So now, in order to start the positive domino effect in motion, there are seven steps to good health that must be followed, more or less in order, as shown by this chart to the right.

What are the advantages of comprehensive health care?

The whole body is involved in most illness, especially chronic illness. In addition, a person with chronic health problems may need expertise from several disciplines such as:

The Seven Steps Back to Health

7. Rebuild / Restore
6. Eliminate microorganisms
5. Align, balance body structures
4. Biochemical, nutritional support
3. Desensitize allergens, unblock pathways
2. Detoxify and cleanse your body
1. Stop bombing your body with toxins and allergens

- *Chiropractic*
- *Immunology*
- *Microbiology*
- *Dental*
- *Others*

- *Nutrition*
- *Toxicology*
- *Allergy*
- *Herbs*
- *Homeopathy*

In this age of specialization and isolation both by body part and by treatment philosophy, it is important to find a clinic that can treat the whole person and use different disciplines in the proper order. This is one of the strengths of Comprehensive Health Centers - Medical Center. It pulls together the expertise of a number of practitioners. In addition, patient health care is coordinated, with all practitioners sharing a similar philosophy, having access to the same patient charts and test results, and meeting to discuss the best way to work together for the individual patient.

Not all clinics have this same philosophy, nor do they have the to resources to do so. Unfortunately, there are many individual practitioners who have their private clinic in which they can offer their own specialty, leading to the promotion of a "silver bullet" solution - the idea that sauna, colonics, chelation, or Rolfing alone can cure everything from herpes to cancer .

What is the <u>real</u> root cause of the illness? - **The truth will set you free!**
The philosophy of Comprehensive Health Centers - Medical Center is to find out and treat the root causes of illness. Sometimes what seems like the apparent root cause may have an even deeper cause. For example, certain symptoms such as fatigue or headache may be treated symptomatically by many doctors. A better doctor may discover the apparent root cause as being a yeast overgrowth, and treat the yeast with diet and medication, with subsequent, if temporary, alleviation of symptoms. A very good doctor or clinic would see the yeast overgrowth as being a symptom of a systemic imbalance in itself and would ask why the body isn't keeping the yeast population under control. Such a doctor or clinic would realize that the mercury in amalgam fillings has an antibiotic effect which can kill the beneficial bacteria in the intestines which control the yeast population, and it is the mercury, not the yeast, which is the root cause that needs to be addressed.

One step toward having an effective clinic
An effective clinic will help stop the influx of, and remove, toxins which can be suppressing your body's systems, and support the body nutritionally and biochemically in healing disease. An effective - and honest - clinic will then admit that the actual healing is outside of their hands.

How does dentistry fit in?
Dental problems such as mercury amalgam fillings, electrical charges (the battery effect) from metal dental work, root canals, and misalignments in the jaw are major players in a surprising number of health problems. A good medical clinic will have an affiliation with a dentist who knows how to remove mercury fillings safely and whose knowledge and methods are known and trusted by the clinic. Ideally, the medical and dental clinics should work together in a supportive manner on diagnosis (medical) and treatment (dental) of such problems as:

- *Whiplash, which can throw the bite off*
- *TMD or cranial sutures out of alignment*
- *Patient sensitivity to some dental materials*
- *Electrical charges from metal dental work*

- *Bite balancing*
- *Infected toxic root canals*

In summary, an effective medical clinic should have knowledgeable practitioners, a comprehensive approach, and be able to refer patients to a dental clinic that understands and practices the kind of non-toxic dentistry that complements and supports what is happening for the patient medically in the ideal clinic.

CHC - Medical is such a place, with Coastal Dental as an adjunct dental practice providing the type of competent dental care that can be trusted to support the patient in a complementary manner.

* * * * * * * * * * * * * * * * * * *

In closing, a personal word of testimony from Dr. Bill Kellas and how the philosophy on which the concept of the ideal clinic was built, came into being -- the key to how you can rebuild and keep your health -- finding the root causes.

This approach of getting to the root of the cause has been the key-note of our success

.. . . . .Folks, it's a little bit like getting rid of the weeds in your garden. Rather than trim back the weeds (suppressing the evidence of their presence) it has been our belief that if you pull the weeds out at the root, starting with the most offensive kind first, then you will be the most effective. And the flowers will have room to bloom, where once the weeds crowded them out.

Once the truth of this concept begins to water the garden you've been laboring in, you will be rid of those weeds once and for all, and the fragrance of beautiful flowers will fill your life.

You will know the truth and the truth will set you free.

References

Abbreviations Used

AAs	Amino acids, protein building blocks
ADD	Attention Deficit Disorder
AIDS	Acquired Immune Deficiency Syndrome
ALS	Amyotrophic Lateral Sclerosis, also called Lou Gehrig's disease
AMAS	Anti-Malignin Antibody in Serum, a cancer test
ASI	Adrenal Stress Index, a test of adrenal function
ATP	Adenosine triphosphate, a cellular form of energy
c-AMP	Cyclic Adenosine Monophosphate, an immune system booster
Ca	Calcium
CAT	Computerized Axial Tomography, an x-ray imaging technique, also called CT scan
CDC	Centers for Disease Control
CEBV	Chronic Epstein-Barr Virus syndrome, old name for Chronic Fatigue Syndrome
CFIDS	Chronic Fatigue Immune Deficiency Syndrome, same as CFS
CFS	Chronic Fatigue Syndrome
CHOs	Carbohydrates
Cl	Chlorine
CNS	Central Nervous System
CO$_2$	Carbon dioxide
CSF	Cerebrospinal Fluid
DHEA	Hormone for adrenal support
DNA	Deoxyribonucleic acid, a genetic component
EBV	Epstein-Barr Virus, which causes mononucleosis
EDTA	Ethylenediaminetetraacetic acid, a chelating agent
EEG	Electroencephalogram, a measure of the brain's electrical activity
EI	Environmental Illness
EKG	Electrocardiogram, a measure of the heart's electrical activity
EMS	Eosinophilia Myalgia Syndrome, caused by a contaminated batch of Tryptophan
ER	Endoplasmic Reticulum, a cellular component
ER	Emergency Room of the hospital
et al	And others, a Latin abbreviation in journal references
FDA	Food and Drug Administration
Fe	Iron
GABA	Gamma-Aminobenzoic Acid, an amino acid and neurotransmitter
GLA	Gamma-linolenic Acid, an essential fatty acid
GTF	Glucose Tolerance Factor, found in brewers yeast
H$_2$O	Water
HCl	Hydrochloric acid
Hct	Hematocrit, a measure of red blood cells
HDL	High Density Lipoprotein, "good" cholesterol
Hg	Mercury
Hgb	Hemoglobin, a measure of the oxygen carrying capacity of red blood cells

Ig	Immunoglobulin, immune system components IgA, IgE, IgM, IgG, and IgD
IM	Intramuscular
IND	Investigational New Drug
IU	International Units, a measure of potency for oil soluble vitamins A, D, E, and K
IUD	Intrauterine Device for birth control
IV	Intravenous
IVF	Intervertebral Foramen, which holds the spinal cord
K	Potassium
LBA	Live Blood Analysis
LDH	Lactose dehydrogenase, a liver enzyme
LDL	Low Density Lipoprotein, "bad" cholesterol
LGB 414	Homeopathic to aid digestion
mcg	Microgram, 1/1,000,000 of a gram (1 gram = 1/28 ounce)
mcg/dl	Micrograms per Deciliter, a measure of concentration
MCS	Multiple Chemical Sensitivity
MD	Medical Doctor
ME	Myalgic Encephalomyelitis, similar to Chronic Fatigue Syndrome
mg	Milligram, 1/1000 of a gram (1 gram = 1/28 ounce)
mg/kg	Milligrams per kilogram, a measure of dosage per unit of body weight
ml	Milliliter, a measure of volume (about 1/1000 of a quart)
MRI	Magnetic Resonance Imaging, a diagnostic technique
MS	Multiple Sclerosis
Na	Sodium
NAET	Nambudripad's Allergy Elimination Technique
NDA	New Drug Application
NET	Neuro-Emotional Therapy
NK	Natural Killer cells of the immune system
NSAIDs	Nonsteroidal Anti-Inflammatory Drugs
PABA	Para-Aminobenzoic Acid, a B vitamin
PCM-4	Immune system support product containing antioxidants thymus and ginseng
PDR	Physician's Desk Reference, a book of drug effects
PET	Positron Emission Tomography, an imaging testing technique
PGE1,2,3	Prostaglandins, hormones which cause or inhibit inflammation
pH	Measure of acidity or alkalinity of a solution
PMS	Premenstrual Syndrome
ppb	Parts Per Billion
ppm	Parts Per Million
PVCs	Premature Ventricular Contractions, irregular heartbeat
RBC	Red Blood Cells
RNA	Ribonucleic acid, a genetic component
SID	Syndrome of Immune Dysregulation
SIDS	Sudden Infant Death Syndrome
SLE	Systemic Lupus Erythematosus, also called lupus, an autoimmune disease
T3	Triiodothyronine, a thyroid hormone
T4	Thyroid hormone; also an unrelated type of immune system cell

472

TIS	Toxic Immune Syndrome
TMD	Temporomandibular joint Dysfunction
TMJ	Temporomandibular joint in the jaw; also used to refer to problems with this joint
TSH	Thyroid Stimulating Hormone
U.S.	United States
UV	Ultraviolet
WBC	White Blood Cells
Zn	Zinc

This glossary contains medical and non-lay terms used throughout the book. *Italicized* words within a definition are themselves defined in this glossary. More detailed definitions, or definitions of words not found here, can be located by using the Index at the end of this book.

Acetaldehyde - A toxic metabolic byproduct of ethanol, or beverage alcohol; also called acetyl aldehyde. Can also be produced by fungus

Acidophilus - Protective (beneficial) bacteria, which is produced in the body and can also be taken as a supplement

Acquired Immune Deficiency Syndrome (AIDS) - System-wide immune suppression caused by the incapacitation of *T cells*

Acute - Referring to illness lasting less than 120 days, or that which has a comparatively sudden onset

Addison's disease - An *autoimmune disease* which affects the adrenal glands

Adrenaline - The fight-or-flight hormone released by the adrenal glands which is responsible for the fight-or-flight reaction to stress and for a feeling of energy or anxiety. Also called epinephrine

Aerobic - Oxygen-using

Aflatoxin - A potent *carcinogen* from the mold that grows on peanuts and potatoes

Agoraphobia - Fear of leaving the house, driving, or shopping

AIDS - *Acquired Immune Deficiency Syndrome*

Alimentary - Referring to the digestive tract

Allergen - Substance which can cause an allergic reaction

Allergy - An excessive immune system response to something which is relatively harmless to most people

Allopathic - The type of medicine most common in the U.S. Also called Western, symptom-suppressing, or drug-oriented medicine.

ALS - Amyotrophic lateral sclerosis, also called Lou Gehrig's disease; a progressive illness involving the nerves and muscles and loss of muscle control

Alzheimer's disease - A brain disease, sometimes called senility, in which the memory becomes progressively worse

Amalgam - Combination; refers in this context to dental fillings made of mercury, silver, and other metals

Amino acid - Basic building block of protein; protein is broken down through digestion into amino acids which are used by the body

Amylase - *Enzyme* which digests starches

Anabolic - Building up

Anaphylaxis - Allergy-induced shock which can be fatal

Angiogenesis - The formation of new blood vessels, usually in a tumor

Angiography - X-ray study of blood vessels

Ankylosing spondylitis - An *autoimmune disease* which causes pain and stiffness of the spine

Anorexia - Loss of appetite

Anosmia - Loss of ability to smell

Antibodies - Immune system components which attack *antigens* and signal other immune system components to attack

Antigens - Foreign protein which stimulates the immune system, including *allergens* and *microbes*

Antihistamines - Medications which suppress the action of *histamines*, reducing uncomfortable symptoms but also reducing immune system function by design

Antioxidant - Substance which counteracts the damaging effects of oxygen and *free radicals*

Aorta - Main artery from the heart, largest blood vessel in the body

Apocrine - Sweat glands associated with hair follicles and under the arms

Arachidonic acid - Substance found in meat and dairy products which stimulates the production of *prostaglandin* E2, which produces inflammation

Arrhythmia - Irregular heartbeat

Arteries - Blood vessels which carry oxygenated blood to organs and tissues

Arteriosclerosis - Hardening of the arteries

Arthritis - Painful inflammation of the joints

Asphyxia - Lack of oxygen

Asthma - An allergic reaction which causes difficulty in breathing

Atherosclerosis - Hardening of the arteries

Autoimmune disease - A disease in which the immune system appears to attack the body, causing symptoms

Autonomic - Part of the nervous system not under conscious control, such as that which controls heartbeat and digestion

B cells - White blood cells which make *antibodies*

BHT - A food preservative containing the toxic solvent toluene

Bifidus - Protective (beneficial) bacteria, which are produced in the body and colonize in the colon. They can also be taken as a supplement. Bifidus has a role in the production of B vitamins, especially biotin, and helps with digestion and keeping fungus under control

Bile - Substance produced by the liver to aid in digestion of fats. It also digests fat, stores *enzymes*, and carries certain toxic wastes out of the body

Bioavailable - Usable by the body

Biopsy - Removal of a small amount of body tissue for diagnostic purposes

Brain fog - Inability to concentrate, impairment of short-term memory, confusion, spaciness, difficulty in thinking

Capillaries - Tiny blood vessels

Carcinogenic - Cancer-causing

Cardiac - Pertaining to the heart

Cardiovascular - Referring to the *circulatory system*

Casein - Milk protein, a common *allergen*

CAT scan - Computerized axial tomography, an x-ray diagnostic technique

Cells - The microscopic building blocks of all living things, including ourselves

Cerebrovascular - Referring to the blood vessels in the brain

Cervical - Referring to the neck bones

Cesarean - Type of birth in which the baby is surgically removed through the abdomen

Chelation - A technique for removing metals from the blood and tissues

Chelator - Substance which latches onto metals and eliminates them from the body

Cholesterol - A fatty component of the blood which helps to build and repair cell membranes and make *hormones*

Choline - B vitamin needed for building *neurotransmitters*

Chromosomes - *Cell* component which contains genetic material

Chronic - Long-term, referring to illness usually defined as lasting over 120 days

Chymotrypsin - An enzyme secreted by the pancreas which has an inhibiting effect on cancer growth

Circulatory system - Heart and blood vessels

Cirrhosis - Hardening and scarring of the liver

Cis - A chemical configuration, referring to oils which are beneficial

CNS - Central Nervous System, which consists of the brain and spinal cord

Coccyx - Tailbone

Colitis - Inflammation of the *colon*, causing diarrhea and malabsorption of food

Collagen - Major structural component of skin and cartilage

Colon - Lower part of the digestive tract

Colostrum - A component of breast milk which contains *antibodies* to help the baby's immune system

Comprehensive health care - Healing based on finding and treating the root causes of disease. Also called holistic or alternative medicine.

Congener - Grain or carbohydrate from which a particular type of beverage alcohol is made. Congeners are often *allergens*.

Coronary - Referring to the heart

Cortisol - An anti-inflammatory substance naturally produced by the adrenal glands

Crohn's disease - An *autoimmune disease* which affects the intestines, causing chronic diarrhea

Cross-linking - Hardening of *collagen*

Cyanocobalamin - Vitamin B12

Cytochrome P450 - One of the body's detoxification systems

Cytoplasm - The jellylike material in the *cell*

Degenerative diseases - Diseases such as cancer and high blood pressure which take a long time to develop (are *chronic*) and tend to worsen without treatment

Denatured - Chemically changed, usually referring to protein

Dentin - Part of tooth

Dermatitis - Skin inflammation and rashes, often caused by allergy

Dermatology - Study of skin diseases

DNA - Deoxyribonucleic acid, which contains information needed for a *cell* to replicate itself

Eccrine - Sweat glands on skin surface

Eczema - An itchy, unsightly skin rash, usually allergic in origin

Edema - Fluid collecting in the body, usually to try to dilute poisons; swelling due to water retention

Eicosanoids - *Hormones* which regulate and balance many body systems. Also called prostaglandins

Electrolyte - A mineral in *ion*ic form necessary to the body

Endocrine - Referring to glands which secrete *hormones*. Endocrine means ductless, and these hormones are secreted directly into the body

Endogenous - Naturally occurring within the body

Environmental Illness (EI) **-** Sensitivity to many chemicals and artificial substances. Sometimes called Multiple Chemical Sensitivity (MCS)

Enzymes - Biological substances which help to speed up biochemical reactions in the body or enable them to occur

Eosinophil - A type of white blood cell

Epidermis - Outer layer of skin

Epinephrine - Another name for *adrenaline*

Epithelium - Top intestinal layer

Erythrocytes - Red blood cells

Ethanol - Beverage alcohol, a poison

Exogenous - Introduced from outside the body

Fatty acids - Components of fats; fats are broken down through digestion into fatty acids which are used by the body

FDA - <u>F</u>ood and <u>D</u>rug <u>A</u>dministration, which monitors drugs and food additives

Fermented - Changed to alcohol or vinegar

Fibromyalgia - Pain throughout the body due to inflamed tissue

Fluoroscope - Imaging technique using x-rays to see moving parts of the body

Free radicals - *Atoms* with unpaired *electrons* which are extremely reactive and damaging in the body

Gastrointestinal - Pertaining to the stomach and digestive tract

Glutathione - Sulfur-containing *amino acid* which detoxifies metals and chemicals

Gluten - Component of many grains which is often allergenic

Glycogen - Form of sugar stored by the body for short term use

Goiter - A form of *hypothyroidism* due to iodine deficiency, characterized by fatigue and swollen neck

Graves' disease - An overactive thyroid gland; Graves' disease causes bulging eyes and fatigue

Hematocrit - Measure of the number of red blood cells

Hemoglobin - The oxygen-carrying component of blood

Hepatic - Pertaining to the liver

Histamines - Immune system components which attack invaders and whose presence causes typical cold or allergy symptoms

Hormone - A substance which helps regulate a cell's activity

Hydrogenation - a process by which beneficial liquid oils are changed to harmful solid or semi-solid fats

Hypercholesterolemia - High blood *cholesterol*

Hypertension - High blood pressure

Hypochlorhydria - Too little hydrochloric acid in the stomach

Hypoglycemia - Low blood sugar

Hypothesis - An assumption to be proven or disproven through experimentation

Hypothyroidism - Underactivity of the thyroid gland, which can cause fatigue

Hysterectomy - Surgical removal of the uterus

Iatrogenic - Caused by doctors or the medical system

Idiopathic - Of unknown cause

Ileocecal valve - Valve in the small intestine

Immunoglobulins - Types of *antibodies*, called IgA, IgG, IgM, IgE, and IgD

Insulin - Hormone which regulates glucose (sugar) metabolism

Integumentary System - Includes skin, hair, nails and glands within skin

Interleukin - Immune system component that acts as a messenger and regulates temperature

Ischemic - Diseased, usually referring to body tissue

Itis - Suffix meaning infection or inflammation

Jaundice - Skin yellowing caused by a liver problem

Junction boxes - Parts of the body which serve as a link between two or more organ systems

Keratin - Calcium-containing material which forms hair and nails

Kinesiology - Refers to muscle testing

Larynx - Voice box in neck

LD50 - Lethal dose for 50% of test animals, a measure of *acute* chemical toxicity

Leaky gut - Condition in which food is not digested, or broken down into small enough component parts, leading to allergy

Leukemia - A type of cancer affecting the bone marrow's production of white blood cells

Libido - Sex drive

Limbic system - Part of brain which helps to regulate the immune system

Lipase - *Enzyme* which digests fats

Lipid - Fat

Lipophilic - Oil soluble

Lupus erythematosus - An autoimmune disease affecting the kidneys, skin, and other parts of the body. Usually just called lupus

Lymph nodes - Collection points in the lymph system, which collect toxins

Lymphocyte - A type of white blood cell and immune system component

Lymphoma - Cancer of the lymph system

Macronutrients - Proteins, carbohydrates, and fatty acids

Macrophages - Immune system components which attack invaders and clean up after a battle with these invaders

Malaise - Fatigue and weakness, flu-like feelings

Malathion - A pesticide

Malignant - Referring to a cancer that can spread to other parts of the body, with the potential for fatal results

Mammography - X-ray examination of the breast

Mastectomy - Breast removal for cancer

Mcg - Microgram, a unit of weight which is one millionth of a gram, or one-thirty-millionth of an ounce

Melatonin - Hormone which regulates sleep cycles and fights cancer

Meningeal system, or meninges - Outer covering of the brain and spinal cord which acts as shock absorber

Meningeal - Referring to the *meninges*

Meninges - The covering of the brain and spinal cord

Meningitis - Inflammation or infection of the *meningeal system*

Mercury - A toxic metal, most commonly found in amalgam tooth fillings

Meridian - Electrical pathway in the body, usually just under the skin

Metallothionein - A sulfur containing *chelator* which clears metals from the body

Metastasis - The spreading of cancer cells to other parts of the body

Micronutrients - Vitamins and minerals

Mineral - A chemical element, usually in charged form, which is necessary for bodily function

Mitochondria - The power plants of the *cell*

Mononucleosis - An acute infectious viral disease

MRI - Magnetic resonance imaging, a diagnostic technique

Multiple sclerosis (MS) - An *autoimmune disease* in which the *myelin sheath* of the nerves is partially dissolved, leading to loss of control of the muscles served by those nerves

Myalgia - Muscle aches

Myelin sheath - The fatty covering around the nerve cell

Myocardial infarction - Heart attack

Necrosis - Cell or tissue death

Neurons - Nerve cells

Neurotoxic - Poisonous to nerves

Neurotransmitters - Biochemicals which transmit nerve impulses across the *synapse*

Nickel - Toxic and allergenic metal, found in root canal posts and dental braces

Noradrenaline - Also called norepinephrine; hormone which allows you to stay asleep and constricts blood vessels in response to shock

Nosocomial - Referring to infections contracted in the hospital

Nucleus - Center, as of a cell or an *atom*

Olfactory - Referring to the nose

Oncologist - Doctor who focuses on treating cancer

Oncology - The medical specialty that studies and treats cancer

Oophorectomy - Surgical removal of the ovaries

Ophthalmic - Relating to the eye

Organic - a.) A chemical compound which contains carbon
b.) Food which is grown without pesticides or artificial fertilizers

Osteoporosis - A condition in which bones become porous and brittle, leading to height loss and fractures

Ozone - Component of smog which can cause *free radical* damage

PABA - Para-aminobenzoic acid, a B vitamin which helps protect against sunburn

Pacemaker - Part of heart which regulates heartbeat; artificial pacemakers can be surgically implanted

Pancreas - Organ which produces both digestive enzymes and insulin to regulate blood sugar

Parasympathetic - The part of the *autonomic* nervous system which is responsible for digestion and for repairing and restoring body function; the opposite of sympathetic

Parotid - Glands in the mouth which produce saliva

Peptides - Small groups of *amino acids*, or small parts of proteins

Periodic Table - A chemical table which is a simplified model of chemical relationships

Peristalsis - Muscular contractions of the digestive tract which move food downward

pH - Measure of the acidity or alkalinity of a solution

Pituitary gland - Small gland in the base of the brain which regulates activity of the other *endocrine* glands

Placebo - An *inert* substance which physically resembles a drug and is used as a control in studies to evaluate drugs. It can have a positive effect due to the mind's effect on the body

Plaque - Calcium-containing substance which forms on artery walls

Plasma - The liquid part of the blood

Platelets - Blood components responsible for clotting

PMS - Premenstrual syndrome, characterized by depression, irritability, breast soreness, cramps, and/or headache

Prostaglandins - *Hormones* which regulate and balance many body systems. Also called eicosanoids

Protease - *Enzyme* which digests proteins

Psoriasis - An itchy, unsightly skin rash, usually allergic in origin

Pulmonary - Pertaining to the lungs

Putrefaction - Rotting

Putrefied - Rotten, usually referring to proteins in the digestive tract

PVCs - Premature ventricular contractions, or irregular heartbeat

Pyridoxine - Vitamin B6

Referred pain - Pain that is perceived by the brain as coming from a site other than its true origin

Renal - Pertaining to kidneys

Respiratory - Referring to breathing; also referring to oxygen-using cells

Rhinorrhea - Nasal discharge

Riboflavin - Vitamin B2

Saturated - Refers to a fat which contains all the hydrogen it can hold. Saturated fats are usually solid at room temperature. They are toxic to the body.

Sebaceous - Oil glands in skin

Secondary toxic suppressor - A *suppressor*, usually a parasite, which gains a foothold in the body once the immune system is compromised by a primary toxic suppressor

Serotonin - *Neurotransmitter* which promotes feeling of well-being and restful sleep

Specialist - Doctor who focuses on one disease or system of the body, such as a heart specialist or *oncologist* (cancer doctor)

Spleen - Makes antibodies and gets rid of old red blood cells

Subcutaneous - Under the skin

Suppressor - Something which decreases the efficiency of the immune system or body systems in general

Sutures - Divide the bony plates of the skull

Sympathetic dominance - A condition in which the adrenal glands are stimulated to release *adrenaline*

Sympathetic - The part of the *autonomic* nervous system which is responsible for fight-or-flight responses to stress

Symptoms - Early warning signs of a problem; examples of symptoms are headaches and rashes

Synapse - Gap between nerve cells

Syndrome - Collection of *symptoms* which usually occur together to form a recognizable entity

Synergism - Working together to form a whole greater than the sum of the parts, as in two chemicals causing more damage than either one.

Synthetic - Human-made, not natural

Tagamet - Ulcer medication

T cells - Immune system components which decide what to attack and convey this information to other parts of the immune system

Thiamine - Vitamin B1

Thymus - Gland behind the breastbone which is part of the immune system and manufactures *lymphocytes*

TMJ - Temporomandibular joint, where the upper and lower jaws meet

Tocopherol - Vitamin E

Toxic Immune Syndrome - A collection of symptoms caused by interference with the function of the immune system

Toxic - Poisonous

Trans - A chemical configuration, referring to oils which are made harmful by heating or *hydrogenation*

Triglycerides - Fats in the blood

Tryptophan - An amino acid which converts to *serotonin*

Tumor - An abnormal growth of cells which forms a mass; some but not all tumors are cancerous

Ultrasound - The part of the electromagnetic spectrum just above sound; can be used for diagnostic testing

Urticaria - Hives, which are an allergic skin swelling

Vascular - Referring to the blood vessels

Vasectomy - The surgical cutting and tying of the vas deferens (sperm duct) in the male as a birth control technique

Veins - Blood vessels which carry deoxygenated blood back to the heart

Verapamil - A drug which regulates the heartbeat by blocking calcium and increasing magnesium uptake

Vertebrae - Bony segments of the spine. Singular form is vertebra

Villi - Fingerlike projections in the *cell* and in the digestive tract which increase surface area

Whiplash - An injury, most common in automobile accidents, in which the neck is snapped back and then forward

Sources for Products Named in This Book

The following are the sources for some of the nutritional and supportive products named in this book. Years of clinical experience have shown these particular brands to be among the best of their type. Most if not all products named can be ordered directly through:

Comprehensive Health Centers
4403 Manchester Avenue, Suite 107
Encinitas CA 92024
Phone 619-632-9042   Fax 619-632-0574

Product	Brand Name	Company
	Fibroplex	Metagenics
Phosphatidyl choline	Maxicholine	Phillips Nutritionals
Ginkgo biloba	Ginkgo Biloba	Enzymatic Therapy
	PCO Phytosome	Phytopharmica
Hormone enhancer	Remifemin	Enzymatic Therapy
Saw palmetto berry	Super Saw Palmetto	Enzymatic Therapy
Wild yam	YamCon Plus	Phillips Nutritionals
Garlic extract	Kyolic	Wakunaga
Chlorophyll	Sun chlorella	Sun Wellness / Integris
Flax oil	Flax Oil	Barleans
GLA oils	GLA Softgels	Carlson / Phillips Nutritionals
Salmon oil	Salmon Oil Softgels	Carlson
Acidophilus	Megadophilus / UltraDophilus	Metagenics / Ethical Nutrients
Acidophilus	Kyodophilus	Wakunaga
Bifidus	Ultra Bifidus / Megabifidus	Metagenics / Ethical Nutrients
Bacteria	Latero-Flora	Metagenics / Ethical Nutrients
Vitamins A, C, E, selenium	ACES	Carlson
Multinutrient preparation, women	Perfect Equation for Women	Professional Preference
Multinutrient preparation, men	Perfect Equation for Men	Professional Preference
Multinutrient preparation, low blood pressure or underweight	Lo-Balance	Professional Preference
Multinutrient preparation, high blood pressure or overweight	Hi-Balance	Professional Preference
Dipeptide mineral chelates		Metagenics
Glutathione complex	Glutathione complex	Professional Preference
Minerals	Kona Gold	Integris
Melatonin		
Air purifier	Alpine Air	Environmental Health Systems

Candida homeopathic	Aqua Flora I and II	Aqua Flora / East West
Nutrient bars	PR Bars	Fitness Awareness
Rice protein	Life Solubles / Life Wafer	Integris
Rice protein with fiber	Life Fiber	Integris
Protein powder	Ultra Balance	Metagenics
Protein powder	Ultra Clear Plus	Metagenics
Protein powder	Ultra Clear Sustain	Metagenics
Aloe vera powder for yeast	OriFresh	Amni
Digestive enzymes	Bio-Zyme	Enzymatic
Pycnogenol		
Vitamin E	E-Gems	Carlson
Milk thistle	Super Thistle X	Enzymatic
Calcium supplement	Osteo-Citrate	Metagenics
Detoxifier	Toxi-Cleanse	Metagenics
Book	Say Goodbye To Illness - Nambudripad	
Cookbook	Toxic Immune Syndrome Cookbook - Kellas	Comprehensive Health Centers

References

Introduction

1. Bergner, P. and K. Kail, "The U.S. Health Care Costs Crisis: A Crisis of Chronic Disease", *American Association of Naturopathic Physicians*, Sept. 1992.

2. The Burton Goldberg Group, *Alternative Medicine: The Definitive Guide*, Future Medicine Publishing, Puyallup WA, 1994.

3. Bergner, P. and K. Kail, "The U.S. Health Care Costs Crisis: A Crisis of Chronic Disease", *American Association of Naturopathic Physicians*, Sept. 1992.

4. Campbell, Joseph D., "Brief Presented to B.C. Royal Commission on Health", *Townsend Letter for Doctors*, No. 101, Dec. 1991, pp. 999-1000.

5. Hattersley, Joseph G., "Heart Attacks and Strokes", *Townsend Letter for Doctors*, No. 103/104, Feb./Mar. 1992, pp. 131-40.

6. Campbell, Joseph D., "Hair Tissue Mineral Analysis: A Review", *Townsend Letter for Doctors*, No. 118, May 1993, pp. 436-44.

7. Lane, William I. and Linda Comac, *Sharks Don't Get Cancer*, Avery Publishing Group, Garden City Park, NY, 1992.

8. Mason, Margaret, "Centering On Alternatives", *Washington Post*, March 3, 1995.

9. "Harvard Considers Alternative Medicine", *Townsend Letter for Doctors and Patients*, No. 147, Oct. 1995, p. 13.

10. Eisenberg, DM et al, "Unconventional Medicine in the United States: Prevalence, Costs and Patterns of Use", *New England Journal of Medicine*, Vol. 328, Jan. 1993, pp. 246-252.

11. Payer, Lynn, *Medicine and Culture: Varieties of Treatments in the United States, England, West Germany and France*, Henry Holt and Co., NY, 1988.

Diseases of the 21st Century

1. Culbert, Michael L., "Chronic and Acute Elements of a Syndrome of Immune Dysregulation - Part 1", *Townsend Letter for Doctors*, Vol. 121/122, Aug./Sept. 1993, pp. 894-902.

2. Culbert, Michael L., "Chronic and Acute Elements of a Syndrome of Immune Dysregulation - Part 2", *Townsend Letter for Doctors*, Vol. 123, Oct. 1993, pp. 962-8.

3. Straus, S., "Chronic Fatigue Syndrome", U.S. Department of Health and Human Services, Public Health Service, NIH Publication No. 90-3059, June 1990, p. 5.

4. Jones, James F., "Chronic Fatigue Syndrome", *The Human Ecologist*, No. 38, pp. 16-19.

5. Rosenbaum, Michael and Murray R. Susser, *Solving the Puzzle of Chronic Fatigue Syndrome*, Life Sciences Press, Tacoma WA, 1992.

6. The Burton Goldberg Group, *Alternative Medicine: The Definitive Guide*, "Chronic Fatigue Syndrome", pp. 616-624, Future Medicine Publishing, Puyallup WA, 1994.

7. Crook, William G., *Chronic Fatigue Syndrome and The Yeast Connection*, Professional Books, Jackson TN, 1984, 1992.

8. "Understanding CFIDS", *The CFIDS Chronicle*, Vol. 8, No. 3, Summer 1995, pp. 74-77.

9. Collins, Huntly, "Salt Studied as a Way to Ease Chronic Fatigue", *The San Diego Union-Tribune*, Sept. 27, 1995, p. A-7.

10. Bralley, JA and RS Lord, "Treatment of Chronic Fatigue Syndrome With Specific Amino Acid Supplementation", *Journal of Applied Nutrition*, Vol. 46, No. 3, 1994, pp. 74-78.

11. Ashford, Nicholas A. and Claudia S. Miller, *Chemical Exposures: Low Levels and High Stakes*, Van Nostrand Reinhold, NY, 1990.

12. Rea, William J., *Chemical Sensitivity*, Volume I, Lewis Publishers, Boca Raton FL, 1992.

13. Rogers, Sherry, *Tired or Toxic?*, Prestige Publishing, Syracuse NY, 1990.

14. Nambudripad, Devi, *Say Goodbye To Illness*, Delta Publishing Company, Buena Park CA, 1993.

15. Nambudripad, Devi, *The NAET Guidebook*, Delta Publishing Company, Buena Park CA, 1994.

16. Bland, Jeffrey, "New Perspectives in Nutritional Therapies", seminar held Feb. 4, 1996, Los Angeles CA.

17. Cathcart, Robert, "The Vitamin C Treatment of Allergy and The Normally Unprimed State of Antibodies", *Medical Hypotheses*, Vol. 21, No. 3, Nov. 1986, pp. 307-332.

18. Yanick, Paul Jr., "Immune Disorders - Allergy", *Townsend Letter For Doctors*, No. 118, May 1993, pp. 498-502.

19. Culbert, Michael L., "Chronic and Acute Elements of a Syndrome of Immune Dysregulation - Part 1", *Townsend Letter for Doctors*, Vol. 121/122, Aug./Sept. 1993, pp. 894-902.

20. "From Los Angeles: Piercing the Smokescreen View of CFIDS", *CFIDS Chronicle*, Spring/Summer 1990.

21. Leek, Richard, "Fibromyalgia", *The HealthKeepers Journal*, No. 4, April 1995, pp. 4-6.

22. McCarty DJ et al "Treatment of Pain Due to Fibromyalgia With Topical Capsaicin: A Pilot Study", *Semin. Arthritis and Rheumatism*, Vol. 23, 1994, pp. 41-47.

23. Deluze, C. et al, "Electroacupuncture in Fibromyalgia: Results of a Controlled Trial", *British Medical Journal*, Vol. 305, 1992, pp. 1249-52.

24. Gaby, Alan R., Electroacupuncture for Fibromyalgia", *Townsend Letter for Doctors*, Vol. 123, Oct. 1993, p. 927.

The Systems of the Body

1. U.S. Department of Health and Human Services, Public Health Service, National Institutes of Health, "Medicine for the Layman: Osteoporosis".

2. Nelson, ME et al, "A 1-Year Walking Program and Increased Dietary Calcium in the Postmenopausal Woman: Effects on Bone", *American Journal of Clinical Nutrition*, Vol. 53, No. 5, May 1991, pp. 1304-11.

3. Coats, C., "Negative Effects of a High-Protein Diet", **Family Practice Recertification**, Vol. 12, No. 12, Dec. 1990, pp. 80-94.

4. Biser, Sam, and Dean Howell, "Cranial Therapy: The Most Neglected Treatment in Natural Healing", *The Last Chance Health Report*, Vol. 4, No. 3, 1994, pp. 1-7.

5. Yiamouyiannis, John, *Fluoride: The Aging Factor*, Health Action Press, Delaware OH, 1986.

6. Balch, James F. and Phyllis A. Balch, *Prescription for Nutritional Healing*, Avery Publishing Group, Garden City Park, NY, 1990.

7. Siegel, George J. et al (editors), *Basic Neurochemistry*, Little, Brown and Co., Boston MA, 1981, 3rd edition.

8. U.S. Department of Health and Human Services, National Institutes of Health, *Heart Attacks*, Pub. No. 86-2700, Sept. 1986.

9. Petersdorf, RG et al, *Harrison's Principles of Internal Medicine*, McGraw Hill, NY, 10th ed., 1983.

10. National Institute of Neurological Disorders and Stroke, National Institutes of Health, *Stroke Research Highlights*, 1990.

11. Dawood, MY, "Current Concepts in the Etiology and Treatment of Primary Dysmennorrhea", *Acta Obstetrica et Gynecologica Scandinavica*, Vol. 138, 1986, pp. 7-10.

12. Pizzorno, Joseph E. and Michael T. Murray, editors, *A Textbook of Natural Medicine*, John Bastyr College Publications, Seattle WA, 1989.

13. Lark, Susan M., *Menstrual Cramps: A Self-Help Program*, Westchester Publishing Co., Los Altos CA, 1993.

14. *Physician's Desk Reference*, Medical Economics Co., Oradell NJ, 1993.

15. The Burton Goldberg Group, *Alternative Medicine: The Definitive Guide*, Future Medicine Publishing, Puyallup WA, 1994.

16. Dienhart, Charlotte M., *Basic Human Anatomy and Physiology*, W.B. Saunders Co., Philadelphia PA, 1973.

The Cell

1. Waterhouse, Debra, *Outsmarting the Female Fat Cell*, Hyperion, NY, 1993.

2. Stonehouse, Bernard, *The Way Your Body Works*, Crown Publishers, Inc., New York, 1974.

3. Bevan, James, *Anatomy and Physiology*, Simon and Schuster, New York, 1978.

The Immune System

1. Kusaka, Y. et al, "Healthy Lifestyles Are Associated With Higher Natural Killer Cell Activity", *Preventive Medicine*, Vol. 21, 1992, pp. 602-615.

2. Glasser, Ronald J, *The Body is the Hero*, Random House, New York, 1976.

3. Berger, Stuart M., *Dr. Berger's Immune Power Diet*, New American Library, New York, 1985.

4. Hill, TL, "The Link Between Breast Cancer and Bras", *Nude and Natural*, Vol. 15, No. 2, 1996, pp. 40-42.

5. Gaby, Alan R., "Does Wearing a Bra Cause Breast Cancer?", *Townsend Letter for Doctors and Patients*, No. 154, May 1996, p. 29.

6. Singer, Sydney Ross and Soma Grismaijer, "Dressed to Kill: The Link Between Breast Cancer and Bras", *Townsend Letter for Doctors and Patients*, No. 151/152, Feb./Mar. 1996, p. 42.

7. Stewart, Stephen R., and M. Eric Gershwin, "Human Immunobiology", *Immunologic and Rheumatic Diseases*.

8. Mizel, Steven B. and Peter Jaret, *The Human Immune System*, Simon and Schuster Inc., New York, 1985.

9. Steinman, Lawrence, "Autoimmune Disease", *Scientific American*, Vol. 269, No. 3, Sept. 1993, pp. 107+.

10. Vojdani, Aristo, *New Immunobiologic Markers for Diagnosis of Toxic Chemical Exposure*, Immunosciences Lab Inc., Los Angeles CA.

11. Von Boehmer, Harald, and Pawel Kisielow, "How the Immune System Learns About Self", *Scientific American*, Oct. 1991, pp. 74-81.

12. Livingston-Wheeler, Virginia, and Edmond G. Addeo, *The Conquest of Cancer*, Franklin Watts Inc., New York, 1984

13. Livingston-Wheeler, Virginia, and Edmond G. Addeo, "The Immune System: Your Total Defense Against Disease", *Your Good Health*, Vol. 2, No. 7, Nov./Dec. 1984, pp. 34-6.

14. Dienhart, Charlotte M., *Basic Human Anatomy and Physiology*, W.B. Saunders Co., Philadelphia PA, 1973.

Cancer

1. U.S. Department of Health and Human Services, *Cancer Rates and Risks*, 1985.

2. American Cancer Society, *Cancer Facts and Figures*, 1991.

3. Watson, RR and TK Leonard, "Selenium and Vitamins A, E and C: Nutrients with Cancer Prevention Properties", *Journal of the American Diet. Assoc.*, Vol. 86, 1986, pp. 505-510.

4. National Research Council, *Diet, Nutrition and Cancer*, National Academy Press, Washington DC, 1982.

5. Stewart, Kim, "Surviving Cancer", *Delicious*, July\Aug. 1993, pp. 16-19.

6. Keller, Jimmy, "A Talk on Cancer" (tape), 1989.

7. "Breast Cancer and PCBs: A Possible Link", *Business Week*, April 6, 1992, p. 36.

8. National Research Council, *Diet, Nutrition and Cancer*, National Academy Press, Washington DC, 1982.

9. Simone, Charles B., *Cancer and Nutrition*, Avery Publishing Group, Garden City Park NY, 1992, p. 15.

10. Enig, MG et al, "Dietary Fat and Cancer Trends", *Federal Proceedings*, Vol. 37, 1978, pp. 2215-20.

11. Simonton, O. Carl and S. Matthews, *Getting Well Again*, Jeremy P. Tarcher, Los Angeles CA, 1978.

12. Balch, James F. and Phyllis A. Balch, *Prescription for Nutritional Healing*, Avery Publishing Group, Garden City Park, NY, 1990.

13. Gofman, John W., *Preventing Breast Cancer: The Story of a Major, Proven, Preventable Cause of the Disease*, Committee for Nuclear Responsibility, San Francisco CA, 1995.

14. Bristol, JB, "Colorectal Cancer and Diet: A Case-Control Study with Special Reference to Dietary Fibre and Sugar", *Proceedings of the American Association of Cancer Research*, Vol. 26, March 1985, p. 206.

15. Bristol, JB et al, "Sugar, Fat and the Risk of Colorectal Cancer", *British Medical Journal* Clinical Research Edition, Vol. 291, No. 6507, Nov. 1985, pp. 1467-70.

16. "Body Iron Stores and the Risk of Cancer", *New England Journal of Medicine*, Vol. 320, No. 15, April 1990, pp. 1012-4.

17. National Research Council, *Diet, Nutrition and Cancer*, National Academy Press, Washington DC, 1982.

18. Simon, D., S. Yen and P. Cole, "Coffee Drinking and Cancer of the Lower Urinary Tract", *Journal of the National Cancer Institute*, Vol. 54, No. 3, March 1975, pp. 587-591.

19. Mulvehill, JJ, "Caffeine as Teratogen and Mutagen", *Teratology*, Vol. 8, No. 1, Aug. 1973, pp. 69-72.

20. Weinstein, D., I. Maurer and HM Solomon, "The Effects of Caffeine on Chromosomes of Human Lymphocytes: In Vivo and In Vitro Studies", *Mutation Research*, Vol. 16, No. 4, Dec. 1972, pp. 391-9.

21. Sandler, RS, "Diet and Cancer: Food Additives, Coffee and Alcohol", *Nutrition and Cancer*, Vol. 4, No. 4, 1983, pp. 273-8.

22. "Beer Drinking and the Risk of Rectal Cancer", *Nutrition Reviews*, Vol. 42, No. 7, July 1984, pp. 244-7.

23. Potter, JD and AJ McMichael, "Alcohol, Beer and Lung Cancer: A Meaningful Relationship?", *International Journal of Epidemiology*, Vol. 13, No. 2, June 1984, pp. 240-2.

24. Phillips, RL, JW Kuzma and TM Lotz, "Cancer Mortality Among Comparable Members Versus Nonmembers of the Seventh-Day Adventist Church", *Banbury Report 4: Cancer Incidence in Defined Populations*, Cold Spring Harbor Laboratory, NY, 1980, pp. 93-107.

25. Goldberg, MJ, JW Smith and RL Nichols, "Comparison of the Fecal Microflora of Seventh-Day Adventists With Individuals Consuming a General Diet: Implications Concerning Colonic Carcinoma", *Annals of Surgery*, July 1977, pp. 97-100.

26. Phillips, RL, "Cancer Among Seventh-Day Adventists", *Journal of Environmental Pathology and Toxicology*, Vol. 3, 1980, pp. 157-169.

27. Null, Gary, "Vegetarianism and Health: What The Studies Show", *Townsend Letter for Doctors and Patients*, No. 150, Jan. 1996, pp. 39-44.

28. "AMAS is the Blood Test For Cancer The World Has Been Waiting For", *The Friend Foundation for Medical Research*, Vol. 6, No. 1, Spring 1995, pp. 1+.

29. McDonagh, Edward W., "Detecting Cancer", *Townsend Letter for Doctors and Patients*, No. 151/152, Feb./Mar. 1996, pp. 108-110.

30. Bogoch, Samuel and ES Bogoch, "Disarmed Anti-Malignin Antibody in Human Cancer", *Lancet*, Vol. 1, 1979, p. 987.

31. Bogoch, Samuel and ES Bogoch, "Increased Accuracy of Anti-Malignin Antibody Determination in Unstored Sera Permits Screening", *Cancer Detection and Prevention*, Vol. 11, 1987, p. 85.

32. Abrams, MB, KT Bednarek and Samuel Bogoch et al, "Early Detection and Monitoring of Cancer with Anti-Malignin Antibody Test", *Cancer Detection and Prevention*, Vol. 18, 1994, pp. 65-78.

33. Moss, Ralph W., *The Cancer Industry: Unraveling the Politics*, Paragon House, New York, 1989.

34. "Progress Against Cancer?", *New England Journal of Medicine*, May 8, 1986.

35. Faber, M. et al, "Lipid Peroxidation Products and Vitamin and Trace Element Status in Patients With Cancer Before and After Chemotherapy", *Biological Trace Element Research*, Vol. 47, 1995, pp. 171-24.

36. Lane, William I. and Linda Comac, *Sharks Don't Get Cancer*, Avery Publishing Group Inc., Garden City Park, NY, 1992.

37. Maugh, TH, "Angiogenesis Inhibitors Link Many Diseases", *Science*, Vol. 212, no. 4501, June 1981, pp. 1374-5.

38. Williams, DG, "The Final Results of the First Cuban Study", *Alternatives Newsletter*, Vol. 4, No. 20, Feb. 1993.

39. Duarte, Alex, *Jaws For Life: The Story of Shark Cartilage*, Duarte, Grass Valley CA, 1993.

40. Crusinberry, R. and R.D. Williams, "Immunotherapy of Renal Cell Cancer", *Semin. Surg. Oncol.* Vol. 7, No. 4, July-August 1991, pp. 221-9.

41. Garewal, H.S. et al, "Emerging Role of Beta Carotene and Antioxidant Nutrients in the Prevention of Oral Cancer", *Arch. Otolaryngology and Head and Neck Surgery*, Vol. 121, Feb. 1995, pp. 141-4.

42. Heinerman, John, *Heinerman's Encyclopedia of Fruits, Vegetables, and Herbs*, Parker Publishing Co., West Nyack, NY, 1988.

43. Bird, Christopher, *The Persecution and Trial of Gaston Naessens*, H.J. Kramer Inc., Tiburon CA, 1991.

44. Bedell, Berkley, "Bedell Continues to Speak Out", *Townsend Letter for Doctors*, No. 131, June 1994, pp. 631-3.

45. The Burton Goldberg Group, "Cancer", *Alternative Medicine: The Definitive Guide*, Future Medicine Publishing, Puyallup WA, 1994.

46. "Special Hearing on Alternative Medicine", Subcommittee of the Committee on Appropriations, United Stated Senate, June 24, 1993, p. 104.

47. Burzynski, Stanislaw, "Antineoplastons", lecture at the World Research Foundation Congress, Los Angeles CA, Oct. 7, 1990.

48. Burzynski, Stanislaw, "Synthetic Antineoplastons and Analogs", *Drugs of the Future*, Vol. 11, No. 8, 1986, p. 679.

49. Moss, Ralph, *The Cancer Industry*, Paragon House, NY, 1991.

50. Walters, R., *Options: The Alternative Cancer Therapy Book*, Avery publishing Group Inc., Garden City Park NY, 1993, p. 26.

51. Filov, V. et al, "Results of Clinical Study of the Preparation Hydrazine Sulfate", *Voprosy Onkologii*, Vol. 36, No. 6, 1990, pp. 721-6.

52. Chlebowski, Rowan T. et al, "Hydrazine Sulfate in Cancer Patients with Weight Loss: A Placebo-Controlled Clinical Experience", *Cancer*, Vol. 59, No. 3, Feb. 1987, pp. 406-410.

53. Chlebowski, Rowan T. et al, "Influence of Hydrazine Sulfate on Abnormal Carbohydrate Metabolism in Cancer Patients with Weight Loss", *Cancer Research*, Vol. 44, No. 2, Feb. 1984, pp. 857-861.

54. Chlebowski, Rowan T. et al, "Hydrazine Sulfate Influence on Nutritional Status and Survival in Non-Small Cell Lung Cancer", *Journal of Clinical Oncology*, Vol. 8, No. 1, Jan. 1990, pp. 9-15.

55. Manner, Harold W. et al, "Amygdalin, Vitamin A and Enzyme Induced Regression of Murine Mammal Adenocarcinomas", *Journal of Manipulative and Physiological Therapeutics*, Vol. 1, No. 4, Dec. 1978, pp. 246-8.

56. Ericson, R., *Cancer Treatment:Why So Many Failures?*, GE-PS Cancer Memorial, Memorial Park Ridge, IL, 1979, p. 68.

57. Quillin, Patrick, *Beating Cancer With Nutrition*, The Nutrition Times Press, Tulsa OK, 1994.

58. Satillaro, Anthony J., *Recalled By Life*, Avon, NY, 1984. *A physician's story of how he healed prostate cancer using a macrobiotic diet.*

59. Nussbaum, Elaine, *Recovery From Cancer*, Avery Publishing Group Inc., Garden City Park NY, 1992. *One woman's story of her healing using a macrobiotic diet.*

60. Rogers, Sherry A., "Macrobiotic Diet Proven to Improve Cancer Survival", *Townsend Letter for Doctors*, Vols. 127/128, Feb./Mar. 1994, pp. 146-7.

61. Carter, JP, GP Saxe, V. Newbold, CE Peres, RJ Campeau and L. Bernal-Green, "Hypothesis: Dietary Management May Improve Survival From Nutritionally Linked Cancers Based on Analysis of Representative Cases", *Journal of the American College of Nutrition*, Vol. 12, No. 3, 1993, pp. 209-226.

62. Austin, Steve, "Steps You Can Take to Prevent Cancer", *Delicious*, July/August 1993, pp. 24+.

63. The Burton Goldberg Group, *Alternative Medicine: The Definitive Guide*, Future Medicine Publishing, Puyallup WA, 1994.

64. "Role of the Antioxidants in Cancer Prevention and Treatment", *Townsend Letter for Doctors*, Vol. 123, Oct. 1993, pp. 1027-32.

65. Watson, RR and TK Leonard, "Selenium and Vitamins A, E and C: Nutrients with Cancer Prevention Properties", *Journal of the American Diet. Assoc.*, Vol. 86, 1986, pp. 505-510.

66. "Study Finds Vitamins Cut Cancer Deaths", *Los Angeles Times*, Sept. 15, 1993.

67. Colditz, GA et al, "Increased Green and Yellow Vegetable Intake and Lowered Cancer Deaths in a Elderly Population", *American Journal of Clinical Nutrition*, Vol. 41, 1985, pp. 32-36.

68. La Vecchia, C. et al, "Dietary Vitamin A and the Risk of Invasive Cervical Cancer", *International Journal of Cancer*, Vol. 34, No. 3, Sept. 1984, pp. 319-322.

69. Menkes, MS et al, "Serum Beta-Carotene, Vitamins A and E, Selenium and the Risk of Lung Cancer", *New England Journal of Medicine*, Vol. 315, 1986, p. 1250.

70. Ramaswamy, P. and R. Natarajan, "Vitamin B6 Status in Patients with Cancer of the Uterine Cervix", *Nutrition and Cancer*, Vol. 6, 1984, pp. 176-180.

71. Stahelin, HB et al, "Cancer, Vitamins and Plasma Lipids: Prospective Basel Study", *Journal of the National Cancer Institute*, Vol. 73, 1984, pp. 1463-8.

72. Willet, WC and B. MacMahon, "Prediagnostic Serum Selenium and the Risk of Cancer", *Lancet*, Vol. 2, No. 8342, July 1983, pp. 130-4.

73. Butterworth, CE et al, "Improvement in Cervical Dysplasia Associated with Folic Acid Therapy in Users of Oral Contraceptives", *American Journal of Clinical Nutrition*, Vool. 35, No. 1, Jan. 1982, pp. 73-82.

74. Slattery, ML, AW Sorenson and MH Ford, "Dietary Calcium Intake as a Mitigating Factor in Colon Cancer", *American Journal of Epidemiology*, Vol. 128, No. 3, Sept. 1988, pp. 504-514.

75. Stadel, VW, "Dietary Iodine and the Risk of Breast, Endometrial and Ovarian Cancer", *Lancet*, Vol. 1, No. 7965, April 1976, pp. 890-1.

76. Whelen, P., BE Walker and J. Kelleher, "Zinc, Vitamin A and Prostatic Cancer", *British Journal of Urology*, Vol. 55, No. 5, Oct. 1983, pp. 525-8.

77. Greenward, P. and E. Lanza, "Dietary Fiber and Colon Cancer", *Contemporary Nutrition*, Vol. 11, No. 1, 1986.

78. Gerson, Max, *A Cancer Therapy: Results of Fifty Cases*, Gerson Institute, Bonita CA, 5th ed., 1990.

79. Davison, Jaquie, *Cancer Winner*, Pacific Press, Pierce City MO, 1977.

80. Walker, Morton, "The GersonTherapy Combats Cancer and Other Pathologies", *Townsend Letter for Doctors and Patients*, No. 153, April 1996, pp. 32-38.

81. Haught, SJ, *Cancer? Think Curable! The Gerson Therapy*, Gerson Institute, Bonita CA, 1983.

82. Hildebrand, GL, LC Hildebrand, K Bradford and SW Cavin, "Five-Year Survival Rates of Melanoma Patients Treated by Diet Therapy After the Manner of Gerson: A Retrospective Review", *Alternative Therapies*, Vol. 1, no. 4, Sept. 1995, pp. 29-37.

83. Gerson, Max, "Dietary Considerations in Malignant Neoplastic Disease: Preliminary Report", *Review of Gastroenterology*, Vol. 12, 1945, pp. 419-425.

84. Gerson, Max, "No Cancer in Normal Metabolism: Outcomes of a Specific Therapy", *Med. Klin.*, Vol. 49, No. 5, 1954, pp. 175-9.

85. Gerson, Max, "Effects of Combined Dietary Regimen on Patients with Malignant Tumors", *Exp. Med. Surg.*, Vol. 7, 1949, pp. 299-317.

86. Gerson, Max, "Cancer, A Problem of Metabolism", *Med. Klin.*, Vol. 49, No. 26, pp. 1028-32.

87. Gerson, Max, "On the Medications of Cancer Management in the Manner of Gerson", *Med. Klin.*, Vol. 49, No. 49, 1954, pp. 1977-8.

88. Cheng, JY, CL Meng et al, "Optimal Dose of Garlic to Inhibit Dimethylhydrazine-Induces Colon Cancer", *World Journal of Surgery*, Vol. 19, 1995, pp. 621-6.

89. You, WC, WJ Blot et al, "Allium Vegetables and Reduced Risk of Stomach Cancer", *Journal of the National Cancer Institute*, Vol. 81, 1989, p. 162.

90. Steinmetz, KA, LH Kushi et al, "Vegetables, Fruit and Colon Cancer in the Iowa Women's Health Study", *American Journal of Epidemiology*, Vol. 139, 1994, pp. 1-5.

91. Brown, Donald J., "Inhibition of Colon Cancer by Garlic", *Townsend Letter for Doctors and Patients*, No. 151/152, Feb./Mar. 1996, p.154.

92. Nanba, Hiroaki, "Maitake D-Fraction: Healing and Preventing Potentials for Cancer", *Townsend Letter for Doctors and Patients*, No. 151/152, Feb./Mar. 1996, pp. 84-85.

93. Mori, K., T. Toyomatsu, Hiroaki Nanba and H. Kuroda, "Antitumor Activities of Edible Mushrooms by Oral Administration", International Symposium Scientific and Technical, The Penn University, July 1986.

94. Nanba, Hiroaki, "Antitumor Activity of Orally Administered 'D-Fraction' from Maitake Mushroom (*Grifola frondosa*)", *Journal of Naturopathic Medicine*, Vol. 4, No. 1, 1993, pp. 10-15.

95. Levitt, Paul M. and Elissa S. Guralnick, *The Cancer Reference Book*, Facts on File Inc., New York, 2nd ed., 1983.

96. Kaura, S.R., *Understanding and Preventing Cancer*, Health Press, Santa Fe NM, 1991.

Treatment-Caused Trauma

1. Chopra, Deepak, quoting from the *New England Journal of Medicine*, David Singer, 1991.

2. Colgan, Michael, *The New Nutrition: Medicine for the New Millenium*, Apple Publishing Co. Ltd., Vancouver BC, 1995.

3. Roehm, Daniel Christian, "Health Insurance Overload", *Townsend Letter for Doctors*, No. 99, Oct. 1991, pp. 789-90.

4. Bluestone, C.D., "Current Indications for Tonsillectomy and Adenoidectomy", *Annals of Otol. Rhinol. Laryngol. Suppl.*, Jan. 1992, Vol. 155, pp. 58-64.

5. Camilleri, A.E., K. MacKenzie, and S. Gatehouse, "The Effect of Recurrent Tonsillitis and Tonsillectomy on Growth in Childhood", *Clinical Otolaryngology*, April 1995, Vol. 20, No. 2, pp. 153-7.

6. Ainsleigh, H. Gordon, "Relationship Between Colon Cancer and Gall Bladder Surgery", *Townsend Letter for Doctors*, No. 99, Oct. 1991, pp. 783-4.

7. Whiteman-Jones, Michael, "New Directions in Health Care", *Delicious*, July/Aug. 1993, pp. 8+.

8. Gillyat, Peta, "Vasectomy Blues", *Harvard Health Letter*, Harvard Medical School, Sept. 1993, p. 5.

9. Bernstein, SJ et al, "The Appropriateness of Hysterectomy: A Comparison of Care in Seven Health Plans", *Journal of the American Medical Association*, Vol. 269, No. 18, May 1993, pp. 2398-2402.

10. Gerdin, E., S. Cnattingius, and P. Johnson, "Complications After Radiotherapy and Radical Hysterectomy in Early-Stage Cervical Carcinoma", *Acta Obstet. Gynecol. Scand.*, Aug. 1995, Vol. 74, No. 7, pp. 554-61.

11. Watson, N.R., J.W. Studd et al, "Bone Loss After Hysterectomy With Ovarian Conservation", *Obstetrics and Gynecology*, July 1995, Vol. 86, No. 1, pp. 72-77.

12. Rodriguez, C., EE. Calle et al, "Estrogen Replacement Therapy and Fatal Ovarian Cancer", *American Journal of Epidemiology*, May 1, 1995, Vol. 141, No. 9, pp. 828-35.

13. Dillerud, E. and L.L. Haheim, "Long-Term Results of Blunt Suction Lipectomy Assessed by a Patient Questionnaire Survey", *Plastic and Reconstructive Surgery*, July 1993, Vol. 92, No. 1, pp. 35-42.

14. Dillerud, E., "Suction Lipoplasty: A Report on Complications, Undesired Results, and Patient Satisfaction Based on 3511 Procedures", *Plastic and Reconstructive Surgery*, Aug. 1991, Vol. 88, No. 2, pp. 239-46.

15. Lewis, C.M., "Comparison of the Syringe and Pump Aspiration Methods of Lipoplasty", *Aesthetic Plastic Surgery*, Summer 1991, Vol. 15, No. 3, pp. 203-8.

16. Gard, Zane R. and Erma J. Brown, "Silicone Breast Implants and Immunological Disease", *Townsend Letter for Doctors*, No. 119, June 1993, pp. 570-2.

17.Bridges, A.J., "Rheumatic Disorders in Patients With Silicone Implants: A Critical Review", *Journal of Biomater. Sci. Polym. Ed.*, 1995, Vol. 7, No. 2, pp. 147-57.

18. Vojdani, A., N. Brautbar and A.W. Campbell, "Antibody to Silicone and Native Macromolecules in Women with Silicone Breast Implants", *Immunopharmacology and Immunotoxicology*, Nov. 1994, Vol. 16, No. 4, pp. 497-523.

19. Freundlich, B., C. Altman et al, "A Profile of Symptomatic Patients with Silicone Breast Implants: A Sjogrens-Like Syndrome", *Semin. Arthritis and Rheumatism*, Aug. 1994, Vol. 24, pp. 44-53.

20. Robinson, O.G., E.L Bradley and D.S. Wilson, "Analysis of Explanted Silicone Implants: A Report of 300 Patients", *Annals of Plastic Surgery*, Jan. 1995, Vol. 34, No. 1, pp. 1-7.

21. Florence, Mari, "Silicone Implants: How to Get Well Again After the Implants Come Out", *Alternative Medicine Digest*, Issue 10, Jan. 1996, pp. 38-41.

22. Buttram, Harold E. "Overuse of Antibiotics and the Need for Alternatives", *Townsend Letter for Doctors*, No. 100, Nov. 1991, pp. 867-72.

23. Mashkian, M.V. and G.H. Stollerman, "Vaccine-Associated Polio: A Case and its Lessons", *Hospital Practice Off. Ed.*, Sept. 15, 1994, vol. 29, No. 9, pp. 69-73+.

22. Biasi, D., A. Carletto et al, "A Case of Reactive Arthritis After Influenza Vaccination", *Clinical Rheumatology*, Dec. 1994, Vol. 13, No. 4, p. 645.

25. Lear, J.T. and J.S. English, "Anaphylaxis After Hepatitis B Vaccination", *Lancet*, May 13, 1995, Vol. 345, No. 8959, p. 1249.

26. "Measles are Back in '90s", *Townsend Letter for Doctors*, No. 118, May 1993, p. 526.

27. Buttram, Harold, "The Story of an Autistic Child With Possible Implication of Childhood Immunizations", *Townsend Letter for Doctors and Patients*, No. 151/152, Feb./Mar. 1996, pp. 106-7.

28. Brody, JA and R. McAlister, "Depression of Tuberculin Sensitivity Following Measles Vaccination, *American Review of Respiratory Diseases*, Vol. 90, 1964, pp. 607-611.

29. Brody, JA et al, "Depression of the Tuberculin Reaction by Viral Vaccines", *New England Journal of Medicine*, Vol. 271, 1964, pp. 1294-6.

30. Eibl, M. et al, "Abnormal T-Lymphocyte Subpopulations in Healthy Subjects After Tetanus Booster Immunization", *New England Journal of Medicine*, Vol. 310, No. 3, jan. 19, 1984, pp. 198-9.

31. Odent, MR et al, "Pertussis Vaccination and Asthma: Is There A Link?", *Journal of the American Medical Association*, Vol. 272, No. 8, Aug. 24/31, 1994, pp. 592-3.

32. Scheibner, Viera, *Vaccination: 100 Years of Orthodox Research Shows that Vaccines Represent a Medical Assault on the Immune System*, New Atlantean Press, Santa Fe NM, 1993.

33. "Are Vaccines Generally Detrimental to the Human Defense System?", *Townsend Letter for Doctors*, Feb./Mar. 1994, pp. 190-6.

34. Buttram, Harold E., "Routine Childhood Vaccinations - A Probable Contributory Cause of the Chronic Fatigue Syndrome in Young Adults", *Townsend Letter for Doctors*, Jan. 1994, p. 60.

35. Koren, Todd, "Crib Death or Vaccine Death?", *Showcase Magazine*, 1993, pp. 10+.

36. Cherry et al, *Pediatrics Supplement*, 1988, p. 973.

37. Kalokerinos, Archie, *Every Second Child*, Keats Publishing, New Canaan CT, 1981.

Test Methods

1. Breggin, Peter R., *Toxic Psychiatry*, St. Martin's Press, New York, 1991.

2. Megalli, Mark, and Andy Friedman, *Masks of Deception: Corporate Front Groups in America*, Essential Information, Washington DC, 1991.

3. Braithwaite, J., *Corporate Crime in the Pharmaceutical Industry*, Routledge and Kegan Paul, Melbourne Australia.

4. "Why Pharmaceutical Drugs Injure and Kill Because They are Fraudulently Tested", *Townsend Letter for Doctors*, Vol. 126, Jan. 1994, pp. 30-36.

5. Gaby, Alan R., "Will Business Interests Overwhelm Science?", *Townsend Letter for Doctors and Patients*, No. 151/152, Feb./Mar. 1996, pp. 120-1.

6. Gaby, Alan R., "The Cult of Modern Medicine", *Townsend Letter for Doctors*, No. 89, Dec. 1990, p. 879.

General Principles of Nutrition

1. Sauberlink, H.E., "Implications of Nutritional Status on Human Biochemistry", *Clinical Biochemistry*, Vol. 17, April 1984, 132-142.

2. Wallach, Joel, "Dead Doctors Don't Lie" [tape].

3. Department of Health and Human Services, Public Health Services, Pub. No. 88-50210, 1988.

4. Stamler, R. et al, "Cardiac Status After Four Years in a Trial on Nutritional Therapy for High Blood Pressure", *Archives of Internal Medicine*, Vol. 149, March 1989, pp. 661-5.

5. The Burton Goldberg Group, *Alternative Medicine: The Definitive Guide*, "Nutritional Supplements", pp. 385-397, Future Medicine Publishing, Puyallup WA, 1994.

6. Ornish, Dean, *Stress, Diet and Your Heart*, Holt, Rinehart and Winston, NY, 1983.

7. Mertz, W., "The Effects of Zinc in Man: Nutritional Considerations", *Clinical Applications of Zinc Metabolism*, W.J Pories et al (editors), Charles C. Thomas Publishing, Springfield IL, 1974.

8. Quillen, Patrick, "The Role of Nutrition in Cancer Treatment", *Health Counselor*, Vol. 4, No. 6, 1992, pp. 14+.

9. Balch, James F. and Phyllis A., *Prescription for Nutritional Healing*, Avery Publishing Group Inc., Garden City Park NY, 1990.

10. Cooter, Stephen, "Top Dogs and the Food Industry", *Townsend Letter For Doctors*, June 1994, pp. 667-8.

11. Denton, D. and G. Roberts, "Effect of Vitamin and Mineral Supplementation on Intelligence of a Sample of School Children", *The Lancet*, Jan. 23, 1988, pp. 140-3.

12. Bogert, L. Jean, *Nutrition and Physical Fitness*, W.B. Saunders Co., 7th ed., 1960.

13. Rose, Mary Swartz, *A Laboratory Handbook for Dietetics*, MacMillan Co., New York, 1921.

Weight and Calories

1. Balch, James F. and Phyllis A. Balch, *Prescription for Nutritional Healing*, Avery Publishing Group, Garden City Park, NY, 1990.

2. Waterhouse, Debra, *Outsmarting the Female Fat Cell*, Hyperion, NY, 1993.

3. Sears, Barry, *The Zone*, HarperCollins, NY, 1995.

4. Roth, Geneen, *Breaking Free from Compulsive Eating*, Signet Books, New York, 1984.

5. Nambudripad, Devi, *Say Goodbye To Illness*, Delta Publishing Company, Buena Park CA, 1993.

6. Nambudripad, Devi, *The NAET Guidebook*, Delta Publishing Company, Buena Park CA, 1994.

7. Kellas, W.R., *Toxic Immune Syndrome Cookbook*, Comprehensive Health Center, Encinitas CA, 2nd ed., 1995.

8. Colvin, Robert, and Susan C. Olson, *Keeping It Off*, Simon and Schuster, NY, 1985.

Carbohydrates

1. Wade, Carlson, "Iceberg Lettuce", *Nutrition and Dietary Consultant*, Dec. 1992, p. 15.

2. Wade, Carlson, "Vegetable Compound Effective Against Cancer", *Nutrition and Dietary Consultant*, July 1991, p. 4.

3. Yiamouyiannis, John, *High Performance Health*, Health Action Press, Delaware OH, 1987.

4. Brody, Jane E., "Kids Really Do Get A Sugar Buzz, New Study Shows", *The Seattle Post-Intelligencer*, March 15, 1995.

5. "Kids and Sugar", *Townsend Letter for Doctors and Patients*, No. 147, Oct. 1995, p. 13.

6. Kennedy, David, *How To Save Your Teeth*, Health Action Press, Delaware OH, 1993.

7. Kruis, W. et al, "Influence of Diets High and Low in Refined Sugar on Stool Qualities, Gastrointestinal Transit Time and Fecal Bile Acid Excretion", *Gastroenterology*, Vol. 92, 1987, p. 1483.

8. Appleton, Nancy, "Diet, Stress, and the Immune System", *Townsend Letter for Doctors*, No. 109/110, Aug./Sept. 1992, pp. 727-8.

9. Harrington, Geri, *Real Food, Fake Food*, MacMillan Publishing Co., New York, 1987.

10. Cheraskin and Ringsdorf, *Psychodietetics*, Stein and Day, 1974.

11. Appleton, Nancy, "How Sweet It Is or Isn't", *Townsend Letter for Doctors*, No. 107, June 1992, pp. 497-8.

12. Cannon, Geoffry and Hetty Einzig, *Dieting Makes You Fat*, Pocket Books, NY, 1983.

13. "A Tangle of Fibers", *Townsend Letter for Doctors*, No. 101, Dec. 1991, pp. 988-9.

14. Walker, Morton, "Health Enhancement With High Fiber Foods", *Townsend Letter for Doctors*, No. 108, July 1992, pp. 580-3.

15. Damen, Betty, *New Facts About Fiber*, Nutrition Encounter Inc., Novato CA, 1991.

16. Murray, Michael and Joseph Pizzorno, *A Textbook of Natural Medicine*, John Bastyr College Publications, 1989.

17. Anderson, JW and J. Tietyen-Clark, :Dietary Fiber: Hyperlipidemia, Hypertension and Coronary Heart Disease", *American Journal of Gastroenterology*, Vol. 81, No. 10, 1986, pp. 907-919.

18. Schlamowitz, P. et al, "Treatment of Mild to Moderate Hypertension With Dietary Fibre, *Lancet*, 1987, pp. 622-3.

19. Belin, LJ, "Vegetarian and Other Complex Diets, Fats, Fiber, and Hypertension", *American Journal of Clinical Nutrition*, Vol. 59, 1994, pp. 1130S-1135S.

Protein

1. Herbert, Victor, and Genell J. Subak-Sharpe (editors), *The Mount Sinai School of Medicine Complete Book of Nutrition*, St. Martin's Press, New York, 1990.

2. Mindell, Earl, *Vitamin Bible*, Warner Books, New York, 1985.

3. Lee, William H., "The Fabulous World of Amino Acids", *Your Good Health*, Vol. 2, No. 7, Nov./Dec. 1984, pp. 43-4.

4. Hills, Sandra, "The Role of the Amino Acid L-Carnitine", *Nutrition and Dietary Consultant*, May 1992, pp. 9+.

5. Braverman, Eric T. and Carl C. Pfeiffer, *The Healing Nutrients Within*, Keats Publishing, New Canaan CT, 1991.

6. "Amino Acid Connection" (chart), Pax Publishing, San Francisco CA, 1985.

7. Integrated Health, Inc. Seminar Information Guide, Integrated Health Inc., Hawthorn CA, 1990.

8. Rogers, Sherry A., *Tired or Toxic?*, Prestige Publishing, Syracuse NY, 1990.

9. Azzara, A. et al, "Effects of Lysine-Arginine Association on Immune Functions in Patients with Recurrent Infections", *Drugs Experimental Clinical Research*, Vol. 21, 1995, pp. 71-78.

10. Gaby, Alan R., "Lysine/Arginine Enhances Immune Function", *Townsend Letter for Doctors and Patients*, No. 151/152, Feb./Mar. 1996, p. 29.

11. Bralley, JA and RS Lord, "Treatment of Chronic Fatigue Syndrome With Specific Amino Acid Supplementation", *Journal of Applied Nutrition*, Vol. 46, No. 3, 1994, pp. 74-78.

12. Liebman, B., "Crying Over Milk", *Nutrition Action*, Vol. 1, Dec. 1992, pp. 6-7.

13. Ursin, G. et al, "Milk Consumption and Cancer Incidence: A Norwegian Prospective Study", *British Journal of Cancer*, Vol. 61, No. 3, March 1990, pp. 456-9.

14. Ratner, D. et al, "Milk Protein-Free Diet for Nonseasonal Asthma and Migraine in Lactase-Deficient Patients", *Isr. Journal of Medical Science*, Vol. 19, 1983, pp. 806-9.

15. Gay, D., G. Dick and G. Upton, "Multiple Sclerosis Associated with Sinusitis: Case-Controlled Study in General Practice", *Lancet*, Vol. 1, No. 8940, April 1986, pp. 815-9.

16. Crook, William G., "The Dangers of Cows' Milk", *Townsend Letter for Doctors and Patients*, No. 147, Oct. 1995, p. 97.

Oils

1. Halme, Erkki, "The Role of Polyunsaturated Fatty Acids in Overcoming Cancer and Immunological Factors in General", *Townsend Letter for Doctors*, No. 87, Oct. 1990, p. 710.

2. Parthasarathy, S., JC Khoo, E. Miller, J. Barnett, JL Witztum et al, "Low Density Lipoprotein Rich In Oleic Acid is Protected Against Oxidative Modification: Implications for Dietary Prevention of Atherosclerosis", *Proc. National Academy of Sciences*, Vol. 87, 1990, pp. 3894-8.

3. Gaby, Alan R., "Olive Oil and Heart Disease", *Townsend Letter for Doctors*, No. 132, July 1994, p. 712.

4. Trevisan, M. et al, "Consumption of Olive Oil, Butter and Vegetable Oils and Coronary Heart Disease Risk Factors", *Journal of the American Medical Association*, Vol. 263, No. 5, Feb. 1990, pp. 688-692.

5. *New England Journal of Medicine*, Vol. 312, 1985, pp. 1250-9.

6. *Atherosclerosis*, Vol. 63, 1987, pp. 137-143.

7. *Hypertension*, Vol. 4, 1982, p. III-34.

8. Yaychuk-Arabei, Irene, "Evening Primrose Oil: King's Cure-All", *Health Naturally*, No. 3, March/April 1993, pp. 39-41.

9. Rogers, Sherry A., *Tired or Toxic?*, Prestige Publications, Syracuse NY, 1990.

10. Rogers, Sherry A., "Is Your Cardiologist Killing You?", *Townsend Letter for Doctors*, No. 101, Dec. 1991, pp. 993-4.

11. "Epidemiologists Link Margarine to Heart Attacks", *Food Chemical News*, March 29, 1993, pp. 22-23.

12. "Margarines Implicated in Heart Disease Among Females", *Food Chemical News*, March 22, 1993, p. 32.

13. "Study Links Heart Disease to Margarine", *New York Times*, March 5, 1993, p. A10.

14. "U.S. Study Says Margarine May Be Harmful", *New York Times*, October 7, 1992.

15. "Trans Fat - Does Margarine Really Lower Cholesterol?", *Scientfic American*, Jan. 1991, p. 34.

16. "Margarine May Boost Cholesterol", *Wall Street Journal*, Aug. 16, 1990.

17. Wertheim, Alfred H., "Trans Fats", *Townsend Letter for Doctors and Patients*, No. 150, Jan. 1996, pp. 106-7.

18. Hill, E.G. et al, "Intensification of Essential Fatty acid Deficiency in the Rat by Dietary Trans Fatty Acids", *Journal of Nutrition*, Vol. 109, 1979, pp. 1759-65.

19. Kellas, William R., *Toxic Immune Syndrome Cookbook*, Comprehensive Health Center, Encinitas CA, 2nd ed., 1995.

20. Peat, Ray, "Aspects of Wholeness", *Townsend Letter for Doctors*, No. 87, Oct. 1990, pp. 688-93.

21. Queen, H.L., "Another Piece of the Puzzle", *Health Talk*, Vol. 11, No. 2, Sept. 1992, pp. 9-16.

22. Dugdale, *Lancet*, Jan. 17, 1987, pp. 155-6.

23. Isles, CG, *British Medical Journal*, April 8, 1989, pp. 920-4.

24. Martin, Wayne, "Cholesterol, heart Attacks and Cancer", *Townsend Letter for Doctors and Patients*, No. 150, Jan. 1996, pp. 105-6.

25. "Studies Link Aggressiveness to Cholesterol", *Townsend Letter for Doctors*, No. 89, Dec. 1990, pp. 851-7.

26. Schuman, Rosette, "Where's the Fat?", *Townsend Letter for Doctors*, No. 114, Jan. 1993, pp. 40-3.

27. Olszewski, AJ et al, "Reduction of Plasma Lipid and Homocysteine Levels by Pyridoxine, Folate, Cobalamin, Choline, Riboflavin and Troxerutin in Atherosclerosis", *Atherosclerosis*, Vol. 75, No. 1, Jan. 1989, pp. 1-6.

28. Mudd, SH et al, "The Natural History of Homocystinuria Due to Cystathionine Beta-Synthose Deficiency", *American Journal of Human Genetics*, Vol. 37, No. 1, Jan. 1985, pp. 1-31.

29. Hattersley, Joseph G., "Preventing Heart Attacks, Strokes, and Sudden Infant Death", *Townsend Letter for Doctors*, No. 101, Dec. 1991, pp. 982-6.

30. Kostner, GM et al, "HMG CoA Reductase Inhibitors Lower LDL Cholesterol Without Reducing Lp(a) Levels", *Circulation*, Vol. 80, No. 5, 1989, pp. 1313-9.

31. Strandberg, TE et al, "Long-Term Mortality After 5-Year Multi-Factorial Primary Prevention of Cardiovascular Diseases in Middle-Agen Men", *Journal of the American Medical Association*, Vol. 266, No. 9, Sept. 1991, pp. 1225-9.

32. Folkers, K. et al, "Lovastatin Decreases Coenzyme-Q Levels in Humans", *Proceedings of the National Academy of Sciences of the United States of America*, Vol. 87, No. 22, Nov. 1990, pp. 8931-4.

33. Erasmus, Udo, *Fats and Oils*, Alive Books, Vancouver Canada, 1986.

Vitamins

1. Loomis, Donald, "Which is Safer: Drugs or Vitamins?", *Townsend Letter for Doctors*, No. 96, July 1991, p. 526.

2. Ellison, JB, "Intensive Vitamin Therapy in Measles", *British Medical Journal*, Vol. 2, 1932, pp. 708-711.

3. Gaby, Alan R., "Vitamin A Prevents Deaths Due To Measles", *Townsend Letter for Doctors and Patients*, No. 150, Jan. 1996, p. 29.

4. La Vecchia, C. et al, "Dietary Vitamin A and the Risk of Invasive Cervical Cancer", *International Journal of Cancer*, Vol. 34, No. 3, Sept. 1984, pp. 319-322.

5. Kime, Zane R., *Sunlight Could Save Your Life*, World Health Publications, Penryn CA, 1980.

6. Lin, David, "Substantiated Clinical Uses of Vitamin E", *Townsend Letter for Doctors*, No. 100, Nov. 1991, pp. 857-64.

7. DiFabio, Anthony, "Psyllium and Vitamin E", *Townsend Letter for Doctors*, No. 89, Dec. 1990, pp. 851-7.

8. Pearson, Durk, and Sandy Shaw, *Life Extension*, Warner Books, NY, 1982.

9. Rogers, Sherry A., *Tired or Toxic?*, Prestige Publishing, Syracuse NY, 1990.

10. Null, Gary, "Vitamin E", *Townsend Letter for Doctors*, No. 132, July 1994, p. 738.

11. Jialal, I and SM Grundy, "Effect of Dietary Supplementation with Alpha-Tocopherol on the Oxidative Modification of Low Density Lipoprotein", *Journal of Lipid Research*, Vol. 33, No. 6, June 1992, pp. 899-906.

12. Steiner, M., "Influence of Vitamin E on Platelet Function in Humans", *Journal of the American College of Nutrition*, Vol. 10, No. 5, Oct. 1991, pp. 466-473.

13. Boscobionik, D., A. Szewczyk and A. Azzi, "Alpha-Tocopherol (Vitamin E) Regulates Vascular Smooth Muscle Cell Proliferation and Protein Kinase C Activity", *Archives of Biochemistry and Biophysics*, Vol 286, No. 1, April 1991, pp. 264-9.

14. Hennig, B. et al, "Protective Effects of Vitamin E in Age-Related Endothelial Cell Injury", *International Journal of Vitamin and Nutrition Research*, Vol. 59, 1989, pp. 273-9.

15. Rimm, E. et al, "Vitamin E Consumption and the Risk of Coronary Heart Disease in Men", *New England Journal of Medicine*, Vol. 328, No. 20, May 1993, pp. 1450-6.

16. Stampfer, MJ et al, "Vitamin E Consumption and the Risk of Coronary Heart Disease in Women", *New England Journal of Medicine*, Vol. 328, No. 20, May 1993, pp. 1444-49.

17. Stampfer, MJ et al, "Vitamin E and Heart Disease Incidence in the Nurses Health Study", *American Heart Association Annual Meeting*, New Orleans, LA, Nov. 18, 1992.

18. Rimm, E. et al, "Vitamin E and Heart Disease Incidence in the Health Professionals Study", *American Heart Association Annual Meeting*, New Orleans, LA, Nov. 18, 1992.

19. Stahelin, HB et al, "Cancer, Vitamins and Plasma Lipids: Prospective Basel Study", *Journal of the National Cancer Institute*, Vol. 73, 1984, pp. 1463-8.

20. Goodman, Sandra, *Vitamin C: The Master Nutrient*, Keats Publishing Inc., New Canaan CT, 1991.

21. Gaby, SK and VN Singh, "Vitamin C", *Vitamin Intake and Health: A Scientific Review*, Marcel Dekker, NY, 1991.

22. Cheraskin, Emmanuel, *Vitamin C: Who Needs It?*, Arlington Press, Birmingham AL, 1993.

23. Pizzorno, Joseph E. and Michael T. Murray, *A Textbook of Natural Medicine*, John Bastyr College Publications, Seattle WA, 1989.

24. Dittrich, S. et al, "Effects of Nitrate and Ascorbic Acid on Carcinogenesis in the Operated Rat Stomach", *Arch. Geschwulstforsch*, Vol. 58, No. 4, 1988, pp. 235-242.

25. Vlasenko, NL et al, "Effect of Different Doses of Ascorbic Acid on the Induction of Tumors with N-Nitroso Compound Precursors in Mice", *Vopr. Onkol.*, Vol. 34, No. 11, 1988, pp. 839-843.

26. Johnston, CS et al, "Vitamin C Elevates Red Blood Cell Glutathione in Healthy Adults", *American Journal of Clinical Nutrition*, Vol. 58, 1993, pp. 103-5.

27. Susick, RL Jr., GD Abrams, CA Zurawski and VG Zannoni, "Ascorbic Acid Chronic Alcohol Consumption in the Guinea Pig", *Toxicology and Applied Pharmacology*, Vol. 84, No. 2, June 30, 1986, pp. 329-335.

28. Osilesi, O. et al, "Blood Pressure and Plasma Lipids During Ascorbic Acid Supplementation in Borderline Hypertensive and Normotensive Adults", *Nutrition Research*, Vol. 11, 1991, pp. 405-412.

29. Dawson, EB et al, "Effect of Ascorbic Acid on Male Fertility", *Annals of the New York Academy of Science*, Vol. 498, 1987, pp. 312-323.

30. Gaby, SK and VN Singh, "Vitamin C", *Vitamin Intake and Health: A Scientific Review*, Marcel Dekker, NY, 1991.

31. Goldberg, J. et al, "Factors Associated with Age-Related Macular Degeneration", *American Journal of Epidemiology*, Vol. 128, No. 4, Oct. 1988, pp. 700-710.

32. Tsao, CS, LF Xu and M. Young, "Effect of Dietary Ascorbic Acid on Heat-Induced Eye Lens Protein Damage in Guinea Pigs", *Ophthalmic Research*, Vol. 22, No. 2, 1990, pp. 106-110.

33. Devamanoharan, PS et al, "Prevention of Selenite Cataract by Vitamin C", *Exp. Eye Research*, Vol. 52, No. 5, May 1990, pp. 563-8.

34. Rubinoff, AB et al, "Vitamin C and Oral Health", *Journal of the Canadian Dental Association*, Vol. 55, No. 9, Sept. 1990, pp. 705-7.

35. Kanofsky, JD et al, "Ascorbate: An Adjunctive Treatment of Schizophrenia", *Journal of the American College of Nutrition*, Vol. 8, 1989, p. 425.

36. Gaby, Alan R., "Vitamin C for Schizophrenics", *Townsend Letter for Doctors and Patients*, No. 151/152, Feb./Mar. 1996, p. 29.

37. Hoffer, Abram, "Schizophrenia: An Evolutionary Defense Against Severe Stress", *Townsend Letter for Doctors and Patients*, No. 151/152, Feb./Mar. 1996, pp. 52-59.

38. Philpott, William H. and Dwight K. Kalita, *Victory Over Diabetes*, Keats Publishing, New Canaan CT, 1983.

39. Altschul, R., Abram Hoffer and JD Stephen, "Influence of Nicotinic Acid on Serum Cholesterol in Man", *Arch. Biochem. Biophys.*, Vol. 54, 1955, pp. 558-9.

40. Hoffer, Abram, *The Schizophrenia, Stress and Adrenochrome Hypothesis*, In Press, 1995.

41. Hoffer, Abram, *Orthomolecular Medicine for Physicians*, Keats Publishing, Inc., New Canaan CT, 1989.

42. Hoffer, Abram, *The Treatment of Schizophrenia*, In Press, 1995.

43. Hoffer, Abram, *The Development of Orthomolecular Medicine*, In Press, 1995.

44. Hoffer, Abram, *Niacin Therapy in Psychiatry*, C. Thomas, Springfield IL, 1962.

45. Wilson, Bill, "The Vitamin B-3 Therapy: The First Communication to A.A.'s Physicians and A Second Communication to A.A.'s Physicians", 1967 and 1968.

46. Smith, RF, "A Five Year Trial of Massive Nicotinic Acid Therapy of Alcoholics in Michigan", *Journal of Orthomolecular Psychiatry*, Vol. 3, 1974, pp. 327-331.

47. Smith, RF, "Status Report Concerning The Use of Megadose Nicotinic Acid In Alcoholics", *Journal of Orthomolecular Psychiatry*, Vol. 7, 1978, pp. 52-55.

48. Jacobson, M. and E. Jacobson, "Niacin, Nutrition, ADP-Ribosylation and Cancer", The 8th International Symptosium on ADP-Ribosylation, Texas College of Osteopathic Medicine, Fort Worth TX, 1987.

49. Titus, K., "Scientists Link Niacin and Cancer Prevention", *The D.O.*, Vol. 28, 1987, pp. 103-4.

50. Hostetler, D., "Jacobsons Put Broad Strokes in the Niacin/Cancer Picture", *The D.O.*, Vol. 28, 1987, pp. 103-4.

51. Chaplin, DJ, MP Horsman and DS Aoki, "Nicotinamide, Fluosol DA and Carbogen: A Strategy to Reoxygenate Acutely and Chronically Hypoxic Cells in Vivo", *British Journal of Cancer*, Vol. 63, 1990, pp. 109-113.

52. Nakagawa, K., M. Miyazaka, K. Okui, N. Kato, Y. Moriyama and S. Fujimura, "N1-Methylnicotinamide Level in the Blood After Nicotinamide Loading as Further Evidence for Malignant Tumor Burden", *Japanese Journal of Cancer Research*, Vol. 82, 1991, pp. 1277-1283.

53. Gerson, Max, "Dietary Considerations in Malignant Neoplastic Disease; A Preliminary Report", *The Review of Gastroenterology*, Vol. 12, 1945, pp. 419-425.

54. Gerson, Max, "Effects of a Combined Dietary Regime on Patients with Malignant Tumors", *Experimental Medicine and Surgery*, Vol. 7, 1949, pp. 299-317.

55. Langer, Stephen, "Power Workouts the Natural Way", *Better Nutrition for Today's Living*, Aug. 1993, pp. 24-30.

56. "A Nutritional Approach to Premenstrual Syndrome", *Karuna Professional Information Series*, Karuna Corporation, 1986.

57. Werbach, Melvyn R., *Nutritional Influences on Illness*, Keats Publishing, New Canaan CT, 1988.

58. Kuzuya, F., "Vitamin B6 and Arteriosclerosis", *Nagoya Journal of Medical Science*, Vol. 55, 1993, pp. 1-9.

59. Gaby, Alan R., "Vitamin B6 and Atherosclerosis", *Townsend Letter for Doctors*, Vols. 127/128, Feb./Mar. 1994, p. 143.

60. Hattersley, JG, "Heart Attacks and Strokes", *Townsend Letter for Doctors*, Vol. 104, Feb./Mar. 1992.

61. "Is Vitamin B6 an Antithrombotic Agent?", *Lancet*, Vol. 1, No. 8233, June 1981, pp. 1299-1300.

62. Imagawa, M. et al, "Coenzyme Q10, Iron, and Vitamin B6 in Genetically Confirmed Alzheimer's Disease", *Lancet*, Vol. 340, No. 8820, Sept. 1992, p. 671.

63. Ramaswamy, P. and R. Natarajan, "Vitamin B6 Status in Patients with Cancer of the Uterine Cervix", *Nutrition and Cancer*, Vol. 6, 1984, pp. 176-180.

64. Ellis, John M., *Vitamin B6, The Doctor's Report*, Harper and Row, NY, 1973.

65. Buist, R., *Intern. Clinical Nutrition Review*, Vol. 4, No. 1, Jan. 1984.

66. Specker, B.L., D. Miller, E.J. Norman, H. Greene, and K.C. Hayes, "Increased Urinary Methylmalonic Acid Excretion in Breastfed Infants of Vegetarian Mothers", *American Journal of Clinical Nutrition*, No. 47, pp. 89-92.

67. Marty H., "Pernicious Anemia As Cause of Secondary Sterility", *Schweiz. Med. Wochenschr.*, Vol. 114, No.; 5, 1984, pp. 178-9.

68. Kumamoto, Y. et al, "Clinical Efficacy of Mecobalamin in Treatment of Oligozoospermia: Results of Double-Blind Comparative Clinical Study", *Acta Urol. Jpn.*, Vol. 34, 1988, pp. 1109-32.

69. Lindenbaum, J. et al, "Neuropsychiatric Disorders Caused by Cobalamin Deficiency in the Absence of Anemia or Macrocytosis", *New England Journal of Medicine*, Vol. 18, No. 6, 1988, pp. 1720-8.

70. Navarro, J., "Folic Acid and Pregnancy", *J. Arch. Pediatr.*, Vol. 2, 1995, pp. 173-181.

71. Giles, W.H et al, "Serum Folate and Risk For Ischemic Stroke", *Stroke*, Vol. 26, 1995, pp. 1166-70.

72. Melamed, E. et al, "Reversible Central Nervout System Dysfunction In Folate Deficiency", *Journal of Neurol. Science*, Vol. 25, 1975, pp. 93-98.

73. Pizzorno, Joseph E. and Michael T. Murray, *A Textbook of Natural Medicine*, John Bastyr College Publications, Seatle WA, 1989.

74. Blasztajn, J.K. and R.J. Wurtman, "Choline and Cholinergic Neurons, *Science*, Vol. 221, 1983, pp. 614-620.

75. Wurtman, R.J., Alzheimer's Disease, *Scientific American*, Vol. 252, 1985, pp. 62-75.

76. Little, A. et al, "A Double-Blind Placebo Controlled Trial of High Dose Lecithin in Alzheimer's Disease", *Journal of Neurol. Neurosurg. Psych.*, Vol. 48, 1985, pp. 736-742.

77. Mindell, Earl, *Vitamin Bible*, Warner Books, New York, 1985.

Minerals

1. Appleton, Nancy, *Secrets of Natural Healing With Food*, Rudra Press, Portland OR, 1995.

2. Mazariegos-Ramos, E. et al, "Consumption of Soft Drinks with Phosphoric Acid as a Risk Factor for the Development of Hypocalcemia in Children: A Case-Control Study", *Journal of Pediatrics*, Vol. 126, 1995, pp. 940-2.

3. Colgan, Michael, *The New Nutrition: Medicine For The New Millenium*, Apple Publishing Co. Ltd., Vancouver BC, Canada, 1995.

4. Rogers, Sherry, *Tired or Toxic?*, Prestige Publishing, Syracuse NY, 1990.

5. Slattery, ML, AW Sorenson and MH Ford, "Dietary Calcium Intake as a Mitigating Factor in Colon Cancer", *American Journal of Epidemiology*, Vol. 128, No. 3, Sept. 1988, pp. 504-514.

6. Henry, HJ et al, "Increasing Calcium Intake Lowers Blood Pressure: The Literature Reviewed", *Journal of the American Dietetic Association*, Vol. 85, No. 2, Feb. 1985, pp. 182-5.

7. Belizam, JM et al, "Reduction of Blood Pressure with Calcium Supplementation in Young Adults", *Journal of the American Medical Association*, Vol. 249, No. 9, March 1983, pp. 1161-5.

8. McCarron, DA, CD Morris and C. Cole, "Dietary Calcium in Human Hypertension", *Science*, Vol. 217, No. 4556, 1982, pp. 267-9.

9. Penland, JG, and PE Johnson, "Dietary Calcium and Manganese Effects on Menstrual Cycle Symptoms", *American Journal of Obstetrics and Gynecology*, Vol. 168, 1993, pp. 1417-23.

10. Gaby, Alan R., "Calcium and Manganese for Premenstrual Syndrome", *Townsend Letter for Doctors and Patients*, No. 151/152, Feb./Mar. 1996, p. 29.

11. "Not All Iron Is The Same", *Health Naturally*, No. 3, Mar./Apr. 1993, p. 21.

12. Newman, et al, "Serum Chromium and Angiographically Determined Coronary Artery Disease", *Clinical Chemistry*, Vol. 24, No. 4, 1978, pp. 541-4.

13. Simonoff, M. et al, "Low Plasma Chromium in Patients with Coronary Artery and Heart Diseases", *Biological Trace Elements Research*, Vol. 6, No. 5, Oct. 1984, pp. 431-9.

14. Newman, HA et al, "Serum Chromium and Angiographically Determined Coronary Artery Disease", *Clinical Chemistry*, Vol. 24, No. 4, April 1978, pp. 541-4.

15. "Setback for Lidocaine", *Cortlandt Forum*, Nov. 1990, p. 22.

16. Hambridge, K.M., "Chromium Nutrition in Man", *American Journal of Clinical Nutrition*, Vol. 27, May 1974, pp. 505-514.

17. Boyle, E., B. Mendschein and H. Dash, "Chromium Depletion in the Pathogenesis of Diabetes and Arteriosclerosis", *South. Medical Journal*, Vol. 70, No. 12, Dec. 1977, pp. 1449-53.

18. Hambridge, K.M., D.D. Rogerson and D. O'Brien, "Concentration of Chromium in the Hair of Normal Children and Children With Juvenile Diabetes Mellitus", *Diabetes*, Vol. 17, No. 8, 1968, pp. 517-8.

19. Schroeder, H.A., *Journal of Nutrition*, Vol. 88, 1966, p. 439.

20. Glinsmann, W.H., *Metabolism*, Vol. 15, 1966, p. 510.

21. Merz, W. and K. Schwarz, "Relation of Glucose Tolerance Factor to Impaired Intravenous Glucose Tolerance of Rats on a Stock Diet", *American Journal of Physiology*, Vol. 196, No. 3, 1959, pp. 614-8.

22. Hambidge, KM, "Chromium Nutrition in Man", *American Journal of Clinical Nutrition*, Vol. 27, No. 5, May 1974, pp. 505-514.

23. Sjogren, A. et al, "Magnesium, Potassium and Zinc Deficiencies in Subjects with Type II Diabetes", *Acta Medica Scandinavica*, Vol. 224, 1988, pp. 461-3.

24. "Test Yourself", *Better Nutrition for Today's Living*, August 1993, p. 58.

25. Hackman, Robert M., "Chromium and Cholesterol", *Townsend Letter for Doctors*, No. 97/98, Aug./Sept. 1991, pp. 623+.

26. Stadel, VW, "Dietary Iodine and the Risk of Breast, Endometrial and Ovarian Cancer", *Lancet*, Vol. 1, No. 7965, April 1976, pp. 890-1.

27. Campbell, Joseph D., "Hair Tissue Mineral Analysis: A Review", *Townsend Letter for Doctors*, No. 118, May 1993, pp. 436-44.

28. Bland, Jeffrey, "Preventive Medicine Update", 1989 [tape].

29. Johnston, Leslie N., "SIDS and Iron Overload", *Townsend Letter for Doctors*, No. 132, July 1994, p. 762.

30. Peat, Ray, "Aspects of Wholeness", *Townsend Letter for Doctors*, No. 87, Oct. 1990, pp. 688-93.

31. Cannon, L.A et al, "Magnesium Levels in Cardiac Arrest Victims: Relationship Between Magnesium Levels and Succesful Resuscitation", *Annals of Emergency Medicine*, Vol. 16, No. 11, Nov. 1987, pp. 1195-9.

32. Vikkanski, L., "Magnesium May Slow Bone Loss", *Medical Tribune*, July 22, 1993, p. 9.

33. Mindell, Earl, *Shaping Up With Vitamins*, Warner Books, New York, 1985.

34. Martin, Wayne, "Cholesterol Debate Continues", *Townsend Letter for Doctors*, No. 99, Oct. 1991, pp. 765-8.

35. *Science News*, Vol. 133, June 1988.

36. Rogers, Sherry A. "Is Your Cardiologist Killing You?", *Townsend Letter for Doctors*, No. 101, Dec. 1991, pp. 993-4.

37. Rosenstein, D.L., R.J. Elin et al, "Magnesium Measures Across The Menstrual Cycle in Premenstrual Syndrome", *Biol. Psychiatry*, Vol. 35, No. 8, April 15, 1994, pp. 557-61.

38. Facchinetti et al, "Oral Magnesium Successfully Relieves Premenstrual Mood Changes", *Obstetrics and Gynecology*, Vol. 78, No. 2, August 1991, pp. 177-81.

39. Seelig, M.S., "Interrelationship of Magnesium and Estrogen in Cardiovascular and Bone Disorders, Eclampsia, Migraine and Premenstrual Syndrome", *Journal of the American College of Nutrition*, Vol. 12, No. 4, August 1993, pp. 442-58.

40. Rea, William J., "Magnesium Deficiency and Chemical Sensitivity", *Clinical Ecology*, Vol. 4, No. 4, 1986.

41. Sacks, J.R., "Interaction of Magnesium With the Sodium Pump of the Human Red Cell", *Journal of Physiology*, Vol. 40, 1988, pp. 575-591.

42. Fiaccadori, E. et al., "Muscle and Serum Magnesium in Pulmonary Intensive Care Patients", *Critical Care Medicine*, Vol. 16, 1988, pp. 751-60.

43. Durlach, J., "Magnesium Depletion and Pathogenesis of Alzheimer's Disease", *Magnesium Research*, Vol. 3, No. 3, Sept. 1990, pp. 217-8.

44. Kobayashi, S. S. Fujiwara et al, "Hair Aluminum in Normal Aged and Senile Dementia of Alzheimer Type", *Progress in Clinical and Biological Research*, Vol. 317, 1989, pp. 1095-1109.

45. Leach, R.M. et al, "Studies in the Role of Manganese in Bone Formation", *Journal of Nutrition*, Vol. 78, 1962, pp. 51-6.

46. Prohaska, J.R., "Functions of Trace Elements in Brain Metabolism", *Physiology Review*, Vol. 67, No. 3, July 1987, pp. 858-901.

47. Wenloch, R.W. et al, "Trace Nutrients. 2. Manganese in British Food", *British Journal of Nutrition*, Vol. 41, 1979, pp. 253-361.

48. *Northeast Center for Environmental Medicine Health Letter*, Fall 1992.

49. Skrabal, F., J. Aubock and H. Hortnagl, "Low Sodium / High Potassium Diet for Prevention of Hypertension: Probable Mechanisms of Action, *Lancet*, Vol. 2, No. 8252, Oct. 1981, pp. 895-900.

50. Armstrong, B. et al, "Urinary Sodium and Blood Pressure in Vegetarians", *American Journal of Clinical Nutrition*, Vol. 32, No. 12, Dec. 1979, pp. 2472-6.

51. Moore, Richard, *The High Blood Pressure Solution: Natural Prevention and Cure with the 'K' Factor*, Healing Arts Press, Rochester VT, 1993.

52. Butterworth, CE et al, "Improvement in Cervical Dysplasia Associated with Folic Acid Therapy in Users of Oral Contraceptives", *American Journal of Clinical Nutrition*, Vol. 35, No. 1, Jan. 1982, pp. 73-82.

53. Salonen, JT et al, " Interactions of Serum Copper, Selenium and Low Density Lipoprotein Cholesterol in Atherogenesis", *British Medical Journal*, Vol. 302, No. 6779, March 1991, pp. 756-760.

54. Stead, NW et al "Effect of Selenium Supplementation on Selenium Balance in the Dependent Elderly", *American Journal of the Medical Sciences*, Vol. 290, No. 6, Dec. 1985, pp. 228-233.

55. Hennig, Bernard and Craig J. McClain, *The Nutrition Report*, Vol. 10, No. 11, Nov. 1992, pp. 1, 88.

56. Cichoke, Anthony J., "Take Zinc to Heart", *Townsend Letter for Doctors*, Vols. 127/128, Feb./Mar. 1994, pp. 170-2.

57. Underwood, EJ, *Trace Elements in Human and Animal Nutrition*, Academic Press, Orlando FL, 1987.

58. Frithrof, L. et al, "The Relationship Between Marginal Bone Loss and Serum Zinc Levels", *Acta. Med. Scand.*, Vol. 207, 1980, pp. 67-70.

59. "Microwave Your Prostate", *Men's Health Newsletter*, June 1991, p. 7.

60. Skandhan, KP et al, "Semen Electrolytes in Normal and Infertile Subjects. II. Zinc", *Experientia*, Vol. 34, No. 11, 1978, pp. 1276-7.

61. Abbasi, AA et al, "Experimental Zinc Deficiency in Man: Effect on Testicular Function", *J. Lab. Clin. Med.*, Vol. 96, No. 3, 1980, pp. 544-550.

62. Hunt, CD, PE Johnson, J. Herbel and LK Mullen, "Effects of Dietary Zinc Depletion on Seminal Volume and Zinc Loss, Serum Testosterone Concentrations, and Sperm Morphology in Young Men", *American Journal of Clinical Nutrition*, Vol. 56, No. 1, 1992, pp. 148-157.

63. Mbtizvo, MT et al, "Seminal Plasma Zinc Levels in Fertile and Infertile Men", *South African Medical Journal*, Vol. 71, 1987, p. 266.

64. Elsborg, L., "The Intake of Vitamins and Minerals by the Elderly At Home", *Int. Journal of Vit. Nutr. Res.*, Vol. 53, 1983, pp. 321-9.

65. Grant and Howard, "Zinc Deficiency in Children With Dyslexia", *British Medical Journal*, Vol. 296, 1988, pp. 607-9.

66. Ward, NI and JA Mason, "Neutron Activation Analysis Techniques for Identifying Elemental Status in Alzheimer's Disease", *Journal of Radioanalytical Nuclear Chemistry*, Vol. 113, No. 2, 1987, pp. 515-526.

67. Wenk, GL and KL Stemmer, "Suboptimal Dietary Zinc Intake Increases Aluminum Accumulation Into the Rat Brain", *Brain Research*, Vol. 288, 1983, pp. 393-5.

68. Bondestam, M., T. Foucard and M. Gebre-Medhin, "Subclinical Trace Element Deficiency in Children with Undue Susceptibility to Infections", *Acta Paediatrica Scandinavica*, Vol. 74, No. 4, July 1985, pp. 515-520.

69. Mindell, Earl, *Vitamin Bible*, Warner Books, New York, 1985.

Supplements

1. FDA, Department of Health and Human Services Public Health Service, "Dietary Supplements Task Force Final Report", May 1992.

2. Lamm, DL, et al, "Megadose Vitamins in Bladder Cancer: A Double-Blind Clinical Trial", *Journal of Urology*, Vol. 151, 1994, pp. 21-26.

3. Mindell, Earl, *Vitamin Bible*, Warner Books, New York, 1985.

Digestion

1. Fox, Elaine, "Good Digestion", *Your Good Health*, Vol. 2, No. 7, Nov./Dec. 1984, pp. 24-5.

2. FitzGerald, Frances, "Healthy Digestion", *Health Counselor*, Vol. 4, No. 6, 1992, pp. 23-7.

3. "Test Yourself", *Better Nutrition for Today's Living*, July 1993, p. 58.

4. Lee, Lita, "Enzyme Nutrition: Nutritional Myths", *PPNF Nutrition Journal*, Vol. 15, Nos. 3 and 4, 1991, pp. 16-18.

5. Katke, Christopher and Michael, and William Shaddle, "The Digestion and Absorption of Food", Metagenics Inc., 1988.

6. Chaitow, Leon and N. Trenev, *Probiotics*, HarperCollins, NY, 1990.

7. The Burton Goldberg Group, *Alternative Medicine: The Definitive Guide*, "Probiotics: The Friendly Bacteria", pp. 1014-16, Future Medicine Publishing, Puyallup WA, 1994.

8. Alm, L. et al, "Effect of Fermentation on B Vitamin Content of Milk in Sweden", *Journal of Dairy Sciences*, Vol. 65, pp. 353-9.

9. Alm, L., *Journal of Dairy Sciences*, Vol. 64, No. 4, pp. 509-514.

10. Friend, B. and K. Shalani, "Nutritional and Therapeutic Aspects of Lactobacilli", *Journal of Applied Nutrition*, Vol. 36, pp. 125-153.

11. Hamdan, I., "Acidolin and Antibiotic Produced by Acidophilus", *Journal of Antibiotics*, Vol. 8, pp. 631-6.

12. Reddy, G., "Antitumour Activity of Yogurt Components", *Journal of Food Protection*, Vol. 46, 1983, pp. 8-11.

13. Shehani, K., "Role of Dietary Lactobacilli in Gastrointestinal Microecology", *American Journal of Clinical Nutrition*, Vol. 33, 1980, pp. 2248-57.

14. Mott, G., "Lowering of Serum Cholesterol by Intestinal Bacteria Lipids", 1973, pp. 4282-4431.

15. Rasic, J., *Bifidobacteria and Their Role*, Birkhauser Verlag, Boston MA, 1983.

16. Simon, G., "Intestinal Flora in Health and Disease", in *Physiology of the Intestinal Tract*, L. Johnson (ed.), Raven Press, NY, 1981, pp. 1361-80.

17. Speck, M., "Interactions Among Lactobacilli and Man", *Journal of Dairy Sciences*, Vol. 59, pp. 338-343.

18. Chaitow, Leon and N. Trenev, *Probiotics*, HarperCollins, NY, 1990.

19. Rogers, Sherry A., *Tired or Toxic?*, Prestige Publishing, Syracuse NY, 1990.

20. *New England Journal of Medicine*, 1973.

21. Pizzorno, Joseph E. and Michael T. Murray, *A Textbook of Natural Medicine*, John Bastyr College Publications, Seattle WA, 1989.

22. Magic Chain Health Products chart, Del Mar CA.

23. Castleman, Michael, *The Healing Herbs*, Rodale Press, Emmaus PA, 1991.

Other Needs

1. LaFee, Scott, "H$_2$O", *The San Diego Union-Tribune*, Nov. 3, 1991, pp. E1+.

2. Diamond, Harvey and Marilyn, *Fit For Life II*, Warner Books, New York, 1987.

3. Batmanghelidj, Fereydoon, *Your Body's Many Cries For Water*, Global Health Solutions, Falls Church VA, 2nd ed., 1992.

4. Batmanghelidj, Fereydoon, "Asthma: Prevention and Cure", *Alive: Canadian Journal of Health and Nutrition*, No. 153, June 1995.

5. McCleary, Kathleen, "Trouble From the Tap", *Health*, May 1990, pp. 32+.

6. Ebbert, Stephanie, and Melissa Meyers, "How Fit is Your Drinking Water", *Prevention*, July 1991, pp. 67+.

7. "Household Air Cleaners", *Consumer Reports*, October 1992, pp. 657-662.

8. Turock, Art, *Getting Physical: How to Stick With Your Exercise Program*, Doubleday, NY, 1988.

9. Dollemore, Doug, "Youth Program", *Men's Health*, Vol. 8, May 1993, pp. 50-2.

10. Cannon, Geoffrey, and Hetty Einzig, *Dieting Makes You Fat*, Pocket Books, NY, 1983.

11. Tulloh, Bruce, *Natural Fitness*, Simon and Schuster, New York, 1977.

12. Passo, MS et al, "Exercise Training Reduces Intraocular Pressure Among Subjects Suspected of Having Glaucoma", *Arch. Ophth.*, Vol. 109, 1991, pp. 1096-8.

13. Gyure, Michelle, "Change of Life", *Women's Sports and Fitness*, Vol. 14, Nov./Dec. 1992, pp. 27-8+.

14. Corelli, Rae, "The Mysteries of Sleep and Dreams", *Maclean's*, April 23, 1990, pp. 36-40.

15. "Sleep: The New Good-Health Priority", *Glamour*, Dec. 1991, pp. 194-7.

16. Alvarez, A., "Sleep", *The New Yorker*, Vol. 67, Feb. 10, 1992, pp. 85-90+.

17. Kinoshita, June, "Dreams of a Rat", *Discover*, Vol. 13, July 1992, pp. 34-41.

18. Winson, Jonathan, "The Meaning of Dreams", *Scientific American*, Vol. 263, pp. 86-8+.

19. The Burton Goldberg Group, *Alternative Medicine: The Definitive Guide*, "Sleep Disorders", pp. 838-848, Future Medicine Publishing, Puyallup WA, 1994.

20. Kahn, A. et al, "Insomnia and Cow's Milk Allergy in Infants", *Pediatrics*, Vol. 76, No. 6, Dec. 1985, pp. 880-4.

21. "Can't Sleep? Tired? Tense?", *Redbook*, May 1990, pp. 159-63.

22. "Fit to Snooze: Regular Exercise Helps You Sleep Better", *Prevention*, Vol. 45, pp. 18+.

23. Paica, Joseph, "Sleep Researchers Awake to Possibilities", *Science*, Vol. 245, July 28, 1989, pp. 351-2.

24. Lader, M., "Rebound Insomnia and Newer Hypnotics", *Psychopharmacology*, Vol. 108, No. 3, 1992, pp. 248-255.

25. Mitchell, W., *Naturopathic Application of the Botanical Remedies*, Mitchell, Seattle WA, 1983, pp. 66-67.

26. Shaffer, M., "Melatonin Could Help The Elderly Sleep Better", *Medical Tribune*, July 22, 1993, p. 15.

27. Moss, Jeffrey, "Sleep - The Great, Overlooked Antioxidant?", *Townsend Letter for Doctors and Patients*, No. 150, Jan. 1996, pp. 120-2.

28. Lewy, Alfred J. et al, "Antidepressant and Circadian Phase-Shifting Effects of Light", *Science*, Vol. 235, Jan. 16, 1987, pp. 352-4.

29. Wurtman, R.J., "Nutrients that Modify Brain Function", *Scientific American*, Vol. 246, No. 4, April 1982, pp. 50-60.

30. Roos, PA, "Light and Electromagnetic Waves: The Health Implications", *Journal of the Bio-Electro-Magnetics Institute*, Vol. 3, No. 2, Summer 1991, pp. 7-12.

31. Ott, John Nash, *Health and Light*, The Devin-Adair Co., Old Greenwich CT, 1973.

32. Jaffe, RM, *National Institute of Health Report*, Dec. 1978.

33. "Excessive Sunlight Exposure, Skin Melanoma, Linked to Vitamin D", *International Journal of Biosocial and Medical Research*, Vol 13, No. 1, 1991, pp. 13-14.

34. Garland, FC et al, "Occupational Sunlight Exposure and Melanoma in the U.S. Navy", *Archives of Environmental Health*, Vol. 45, 1990, pp. 261-7.

35. Kime, Zane R., *Sunlight Could Save Your Life*, World Health Publications, Penryn CA, 1980.

507

Emotions Plus

1. Koenenn, Connie, "Doctor Bridges the Gap Between Healing, Prayer", *Los Angeles Times*, Oct. 30, 1993, p. B4.

2. Siegel, Bernie S., *Peace, Love, and Healing*, Harper and Row, New York, 1989.

3. Idler, EL, SV Kast and JH Lemke, "Self-Evaluated Health and Mortality Among the Elderly in New Haven, Connecticut, and Iowa and Washington Counties, Iowa, 1982-1986", *American Journal of Epidemiology*, Vol. 13, No. 1, Jan. 1990, pp. 91-103.

4. Rosen, G., A. Kleinman and W. Katon, "Somatization in Family Practive: A Biopsychosocial Approach", *Journal of Family Practice*, Vol. 14, No. 3, March 1982, pp. 493-502.

5. Stoeckle, JD, IK Zola and GE Davidson, "The Quantity and Significance of Psychological Distress in Medical Patients: Some Preliminary Observations About the Decision to Seek Medical Aid", *Journal of Chronic Disease*, Vol. 17, Oct. 1964, pp. 959-970.

6. Smalley, Gary, and John Trent, *The Two Sides of Love*, Pocket Books, New York, 1992.

7. Alessandra, Tony, *How to Read People* (video and workbook).

8. Miller, D. Patrick, *A Little Book of Forgiveness*, Viking Penguin, 1994.

A Visit To The Doctor

1. Rogers, Sherry, *Tired or Toxic*, Prestige Publishing, Syracuse NY, 1990.

2. Miller, JB, "Intradermal Provocative/ Neutralizing Food Testing and Subcutaneous Food Extract Injection Therapy", in *Food Allergy and Intolerance*, J. Brostoff and S. Challacombe (eds.), Bailliere Tindall Publishers, London England, 1987, pp. 932-947.

3. Nambudripad, Devi, *Say Goodbye To Illness*, Delta Publishing Company, Buena Park CA, 1993.

4. Nambudripad, Devi, *The NAET Guidebook*, Delta Publishing Company, Buena Park CA, 1994.

Exiting the Road To Bad Health

1. Crook, William G., *Chronic Fatigue Syndrome and The Yeast Connection*, Professional Books, Jackson TN, 1984, 1992.

2. Sinclair, L., "Entrepreneurs Tackle Electromagnetic Fields", *Business*, March/April 1993, pp. 34-35.

-T-